# Food Additives and Human Health

## Edited by

### Seyed Mohammad Nabavi
### Seyed Fazel Nabavi

*Applied Biotechnology Research Center,*
*Baqiyatallah University of Medical Sciences, Tehran, Iran*

### Monica Rosa Loizzo
### Rosa Tundis

*Department of Pharmacy,*
*Health, and Nutritional Sciences, University of Calabria, Rende, Italy*

### K. Pandima Devi

*Faculty in Department of Biotechnology,*
*Alagappa University, Karaikudi, Tamil Nadu, India*

### Ana Sanches Silva

*National Institute for Agricultural and Veterinary Research*
*(INIAV), I.P., Vairão, Vila do Conde, Portugal*
*Center for Study in Animal Science (CECA),*
*University of Oporto, Oporto, Portugal*

# Food Additives and Human Health

Editors: Seyed Mohammad Nabavi, Seyed Fazel Nabavi, Monica Rosa Loizzo, Rosa Tundis, K. Pandima Devi and Ana Sanches Silva

ISBN (Online): 978-981-14-4613-9

ISBN (Print): 978-981-14-4611-5

ISBN (Paperback): 978-981-14-4612-2

need for a court order if at any point you breach any terms of this License Agreement. In no event will any delay or failure by Bentham Science Publishers in enforcing your compliance with this License Agreement constitute a waiver of any of its rights.

3. You acknowledge that you have read this License Agreement, and agree to be bound by its terms and conditions. To the extent that any other terms and conditions presented on any website of Bentham Science Publishers conflict with, or are inconsistent with, the terms and conditions set out in this License Agreement, you acknowledge that the terms and conditions set out in this License Agreement shall prevail.

**Bentham Science Publishers Pte. Ltd.**
80 Robinson Road #02-00
Singapore 068898
Singapore
Email: subscriptions@benthamscience.net

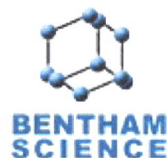

**BENTHAM SCIENCE**

# CONTENTS

# PREFACE

There is an exponential use of food additives, especially processed food, due to the impressive world population growth, changes in lifestyle patterns and demand for high-quality standards including nutritious, safe, colourful, flavourful, affordable and convenient food. Although it is common to add additives to food, it is highly controversial due to the relation of some additives to adverse health effects. This is especially relevant concerning synthetic additives.

This book assesses food additives to be a valuable tool for their rational and safe use. It provides insight into the impact of food additives on human health in the light of recent scientific information. This book is a valuable instrument for researchers, health professionals, students, laypeople, industry and government regulatory agencies.

The book is composed of 16 chapters. Chapters 1 and 2 give out an introduction to food additives. Chapter 1 is dedicated to the background of food additives and their advantages and drawbacks and chapter 2 focuses on Human Health implications of specific groups of food additives. Chapters 3 to 13 are related to different sub-groups of food additives, including preservatives (antibrowning agents, antioxidant agents, antimicrobials and essential oils), natural and synthetic colouring agents, flavouring agents (flavour enhancers, flavours and sweeteners), emulsifiers, stabilisers and indirect additives. When possible, chapters 3 to 13 include information on the intended use of the sub-group of food additives, physicochemical properties of the main representatives of the group, legislation, origin/synthesis, maximum levels, toxicological data and positive/adverse health effects.

Chapter 14 is dedicated to the relation of food additives to adverse health effects, including allergic and immunologic reactions, asthma, autoimmune diseases, cancer, diabetes, hyperkinesis and cardiovascular diseases. Chapter 15 addressed technologies applied to functional foods and food ingredients. Finally, the controversies on food additives are discussed in chapter 16 and foresight is presented.

We are aware of other food additives that could have been addressed, like nutritional additives. We look forward to this edition being well received and that in the future, other food additives can be addressed.

Ana Sanches Silva and Seyed Mohammad Nabavi on behalf of all co-editors.

**Seyed Mohammad Nabavi**
Applied Biotechnology Research Center,
Baqiyatallah University of Medical Sciences,
Tehran,
Iran

**Ana Sanches Silva**
Center for Study in Animal Science (CECA),
University of Oporto,
Oporto,
Portugal

# List of Contributors

**Shafaq Asif**  Faculty of Bioscience and Agri-Food and Environmental Technology, University of Teramo-64100, Italy

**Bule Muhammed**  Department of Pharmacy, College of Medicine and Health Sciences, Ambo University, Ambo, Ethiopia

**Fazlullah Khan**  The Institute of Pharmaceutical Sciences, Faculty of Pharmacy, Tehran University of Medical Sciences, Tehran, Iran

**Kamal Niaz**  Department of Pharmacology and Toxicology, Faculty of Bio-Sciences, Cholistan University of Veterinary and Animal Sciences (CUVAS), Bahawalpur, Pakistan

**Maria Concetta Tenuta**  Department of Pharmacy, Health and Nutritional Sciences, University of Calabria, Arcavacata di Rende (CS), Italy

**Mariarosaria Leporini**  Department of Pharmacy, Health and Nutritional Sciences, University of Calabria, Arcavacata di Rende (CS), Italy

**Faiza Mumtaz**  Department of Pharmacology, School of Medicine, Tehran University of Medical Sciences, Tehran, Iran
Experimental Medicine Research Center, Tehran University of Medical Sciences, Tehran, Iran

**Fazlullah Khan**  International Campus, Tehran University of Medical Sciences (IC-TUMS), Tehran, Iran
Department of Toxicology and Pharmacology, Faculty of Pharmacy, Tehran University of Medical Science, Tehran, Iran

**Ilias Marmouzi**  Biopharmaceutical and Toxicological Analysis Research Team, University Mohammed V-Rabat, Morocco

**Shahira M Ezzat**  Pharmacognosy Department, Faculty of Pharmacy, Cairo University, Cairo, Egypt
Department of Pharmacognosy, University for Modern Science and Arts (MSA), Egypt

**Mourad Kharbach**  Biopharmaceutical and Toxicological Analysis Research Team, University Mohammed V-Rabat, Morocco
Department of Analytical Chemistry, Vrije Universiteit Brussel (VUB), Brussels, Belgium

**Abdelhakim Bouyahya**  Department of Biology, Genomic Center of Human Pathology, Mohammed V University in Rabat, Morocco

**Ovais Sideeq**  School of Medicine, Tehran University of Medical Sciences(TUMS), Tehran, Iran
International Campus, Tehran University of Medical Sciences(TUMS), Tehran, Iran

**Regiane Ribeiro-Santos**  Department of Food Technology, Federal Rural University of Rio de Janeiro, Seropédica, Brazil

**Mariana Andrade**  Department of Food and Nutrition, National Institute of Health Dr. Ricardo Jorge, Lisbon, Portugal

| | |
|---|---|
| **Ana Sanches-Silva** | National Institute for Agricultural and Veterinary Research (INIAV), Vairão, Vila do Conde, Portugal<br>Center for Study in Animal Science (CECA), University of Oporto, Oporto, Portugal |
| **Natália Martins** | Centro de Investigação de Montanha (CIMO), Instituto Politécnico de Bragança, Bragança, Portugal |
| **Isabel C.F.R. Ferreira** | Centro de Investigação de Montanha (CIMO), Instituto Politécnico de Bragança, Bragança, Portugal |
| **Mahalingam Jeyakumar** | Department of Biotechnology, Alagappa University, Tamil Nadu, India |
| **Kasi Pandima Devi** | Department of Biotechnology, Alagappa University, Tamil Nadu, India |
| **Raees Khan** | Quaid-i-Azam University, Islamabad, Pakistan<br>Zoological Survey of Pakistan, Ministry of Climate Change, Islamabad, Pakistan |
| **Faiz-ur Rehman** | Quaid-i-Azam University, Islamabad, Pakistan |
| **Shehzad Mehmood** | Quaid-i-Azam University, Islamabad, Pakistan |
| **Saima Ali** | Quaid-i-Azam University, Islamabad, Pakistan |
| **Sheikh Zain Ul Abidin** | Quaid-i-Azam University, Islamabad, Pakistan |
| **Abdul Samad Mumtaz** | Quaid-i-Azam University, Islamabad, Pakistan |
| **Ejaz Aziz** | Quaid-i-Azam University, Islamabad, Pakistan |
| **Riffat Batool** | Quaid-i-Azam University, Islamabad, Pakistan |
| **Hussain Badshah** | Quaid-i-Azam University, Islamabad, Pakistan |
| **Ömer Kiliç** | Bingol University, Bingöl, Turkey |
| **Francesca Aiello** | Department of Pharmacy, Health and Nutritional Sciences, University of Calabria, Arcavacata di Rende (CS), Italy |
| **Devasahayam Jaya balan** | Department of Biotechnology, Alagappa University, Tamil Nadu, India |
| **Tarun Belwal** | G.B. Pant National Institute of Himalayan Environment and Sustainable Development, Uttarakhand, India |
| **Hari Prasad Devkota** | School of Pharmacy, Kumamoto University, Kumamoto, Japan |
| **Hari Prasad Devkota** | School of Pharmacy, Kumamoto University, Kumamoto, Japan<br>Program for Leading Graduate Schools, Kumamoto University, Kumamoto, Japan |
| **Ankur Kumar Goel** | Jubilant Generics Limited, Uttarakhand, India |
| **Indra D. Bhatt** | G.B. Pant National Institute of Himalayan Environment and Sustainable Development, Uttarakhand, India |
| **Seyed M. Nabavi** | Applied Biotechnology Research Center, Baqiyatallah University of Medical Sciences, Tehran, Iran |
| **Devesh Tewari** | Department of Pharmacognosy, Lovely Professional University, Punjab, India |
| **Pooja Patni** | Institute of Pharmaceutical Research, GLA University, Mathura, India |
| **Sweta Bawari** | Department of Pharmaceutical Sciences, Kumaun University Nainital, Uttarakhand, India |

**Archana N. Sah**          Department of Pharmaceutical Sciences, Kumaun University, Uttarakhand, India

**Archana N. Sah**          Department of Pharmaceutical Sciences, Kumaun University, Uttarakhand, India

**Carmela Conidi**          Institute on Membrane Technology, National Research Council, Cosenza, Italy

**Francesco Galiano**          Institute on Membrane Technology, National Research Council, Cosenza, Italy

**Cassano Alfredo**          Institute on Membrane Technology, National Research Council, Cosenza, Italy

**Figoli Alberto**          Institute on Membrane Technology, National Research Council, Cosenza, Italy

**Dalia Sánchez-Machado**          Instituto Tecnológico de Sonora, Sonora, Mexico

**Jaime López-Cervantes**          Instituto Tecnológico de Sonora, Sonora, Mexico

# DEDICATION

*With memory of Seyed Ali Asghar Nabavi, I dedicate this book to my family*

*Seyed Mohammad Nabavi and Seyed Fazel Nabavi*

*To my grandfather, José Sanches*

*Ana Sanches Silva*

*I dedicate this book to my family*

*Kasi Pandima Devi*

*To my little Ludovica light of my eyes*

*Monica Rosa Loizzo*

*To Andrea e Maria Francesca Bonesi*

*Rosa Tundis*

## CHAPTER 1

# Historical Background of Food Additives, Their Advantages and Drawbacks

**Shafaq Asif[1], Muhammed Bule[2], Fazlullah Khan[3] and Kamal Niaz[4,\*]**

[1] *Faculty of Bioscience and Agri-Food and Environmental Technology, University of Teramo-64100, Italy*

[2] *Department of Pharmacy, College of Medicine and Health Sciences, Ambo University, Ambo, Ethiopia*

[3] *The Institute of Pharmaceutical Sciences, Faculty of Pharmacy, International campus, Tehran University of Medical Sciences, Tehran-1417614411, Iran*

[4] *Department of Pharmacology and Toxicology, Faculty of Bio-Sciences, Cholistan University of Veterinary and Animal Sciences (CUVAS), Bahawalpur-63100 Pakistan*

**Abstract:** Food additives have been used since primordial times. They are the most important to impart artificial flavors and improve the quality of food and drinks. The earliest record in the history of adding additives to food dates back to Ancient Egyptian papyri circa 1500 BC. Food additives are added to food during preparation, processing manufacturing, treatment or packaging to modify chemical, biological, sensory or physical characteristics, and most of them do not have any nutritional value. They play a very important role as colorants, preservatives, antioxidants, acidity regulators, thickeners, stabilizers, emulsifiers, anti-caking agents and flavor enhancers. In addition, the demand of food additives in the food processing industries has sharply increased due to consumers' preferences and commercial advantage they provide to the manufactured food because of longer shelf-life, standardized composition and convenience in processing. Dietary fibers play a vital role in weight management, diabetes, immune regulation, promoting dental health, colonic health, cardiovascular disease prevention and functions as dietary fiber and also support digestion in both animals and human beings. On the other hand, the use of food additives has been criticized for multiple health impacts such as cancer, asthma, allergies, and behavioral disorders in children. Therefore, regulatory authorities and law enforcement agencies have passed strict laws regarding food additives' approval and control. Nevertheless, in the last few decades, the food science and technology has swiftly advanced, resulting in an increased number and variety of food additives. Moreover, the quality and safety of food additives have developed as well.

\* **Corresponding author Dr. Kamal Niaz:** Department of Pharmacology and Toxicology, Faculty of Bio-Sciences, Cholistan University of Veterinary and Animal Sciences (CUVAS), Bahawalpur-63100 Pakistan; Tel: +923129360054; E-mail: kamalniaz1989@gmail.com

**Seyed Mohammad Nabavi *et al*. (Eds.)**

**Keywords:** Disease, Food additives, Health.

# INTRODUCTION

Food additives are added to food during preparation, processing, manufacturing, treatment or packaging to modify chemical, biological, sensory or physical characteristics, and most of them do not have any nutritional value [1]. In the last few decades, changes in food technology and dietary pattern have brought about increased development and consumption of various processed food items. Food additives have become crucial in satisfying consumer demand [2]. The European regulation (EC) No. 1333/2008, defines food additives as any substance not normally consumed as a food itself but is utilized for a technological purpose, *e.g.* preservation. This regulation comprises 26 categories of food additives, which fall mainly into two categories based on their purpose: (I). Safety and prevention of the degradation of food by bacteria, oxidation or chemical reactions and/or (II). Improvement of the taste, appearance or mouth-feel of the product [3, 4]. In addition to their basic functions, food additives are used as non-nutritive sweeteners to replace sugar in food, thus minimizing the risk of dental decay and reducing the energy content of the food. In food industries, additives are quite important for producing a variety of consistently nutritious, safe and appealing products [3]. Maintaining the standards of safety, selection and convenience of processed food products is unthinkable without food additives [2]. Besides, the basic principle of additive use is safety, hence, prior to its approval for use; an additive must fulfill the toxicological evaluation requirements, considering any synergistic, cumulative and protective effects resulting from its use [1]. As a result, the acceptable maximum permitted levels have been set by authorities, but there are variations among countries. For instance, in the European Union, the daily intake threshold values of authorized food additives are listed in the annexes of council directives [5].

Improving the taste of food products *via* flavoring additives that can enhance or provide flavor and aroma without any nutritional value is a common practice. These flavoring agents are classified based on their sources as natural, synthetic nature-identical and synthetic artificial. Their chemical composition is complex and consists of various classes of compounds like antioxidants, preservatives, defoamers, emulsifiers, diluents, flavor enhancers, stabilizers, dyes, acidity regulators, anti-caking agents, and solvents used for the purpose of extraction and processing [6]. The other important feature of food additives is providing a desired appearance to the food item. Dyes are a group of food additives that are used in a wide variety of foods to enhance their appearance [7]. In this regard, natural colors such as chlorophyll, saffron, caramel, β-carotene, and annatto and synthetic colorants like tartrazine, ponceau 4R, permitted organic synthetic dyes, allura red, Brilliant blue, orange GGN and sunset yellow are the most commonly used colorants. Moreover, synthetic colorants are preferred because of their stability, coloring properties, uniformity and low cost [8]. The US Food and Drug Administration (USFDA) has approved 12 synthetic food colorant additives (referred to as 'certified' or 'FD&C') which are subject to 'batch certification', that requires undergoing chemical analysis at the USFDA laboratory for every batch produced, to confirm the quality and purity standards [9, 10]. Artificial food coloring additives (AFCAs) have been studied for their health effects and are associated with systemic, cognitive, behavioral, and skin related effects. Their action against antioxidative enzymes and endogenous antioxidants in the skin has also been recorded [11].

The other major and important groups of food additives that serve the protective and safety role in processed food by preventing food degradation by microorganisms, oxidative, and chemical processes are the preservatives and antioxidants. Preservatives are food additives that prolong the shelf life by preventing the biodegradation of food. The ester of *p*-hydroxybenzoic acid (parabens), sorbic acid, benzoic acid and sulfites are among the most commonly utilized preservatives [7]. Various compounds, some with OH groups, are added to food to prevent degradation due to microorganisms and oxygen, or to improve the color, taste, and aroma. However, the added amount will be considered not to exceed the allowed daily intake value of food additives [12]. Essential oils are commonly used as flavoring agents, nevertheless, their antimicrobial effects against foodborne pathogens have made them a significant source of natural preservatives. Particularly in dry-cured meat products, their use has gained interest in the control of microorganisms [13]. Furthermore, natural antioxidant food additives, which comprise extracts and their diverse ingredients, are extensively used to prevent deterioration due to oxidation and control the quality and safety of processed food [14]. Antioxidants mostly used are synthetic antioxidants such as the propyl gallate (PG), dodecyl gallate (DG), octyl gallate (OG), *tert*-butyl hydroquinone (TBHQ), butylated hydroxyanisole (BHA) and butylated hydroxytoluene (BHT). In addition, ascorbic acid and its L isomer, and isoascorbic acid, are natural antioxidants particularly used in beverages [7]. However, there is a strict regulation on the use of synthetic antioxidants because of their likely health hazard leading to carcinogenesis and consumers' rejection of synthetic food additives. Besides, only a limited number of natural food additives are available to be used as an alternative to replace the synthetic ones. Thus, the demand for the search of more effective natural antioxidants, their development and use is high among researchers in the area [15].

Generally, food additives have been utilized to speed up and complement the production process in the contemporary food supply chain. However, every consumer is unavoidably exposed to the potential allergens in the food additives [16]. Although there are thousands of food additives, fairly few have been associated with serious adverse reactions. Some of the additives indicated to have potential adverse reactions are monosodium glutamate, tartarazine, sulphite, salycilate, benzoate, nitrites, aspartame and some colorants [2]. As a matter of fact these additives in food may cause adverse reactions in sensitive individuals with preexisting allergies like hay fever and asthma [5]. Coupled with a significantly increased risk of long-term effects such as cancer, certain consumers have shown acute intolerance and allergic reactions to approximately 200 food additives [17].

Allergy due to food additives is a widely studied and well-recorded phenomenon [18]. Side effects related to food additives may result in one or more types of health risks [19]. The natural dye cochineal extract, which is obtained from dried female insects of the *D. coccus*, is hydrophilic, stable to heat and light and changes color with a change in pH without forming sediment. It has been widely used as a food additive but allergic reactions have been reported in relation to its use, probably arising from proteins and peptide contents of the extract [20]. In one study, it is indicated that carmine, a natural food colorant and cochineal extract, plays a role in atopic eczema. Furthermore, carmine-induced occupational asthma and anaphylaxis after consuming carmine containing products have been reported [21]. Additionally, high fructose corn syrup (HFCS), which is a well-refined sweetener and a leading source of calories in the USA, is believed to increase LDL cholesterol level, and the risk of diabetes and obesity. Moreover, the widely used preservatives BHA and BHT, which are added to maintain food color, flavor, and prevent rancidity are liable for the cancer causing reactive compounds in the body [19]. Another notable heterocyclic compound 4(5)-methylimidazole is formed during the thermal processing of food spontaneously *via* Millard reaction. The 4(5)-methylimidazole, which is commonly found in brown foods such as coffee, backed food, processed sauces, roasted food, beer and soft drinks, has been classified as a carcinogen by the Office of Environmental Health Hazard Assessment (OEHHA) and California Environmental Protection Agency (EPA) [22, 23]. As a result, the European Commission (EC) and the Joint FAO/WHO Expert Committee on Food Additives (JECFA) have recommended limiting class III and IV caramel concentration to 250 mg/kg and 300 mg/kg, respectively [24, 25]. In general, the relevance of food additives used for various purposes in present-day food processing industries is quite obvious. However, their use should be strictly consulted to minimize direct and indirect health hazards.

## BACKGROUND OF FOOD ADDITIVES

The earliest record in the history of the addition of additives to food dates back to Ancient Egyptian papyri circa 1500 BC. In addition to adding spices in food to improve the flavor and make it more appealing, the Egyptians also utilized yeast in baking to allow the bread to rise. Later, in the nineteenth century, the invention of a leavening substance containing bicarbonate of soda (E500) replaced yeast. In the last few decades, food science and technology has swiftly advanced, resulting in an increased number and variety of food additives. Currently, there are more than 320 food additives approved for use in the European Union [3, 26, 27]. The dynamics of the human diet have changed significantly since the mid-twentieth century due to a rise in food additives consumption. The basic concern in the approval process of food additives is the idea that they do not lead to acute toxicity at a concentration fairly greater than the approved amount [28]. The Joint FAO/WHO Expert Committee on Food Additives (JECFA) is an international scientific expert committee that is administered jointly by the Food and Agriculture Organization of the United Nations (FAO) and the World Health Organization (WHO). With the primary idea of evaluating the safety of food additives, the JECFA has been conducting meetings since 1956. Currently, the JECFA is responsible for the evaluation of naturally occurring toxicants, contaminants and veterinary drugs in food [25, 29]. Moreover, there are a number of institutions which perform in a similar manner, for instance, the USFDA, the EC and the JECFA, Australia and New Zealand are few among many [3, 4, 10, 25].

Throughout the history, numerous legislations about the use of food additives have been passed to ensure their safety. Being the first of its kind, the German Beer Purity law of 1516 was enacted in order to control the purity of beer ingredients and substances that could be added to food and beverages. Thenceforth, legislation has been enforced to control the actions of processed food manufacturers and prevent public health threats [3]. With the aim of prolonging shelf life, improving flavor and appearance, food additives have been used for centuries. In 1958, there were only about 800 food additives when the US Congress first g authorized the use of food additives by the USFDA. Since then, the FDA has registered quite a large number of food additives of B class generally recognized as safe (GRAS). Currently, the figure continues to grow faster and there are more than 10,000 food additives in use [19]. In accordance with the US FDA 1958 amendment of food additives, manufacturers are allowed to determine GRAS food additives under the 'GRAS determination'. Once the GRAS determination is concluded, except in some instances, the producers are not obliged to notify the FDA. However, the agency ruled out this option in 1997 and considered sending a letter to the producers in case there appears an insufficient ground for GRAS determination, whenever the agency disagreed. Later in 2010, the US Government Accountability Office (GAO) inspected the GRAS determination, and recommended that the FDA should minimize the potential for conflicts of interest in companies, GRAS determinations and inquire any company that conducts a GRAS determination to provide the FDA with basic information- as defined by the agency to allow for adequate oversight about this determination [30].

Furthermore, the Legislation passed by the US Congress in 1958, which is referred to as the Delaney Clause, prohibits the use of any food additive proved to be carcinogenic in any species of animal or humans. However, it has been blamed for being too restrictive with zero tolerance to any level of risk [31]. In addition to the Delaney Clause, various amendments have been made to the Federal Food, Drug, and Cosmetic Act since the 1960's. The FDA has recently adopted a review of direct food additives to satisfy the demand to obtain better data and to standardize the criteria for acceptability and the testing procedures. Likewise, the JECFA has also recognized the reevaluation or examination of the safety of numerous food additives [32]. On the other hand, the EFSA and JECFA highlighted children as the most vulnerable to the impact related to food additives due to their dietary behavior and the fact that their physiological reactions may differ greatly from adults [33]. In this regard, the EU legislation of food additives, published in October 2008 and enforced in January 2009 (regulation EC No. 1333/2008; and European Commission 2008), insists on labeling any food on sale to indicate food that contains particular food additives (Sunset Yellow, Carmoisine, Tartrazine, Ponceau 4R, Allura Red, and Quinoline Yellow) that it 'may have an adverse effect on activity and attention in children' [4, 26, 34]. Besides, the European Commission published Regulation (EU) No [4], which entered into force in June 2013, produced a system for categorizing foods on the basis of Codex Alimentarius General Standard for Food Additives and the maximum allowed level of food additives [33]. Despite the tight regulatory process that rules out most of the potentially harmful food additives, there still exists a small amount of uncertainty. Thus, consumers who are frequently exposed to misleading information might assume that food additives are associated with a high level of risk. Such misconceptions could cause disbelief and a sense of anxiety among the consumers and the producers [2]. Although inappropriate use may result in carcinogenesis or other toxicity, most food additives are regarded as safe for daily uses. Additionally, hyperactivity in children, migraines, asthma, and allergies are adverse reactions often caused by food additives [35]. However, regardless of all these, food additives have been the heart of the global food industry in the last few decades, represented by terms like 'food is processing' and 'agribusiness'. Therefore, food additives that provide a commercial advantage to manufactured food because of longer shelf-life, standardized composition and convenience in the processing are still demanded in the food processing industry [17].

## ADVANTAGES AND DISADVANTAGES OF FOOD ADDITIVES

Food additives have been used since primordial times. They are important in order to impart artificial flavors and improve the quality of food and drinks. They play very important roles as they are not food themselves but being colorants, preservatives, antioxidants, acidity regulators, thickeners, stabilizers, emulsifiers, acidity regulators, anti-caking agents and flavor enhancers, they are the major constituents of the food [36, 37].

Before pondering over the current sufferings and benefits, just have a look on the list of additives, issued by the secretariat of the joint FAO/WHO. They are also given E number by the European Union committee [38, 39].

### Groups of Food Additives

1. Acids, bases and salts such acetic acid, citric acid, calcium carbonate and sodium chloride.
2. Anti-caking agents such as magnesium carbonate and calcium silicate.
3. Antioxidants and antioxidant synergists such as ascorbic acid and BHA.
4. Carrier solvents such as glycerin and propylene glycol.
5. Colors such as amaranth and tartrazine.
6. Emulsifiers, stabilizers and thickening agents such as lecithin, propylene glycol esters of fatty acids, and modified starches.
7. Enzyme preparations such as rennet.
8. Extraction solvents such as ethanol, ethyl acetate *etc*.
9. Flavors such as mint flavor (mint oil).
10. Flavors enhancers such as glutamic acid.
11. Flour-treatment agents such as ascorbic acid, chlorine dioxide.
12. Miscellaneous such as mineral oil.
13. Non-nutritive sweeteners such as saccharin.

The major classes of food additives, along with their effects, have been mentioned in Fig. (**1**). The major purpose of the food additives as acid and alkalis (bases) is to prevent the growth of bacteria and other harmful microbes in food in order to preserve their characteristics as acidity regulators and pH control agents (Fig. **1**). Moreover, they are important to increase food's shelf life. Oxidative stress gives an impression of being responsible for numerous human disorders; therefore, frequently used antioxidants are indicated in the pharmacological treatment or as dietary supplements for stroke, reproductive and neurodegenerative ailments and even altitude or height phobia [40]. In addition, oxidative stress is both the reason and the result of the disorder. It has been well-established that the body has own self mechanism to secrete cytokines and enzymes which help in the prevention of cancer and improve health safety. They act to prevent healthy cells from apoptosis, DNA damage and oxidative stress caused by the high production of free radicals produced by polycyclic aromatic hydrocarbons and smoke flavorings foods additives [41]. Vast clinical trials with a predetermined number of reinforcements identified no advantage and even recommended that abundant supplementation with certain putative cancer prevention agents might be dangerous.

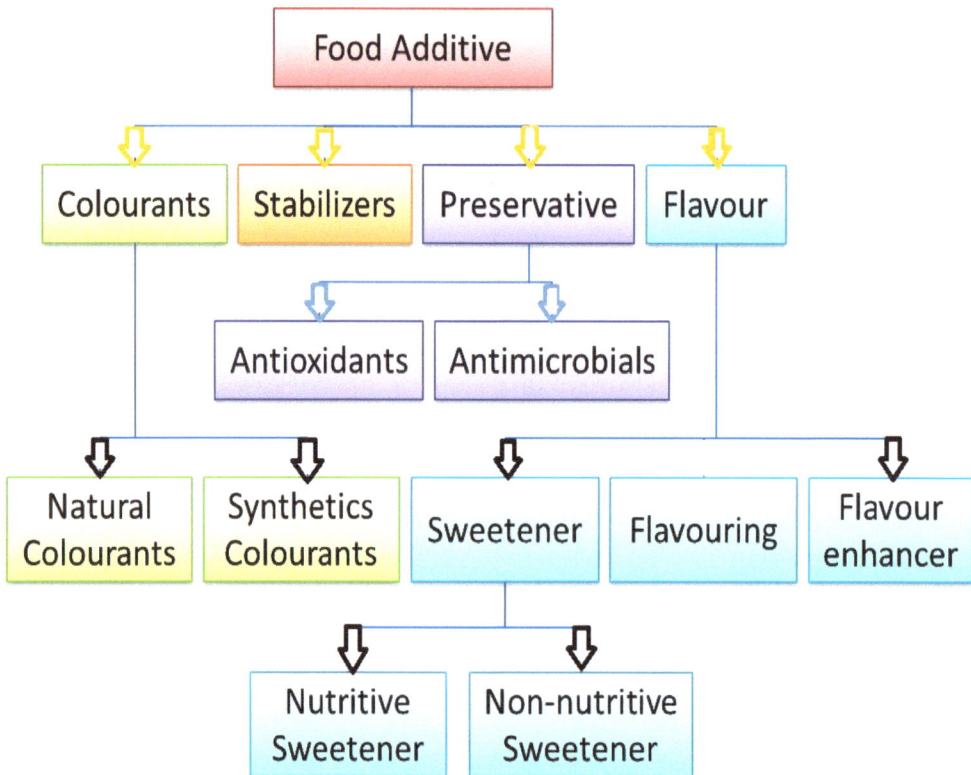

**Fig. (1).** Flow chart illustrate various food additives effect categories.

Food preservatives can cause allergies to skin, nausea, vomiting and irritation of the eyes and nose [42 - 44].

Anti-caking agents are anhydrous mediators that are incorporated in little amounts, to keep food and pharmaceuticals dry, to prevent the particles coagulating due to moisture and to ensure that the item stays dry and free-streaming. Calcium silicate is the most well-known anti-caking agent available [45, 46]. A study explored that anticaking agents are broken in the gastrointestinal tract (GIT) and absorb as broken silicates, however, the body also absorbs nano-silica particles themselves from the GIT. For stimulating infants' lung and gut maturation, a nutritional composition containing 3-20% weight phospholipids based on total fat is needed to be administered [47]. For the first scenario, nearly 100 food additives products were reviewed and observed for toxicological data. In the meeting, where possible, acceptable daily intakes (ADI) were checked for human additives, however, for 14 food additives, no ADI were recommended due to limited data. The adverse effect was found of nano-silica, while for the second situation; hazardous effects of nano-silica are yet to be explored, as anti-caking agents cause liver damage but still studies are in progress [48].

Food colorants are substances that give colors to food in order to enhance the appearance of food. Different studies have been dedicated to evaluate the toxicity of additives to foods, specifically to azo-colors. This group of colorants normally comprises splendid and bright colors [49 - 51]. After banning cyclamates in the United State and Britain, the alternative artificial sweetener saccharin was used and it has potential cancer-causing nature and later on, it was declared as a carcinogen due to unique urine chemistry.

Previous studies (2014-16) have found that children consume more food colorants and they are more affected in order to undergo behavioral disorders, psychological problems which interfere in their activity, produce attention disorders and intolerant reactions in small populations [52 - 56]. *In vitro* studies have also remarked the adverse effect of food colorants on the neural cell differentiation but till that time, the mechanism and action of this particular disability were unknown. The common examples are alginic acid (E400) and sodium alginate (E401). Hydrocolloids are miraculous because they exhibit the useful properties relevant to the foodstuff colloidal frameworks. They work as food thickeners, gelling initiators, foaming agents, delicious and attractive coatings for food, emulsifiers, stabilizers, and so on [57 - 59]. The primary drawback besides the broad use of hydrocolloids in the food industry is their capacity to bind with water and alter the properties of food and its fixation. They also function as dietary fiber and support digestion both in the animals and human beings. Food additives' consumption provides unlimited benefits such as weight management, immune regulation, colonic health, and cardiovascular disease prevention. It plays a vital role in glycaemia and insulinaemic control in type-2 diabetes [60]. Generally, enzymes/proteins are not added to food but they are the major part of the food in the form of essential amino acids. Numerous enzymes have been widely utilized as a part of nutrition in the food industry [61]. Soybean proteins are incorporated into a wide range of eatables as a food source and nowadays, as an essential protein for vegetarians [62, 63]. Enzymes actively play a role in the preservation of food. The use of biofilm for packaging foodstuff which has an antimicrobial activity enhances the shelf life, maintains the packaging of food fresh and lessens the risk of pathogens attack and their growth. The application of high-grade antimicrobial packaging films is due to biodegradability which reduces the use of drugs/chemicals as antibiotics and decreases economic loss as they are compatible with the modern community [64, 65]. Transformation or preservations have both good and bad aspects. The use of combined and pulse electric field treatment inactivates the endospore, however, in the industrial application, optimization of the treatment chamber design has to be monitored for inhomogeneous temperature fields [66].

Flavor agents have the capability to restore the taste and to improve aroma or maintain nourishment. Two additive enhancers L-glutamic acid (mono-sodium glutamate) and also aspartame (1-methyl N-L-alpha-aspartyl-phenylalanine) have been analyzed regarding their safety for the purpose of enhancing the taste of food. Since the excitotoxic effects are noteworthy, the possibility to alter central neurons by excessive stimulation of postsynaptic excitatory membrane receptors, predominantly the NMDA subtype of glutamate receptor is obvious [67]. The use of food additives such as acesulfame-K, saccharin, caffeine, benzoic acid and sorbic acid in different beverages, soft drinks and nectars did not establish ADIs in Portuguese people.

Diabetes and obesity are common problems of modern world that are the consequence of the life style adapted and the intake of unhealthy food. The food industries are obliged to satisfy their customers by fulfilling their demands. To achieve their goals, they prefer to produce products with low energy content, sugar control and dietary products with sugar alcohols and sweeteners. Hydrogenation of carbohydrates with the help of a catalyst promotes the production of such kind of products. Naturally, such sweeteners are found in vegetables, mushrooms and fruits. Human bones ligaments and other organs are also the source of such sweeteners after degradation [68]. Sugar alcohols are supportive towards the enhancement of dental health and as prebiotics [69, 70]. Such food sweeteners are being used in food products, drinks, *i.e.* colas, medicinal drugs and powdered sweeteners products. Such artificial sugars are expected to control and reduce the intake of calories. Consumption of low-calorie food eventually leads to calorie-controlled diet around the world that results in a dramatically increased population; however, concerns arise in the use of sweeteners. Many surveys highlight the regular use of sugar alcohols, for example, erythritol, isomalt, lactitol, maltitol, mannitol, sorbitol and xylitol as sugar substitutes by the food industry [71 - 73].

Some food additives can possibly cause unsafe symptoms. For instance, butylated hydroxyanisole, generally known as BHA, is an additive utilized as a part of food items such as potato chips, wafers, lager, prepared products and oat. It has been certified by the U.S. Bureau of Health and Human Services as an additive "sensibly foreseen to be a human cancer-causing agent." Sulfites, which are added to prepared products, wine, sauces and nibble agents, could cause hives, diarrhea, nausea, and shortness of breath in a few people.

Food additives' consumption improves the quality and quantity of food according to the consumers' demands. This is achieved by flavoring, coloring, emulsification, and stabilization from a medicinal point of view or due to longer preservation and improvement of quality to increase importations/exportations. Furthermore, the advancement in food due to science technology is nowadays noteworthy economic progress [74]. The interesting properties of food additives need special attention to protect nutritive value according to the needs of customers around the globe. Numerous food additives are known to have antimicrobial potential against the most common bacteria found in food, such as *L. monocytogenes, E. coli* and *Salmonella* [75]. For some foods, (*e.g.* meat, poultry, dairy products, vegetables and fruits), both quality and quantity are important and food preservatives enhance as analogous to the conventional synthetic preservative effect for each food, so food preservatives have a vital role in the commercial world. The food scientist usually deals with the challenge of modifying the formulation of food products to enhance taste, texture or appearance of food and to obtain a healthier product or food with longer shelf-life. The objectives are to reduce production cost by incorporating cheaper ingredients or to improve manufacturing efficiency by bringing in new processing technology.

As mentioned earlier, all perspectives are of greater importance to enhance the value of eatables such as food and drinks at both edges *i.e.* for seller and buyer. The advancement in food science and technology cannot be underestimated but the major concern is about the original texture and the organic nature of the food. As it is worthy that food is valuable when it is according to the consumer's choice and nutritional benefits. The more artificial is the food; the more prone it is to have adverse health effects. Food additives have adverse effects particularly on the nervous system, of both children and adults. They are causative agents of psychological disorders [76 - 79]. They lead to vulnerable mental problems. On one hand, from the industrial point of view, additives in the form of preservatives, and flavors improve the number of consumers and improve business, on the other hand, they can be detrimental to the life of consumers, therefore it is essential to ensure their safe use.

## CONCLUSION AND FUTURE ASPECTS

Food additives with all their pros and cons are important ingredients of modern food and drinks. Worldwide, they are constantly being used as the major constituents of diet. In the current scenario, global warming is a major threat to climate and drastic changes, which has been observed across the planet in the shape of unexpected drought and food shortage. Hence those substances that are used to ensure the long and safer shelf life of food must be appreciated. Such food additives will improve the quality of stored food and increase their shelf life. However, it should be kept in mind that the application of food additives would be an ideal alternative if the adverse effects of these additives were minimum. The addition of food additives leads to the improvement of the food quality that fulfills the demand of consumers according to their needs. It is noteworthy that food additives' intake should provide the basis for productive food and nutritional scrutiny policy to aid in developing healthy eating habits. Preliminary utilization of food additives was a great improvement as they enhanced the quantity and quality of food [80]. These chemicals or preservatives are used in order to extend the life of available food and preserve food for longer periods. By providing easy access to consumers of food in adequate quantities by enhancing the shelf life of food, these profits significantly exceed the losses and threats distinguished by the advanced systems of food science and biotechnology. It will be a major breakthrough if the food additives are used under standard conditions of quality and controlled worldwide with greater benefits to the health and economy of the consumers.

## AUTHOR CONTRIBUTIONS

All authors have directly participated in the planning or drafting of the chapter, read and approved the final version.

## CONSENT FOR PUBLICATION

Not applicable.

## CONFLICT OF INTEREST

The author confirms that this chapter contents have no conflict of interest.

## ACKNOWLEDGEMENTS

This chapter is the outcome of an in-house financially non-supported study.

## REFERENCES

[1]    Campos JM, Stamford TL, Sarubbo LA, de Luna JM, Rufino RD, Banat IM. Microbial biosurfactants as additives for food industries. Biotechnol Prog 2013; 29(5): 1097-108.
[http://dx.doi.org/10.1002/btpr.1796] [PMID: 23956227]

[2]    Kang MG, Song WJ, Park HK, *et al.* Basophil activation test with food additives in chronic urticaria

patients. Clin Nutr Res 2014; 3(1): 9-16.
[http://dx.doi.org/10.7762/cnr.2014.3.1.9] [PMID: 24527415]

[3]     Martyn DM, McNulty BA, Nugent AP, Gibney MJ. Food additives and preschool children. Proc Nutr
        Soc 2013; 72(1): 109-16.
        [http://dx.doi.org/10.1017/S0029665112002935] [PMID: 23336563]

[4]     Regulation (EC) no 1333/2008 of the European Parliament and of the council of 16 December 2008 on
        food additives Official Journal of the European Union 2008; 354(16)

[5]     Aşçı B, Dinç Zor Ş, Aksu Dönmez Ö. Development and Validation of HPLC Method for the
        Simultaneous Determination of Five Food Additives and Caffeine in Soft Drinks. Int J Anal Chem
        2016; 20162879406
        [http://dx.doi.org/10.1155/2016/2879406] [PMID: 26989415]

[6]     Nunes RD, Sales IM, Silva SI, Sousa JM, Peron AP. Antiproliferative and genotoxic effects of nature
        identical and artificial synthetic food additives of aroma and flavor. Braz J Biol 2016; 0: 0.
        [http://dx.doi.org/10.1590/1519-6984.12115]

[7]     Boyce MC. Determination of additives and organic contaminants in food by CE and CEC.
        Electrophoresis 2007; 28(22): 4046-62.
        [http://dx.doi.org/10.1002/elps.200700280] [PMID: 17948272]

[8]     El-Wahab HM, Moram GS. Toxic effects of some synthetic food colorants and/or flavor additives on
        male rats. Toxicol Ind Health 2013; 29(2): 224-32.
        [http://dx.doi.org/10.1177/0748233711433935] [PMID: 22317828]

[9]     Bastaki M, Codrea S. Article on food color additives analysis is invalid and misleading. Clin Pediatr
        (Phila) 2014; 53(13): 1308.
        [http://dx.doi.org/10.1177/0009922814551126] [PMID: 25238777]

[10]    US FDA. Food Additive and Color Additive Petitions Under Review or Held in Abeyance. FDA 2018.

[11]    Başak K, Başak PY, Doğuç DK, *et al.* Does maternal exposure to artificial food coloring additives
        increase oxidative stress in the skin of rats? Hum Exp Toxicol 2017; 36(10): 1023-30.
        [http://dx.doi.org/10.1177/0960327116678297] [PMID: 27852938]

[12]    Aoshima H, Mitsusada N, Nishino T. Effects of aliphatic alcohols and food additives on nicotinic
        acetylcholine receptors in Xenopus oocytes. Biosci Biotechnol Biochem 1994; 58(10): 1776-9.
        [http://dx.doi.org/10.1271/bbb.58.1776] [PMID: 7765504]

[13]    García-Díez J, Alheiro J, Pinto AL, *et al.* Influence of Food Characteristics and Food Additives on the
        Antimicrobial Effect of Garlic and Oregano Essential Oils. Foods 2017; 6(6): 44.
        [http://dx.doi.org/10.3390/foods6060044] [PMID: 28604598]

[14]    Amakura Y, Yoshimura M, Sugimoto N, Yamazaki T, Yoshida T. Marker constituents of the natural
        antioxidant Eucalyptus leaf extract for the evaluation of food additives. Biosci Biotechnol Biochem
        2009; 73(5): 1060-5.
        [http://dx.doi.org/10.1271/bbb.80832] [PMID: 19420705]

[15]    Maqsood S, Benjakul S, Shahidi F. Emerging role of phenolic compounds as natural food additives in
        fish and fish products. Crit Rev Food Sci Nutr 2013; 53(2): 162-79.
        [http://dx.doi.org/10.1080/10408398.2010.518775] [PMID: 23072531]

[16]    Gultekin F, Doguc DK. Allergic and immunologic reactions to food additives. Clin Rev Allergy
        Immunol 2013; 45(1): 6-29.
        [http://dx.doi.org/10.1007/s12016-012-8300-8] [PMID: 22278172]

[17]    Mepham B. Food additives: an ethical evaluation. Br Med Bull 2011; 99: 7-23.
        [http://dx.doi.org/10.1093/bmb/ldr024] [PMID: 21725085]

[18]    Myles IA, Beakes D. An Allergy to Goldfish? Highlighting the Labeling Laws for Food Additives.
        World Allergy Organ J 2009; 2(12): 314-6.

[http://dx.doi.org/10.1097/WOX.0b013e3181c5be33] [PMID: 20076772]

[19]   Çelik Ertuğrul D. FoodWiki: a Mobile App Examines Side Effects of Food Additives *Via* Semantic Web. J Med Syst 2016; 40(2): 41.
[http://dx.doi.org/10.1007/s10916-015-0372-6] [PMID: 26590979]

[20]   Ito Y, Harikai N, Ishizuki K, Shinomiya K, Sugimoto N, Akiyama H. Spiroketalcarminic Acid, a Novel Minor Anthraquinone Pigment in Cochineal Extract Used in Food Additives. Chem Pharm Bull (Tokyo) 2017; 65(9): 883-7.
[http://dx.doi.org/10.1248/cpb.c17-00404] [PMID: 28674282]

[21]   Catli G, Bostanci I, Ozmen S, Dibek Misirlioglu E, Duman H, Ertan U. Is Patch Testing with Food Additives Useful in Children with Atopic Eczema? Pediatr Dermatol 2015; 32(5): 684-9.
[http://dx.doi.org/10.1111/pde.12588] [PMID: 25873103]

[22]   Adams LS, Schwarzenegger A. Office of Environmental Health Hazard Assessment. 2009.

[23]   Lee KG, Jang H, Shibamoto T. Formation of carcinogenic 4(5)-methylimidazole in caramel model systems: a role of sulphite. Food Chem 2013; 136(3-4): 1165-8.
[http://dx.doi.org/10.1016/j.foodchem.2012.09.025] [PMID: 23194510]

[24]   Lee S, Lee JB, Hwang J, Lee KG. Effect of Various Food Additives on the Levels of 4(5)-Methylimidazole in a Soy Sauce Model System. J Food Sci 2016; 81(1): T262-7.
[http://dx.doi.org/10.1111/1750-3841.13183] [PMID: 26661512]

[25]   Food RO. Joint FAO/WHO expert committee on food additives (JECFA)

[26]   Commission Regulation EU. Commission Regulation (EU) No 1129/2011 of 11 November 2011 amending Annex II to Regulation (EC) No 1333/2008 of the European Parliament and of the Council by establishing a Union list of food additives Official Journal of the European Union L, 2011; 295(4): 12.11.

[27]   Commission EU. EU Commission. Amending Annex II to Regulation (EC) No 1333/2008 of the European Parliament and of the Council by establishing a Union list of food additives 1129/2011

[28]   Roca-Saavedra P, Mendez-Vilabrille V, Miranda JM, *et al.* Food additives, contaminants and other minor components: effects on human gut microbiota-a review. J Physiol Biochem 2018; 74(1): 69-83.
[http://dx.doi.org/10.1007/s13105-017-0564-2] [PMID: 28488210]

[29]   Boobis A, Cerniglia C, Chicoine A, *et al.* Characterizing chronic and acute health risks of residues of veterinary drugs in food: latest methodological developments by the joint FAO/WHO expert committee on food additives. Crit Rev Toxicol 2017; 47(10): 885-99.
[http://dx.doi.org/10.1080/10408444.2017.1340259] [PMID: 28691548]

[30]   Neltner TG, Alger HM, O'Reilly JT, Krimsky S, Bero LA, Maffini MV. Conflicts of interest in approvals of additives to food determined to be generally recognized as safe: out of balance. JAMA Intern Med 2013; 173(22): 2032-6.
[http://dx.doi.org/10.1001/jamainternmed.2013.10559] [PMID: 23925593]

[31]   Ashby J. Change the rules for food additives. Nature 1994; 368(6472): 582.
[http://dx.doi.org/10.1038/368582a0] [PMID: 8145840]

[32]   Council NR. Diet, nutrition, and cancer. National Academies Press 1982.

[33]   Diouf F, Berg K, Ptok S, Lindtner O, Heinemeyer G, Heseker H. German database on the occurrence of food additives: application for intake estimation of five food colours for toddlers and children. Food Addit Contam Part A Chem Anal Control Expo Risk Assess 2014; 31(2): 197-206.
[http://dx.doi.org/10.1080/19440049.2013.865146] [PMID: 24229358]

[34]   Connolly A, Hearty A, Nugent A, *et al.* Pattern of intake of food additives associated with hyperactivity in Irish children and teenagers. Food Addit Contam Part A Chem Anal Control Expo Risk Assess 2010; 27(4): 447-56.
[http://dx.doi.org/10.1080/19440040903470718] [PMID: 20013441]

[35] Park M, Park HR, Kim SJ, *et al.* Risk assessment for the combinational effects of food color additives: neural progenitor cells and hippocampal neurogenesis. J Toxicol Environ Health A 2009; 72(21-22): 1412-23.
[http://dx.doi.org/10.1080/15287390903212816] [PMID: 20077213]

[36] Saltmarsh M. Recent trends in the use of food additives in the United Kingdom. J Sci Food Agric 2015; 95(4): 649-52.
[http://dx.doi.org/10.1002/jsfa.6715] [PMID: 24789520]

[37] Carocho M, Barreiro MF, Morales P, Ferreira IC. Adding molecules to food, pros and cons: A review on synthetic and natural food additives. Compr Rev Food Sci Food Saf 2014; 13(4): 377-99.
[http://dx.doi.org/10.1111/1541-4337.12065]

[38] Joint FA. World Health Organization, Evaluation of Certain Veterinary Drug Residues in Food: Eighty-first Report of the Joint FAO/WHO Expert Committee on Food Additives. World Health Organization 2016; Vol. 81.

[39] Sarıkaya R, Selvi M, Erkoç F. Evaluation of potential genotoxicity of five food dyes using the somatic mutation and recombination test. Chemosphere 2012; 88(8): 974-9.
[http://dx.doi.org/10.1016/j.chemosphere.2012.03.032] [PMID: 22482698]

[40] Carocho M, Ferreira IC. A review on antioxidants, prooxidants and related controversy: natural and synthetic compounds, screening and analysis methodologies and future perspectives. Food Chem Toxicol 2013; 51: 15-25.
[http://dx.doi.org/10.1016/j.fct.2012.09.021] [PMID: 23017782]

[41] Šimko P. Determination of polycyclic aromatic hydrocarbons in smoked meat products and smoke flavouring food additives. J Chromatogr B Analyt Technol Biomed Life Sci 2002; 770(1-2): 3-18.
[http://dx.doi.org/10.1016/S0378-4347(01)00438-8] [PMID: 12013240]

[42] Zaknun D, Schroecksnadel S, Kurz K, Fuchs D. Potential role of antioxidant food supplements, preservatives and colorants in the pathogenesis of allergy and asthma. Int Arch Allergy Immunol 2012; 157(2): 113-24.
[http://dx.doi.org/10.1159/000329137] [PMID: 21986480]

[43] Ho MHK, Wong WH, Chang C. Clinical spectrum of food allergies: a comprehensive review. Clin Rev Allergy Immunol 2014; 46(3): 225-40.
[http://dx.doi.org/10.1007/s12016-012-8339-6] [PMID: 23229594]

[44] Silva MM, Lidon FC. Food preservatives-An overview on applications and side effects. Emir J Food Agric 2016; 28(6): 366.
[http://dx.doi.org/10.9755/ejfa.2016-04-351]

[45] Abad E, Llerena JJ, Sauló J, Caixach J, Rivera J. Comprehensive study on dioxin contents in binder and anti-caking agent feed additives. Chemosphere 2002; 46(9-10): 1417-21.
[http://dx.doi.org/10.1016/S0045-6535(01)00274-0] [PMID: 12002470]

[46] Martin KR. The chemistry of silica and its potential health benefits. J Nutr Health Aging 2007; 11(2): 94-7.
[PMID: 17435951]

[47] Lai CS, Buddington R. Methods of stimulating infant lung and gut maturation. Google Patents 2014.

[48] Monopalmitate S. Toxicological evaluation of some food colours, emulsifiers, stabilizers, anti-caking agents and certain other substances. 1969.

[49] Wada M, Kido H, Ohyama K, *et al.* Chemiluminescent screening of quenching effects of natural colorants against reactive oxygen species: Evaluation of grape seed, monascus, gardenia and red radish extracts as multi-functional food additives. Food Chem 2007; 101(3): 980-6.
[http://dx.doi.org/10.1016/j.foodchem.2006.02.050]

[50] Branen AL, Davidson PM, Salminen S, Thorngate J, Eds. Food additives. CRC Press 2001.

[51]    Puttemans M, Dryon L, Massart D. Ion-pair high performance liquid chromatography of synthetic water-soluble acid dyes Food dyes, food additives, food colorants, food technology, toxicity, chemical analysis. J Asso Official Ana Chem 1981.

[52]    Heilskov Rytter MJ, Andersen LB, Houmann T, *et al.* Diet in the treatment of ADHD in children - a systematic review of the literature. Nord J Psychiatry 2015; 69(1): 1-18.
        [http://dx.doi.org/10.3109/08039488.2014.921933] [PMID: 24934907]

[53]    Stevens LJ, Burgess JR, Stochelski MA, Kuczek T. Amounts of artificial food dyes and added sugars in foods and sweets commonly consumed by children. Clin Pediatr (Phila) 2015; 54(4): 309-21.
        [http://dx.doi.org/10.1177/0009922814530803] [PMID: 24764054]

[54]    Vojdani A, Vojdani C. Immune reactivity to food coloring. Altern Ther Health Med 2015; 21 (Suppl. 1): 52-62.
        [PMID: 25599186]

[55]    Stevens LJ, Burgess JR, Stochelski MA, Kuczek T. Amounts of artificial food colors in commonly consumed beverages and potential behavioral implications for consumption in children. Clin Pediatr (Phila) 2014; 53(2): 133-40.
        [http://dx.doi.org/10.1177/0009922813502849] [PMID: 24037921]

[56]    Amchova P, Kotolova H, Ruda-Kucerova J. Health safety issues of synthetic food colorants. Regul Toxicol Pharmacol 2015; 73(3): 914-22.
        [http://dx.doi.org/10.1016/j.yrtph.2015.09.026] [PMID: 26404013]

[57]    Hardy Z, Jideani VA. Foam-mat drying technology: A review. Crit Rev Food Sci Nutr 2017; 57(12): 2560-72.
        [http://dx.doi.org/10.1080/10408398.2015.1020359] [PMID: 26167878]

[58]    Dourado F, Leal M, Martins D, Fontão A, Rodrigues AC, Gama M. Celluloses as food ingredients/additives: Is there a room for BNC?, in Bacterial Nanocellulose 2017; 123-33.

[59]    Leser M, Bezelgues JB, Kolodziejczyk E, Michel M. inventors; Nestec SA, assignee. Aqueous foams, food products and a method of producing same 2014. Google Patents

[60]    Li JM, Nie SP. The functional and nutritional aspects of hydrocolloids in foods. Food Hydrocoll 2016; 53: 46-61.
        [http://dx.doi.org/10.1016/j.foodhyd.2015.01.035]

[61]    Nunes CS, Kunamneni A, Kumar V, Habte-Tsion HM. Registration of food and feed additives (enzymes) in the United States, Canada, and China, in Enzymes in Human and Animal Nutrition 2018; 457-80.

[62]    Greco E, Winquist A, Lee TJ, Collins S, Lebovic Z. The Role of Source of Protein in Regulation of Food Intake, Satiety, Body Weight and Body Composition. J Nutr Health Food Eng 2017; 6(6): 00223.

[63]    Augustin MA, Riley M, Stockmann R, *et al.* Role of food processing in food and nutrition security. Trends Food Sci Technol 2016; 56: 115-25.
        [http://dx.doi.org/10.1016/j.tifs.2016.08.005]

[64]    Kaewprachu P, Rawdkuen S. Application of Active Edible Film as Food Packaging for Food Preservation and Extending Shelf Life, in Microbes in food and health 2016; 185-205.

[65]    Zocca RO, Gaspar PD, da Silva PD, Nunes J, de Andrade LP. Introduction to Sustainable Food Production, in Sustainable Food Systems from Agriculture to Industry 2018; 3-46.

[66]    Reineke K, Schottroff F, Meneses N, Knorr D. Sterilization of liquid foods by pulsed electric fields-an innovative ultra-high temperature process. Front Microbiol 2015; 6: 400.
        [http://dx.doi.org/10.3389/fmicb.2015.00400] [PMID: 25999930]

[67]    Diogo JS, Silva LS, Pena A, Lino CM. Risk assessment of additives through soft drinks and nectars consumption on Portuguese population: a 2010 survey. Food Chem Toxicol 2013; 62: 548-53.
        [http://dx.doi.org/10.1016/j.fct.2013.09.006] [PMID: 24036138]

[68]    Grembecka M. Sugar alcohols—their role in the modern world of sweeteners: a review. Eur Food Res Technol 2015; 241(1): 1-14.
[http://dx.doi.org/10.1007/s00217-015-2437-7]

[69]    Wang W, Kannan P, Xue J, Kannan K. Synthetic phenolic antioxidants, including butylated hydroxytoluene (BHT), in resin-based dental sealants. Environ Res 2016; 151: 339-43.
[http://dx.doi.org/10.1016/j.envres.2016.07.042] [PMID: 27522571]

[70]    McCarthy M. Industry influence moved focus of US dental research away from sugar, documents indicate. BMJ 2015; 350: h1322.
[http://dx.doi.org/10.1136/bmj.h1322] [PMID: 25762512]

[71]    Chen J, Zhu Y, Liu S. Functional carbohydrates: development, characterization, and biomanufacturing of sugar alcohols guoqi a ng zha ng and qi n hong wa ng.Functional Carbohydrates. CRC Press 2017; pp. 283-312.
[http://dx.doi.org/10.1201/9781315371061]

[72]    Schorin MD, Sollid K, Edge MS, Bouchoux A. The Science of Sugars, Part I: A Closer Look at Sugars. Nutr Today 2012; 47(3): 96-101.
[http://dx.doi.org/10.1097/NT.0b013e3182435de8]

[73]    Inagaki T, Ishida T. Computational design of non-natural sugar alcohols to increase thermal storage density: beyond existing organic phase change materials. J Am Chem Soc 2016; 138(36): 11810-9.
[http://dx.doi.org/10.1021/jacs.6b05902] [PMID: 27505107]

[74]    Russell NJ, Gould GW. Food preservatives. Springer Science & Business Media 2003.
[http://dx.doi.org/10.1007/978-0-387-30042-9]

[75]    Si W, Gong J, Tsao R, *et al*. Antimicrobial activity of essential oils and structurally related synthetic food additives towards selected pathogenic and beneficial gut bacteria. J Appl Microbiol 2006; 100(2): 296-305.
[http://dx.doi.org/10.1111/j.1365-2672.2005.02789.x] [PMID: 16430506]

[76]    Tuormaa TE. The adverse effects of food additives on health: a review of the literature with a special emphasis on childhood hyperactivity. J Orthomol Med 1994; 9: 225-5.

[77]    Conners CK. Food additives and hyperactive children. Springer Science & Business Media 2012.

[78]    Fuglsang G, Madsen G, Halken S, Jørgensen S, Østergaard PA, Østerballe O. Adverse reactions to food additives in children with atopic symptoms. Allergy 1994; 49(1): 31-7.
[http://dx.doi.org/10.1111/j.1398-9995.1994.tb00770.x] [PMID: 8198237]

[79]    Wilson BG, Bahna SL. Adverse reactions to food additives. Ann Allergy Asthma Immunol 2005; 95(6): 499-507.
[http://dx.doi.org/10.1016/S1081-1206(10)61010-1] [PMID: 16400887]

[80]    Polônio MLT, Peres F. [Food additive intake and health effects: public health challenges in Brazil]. Cad Saude Publica 2009; 25(8): 1653-66.
[PMID: 19649407]

# CHAPTER 2

# Human Health Implications of Specific Group of Food Additives

**Maria Concetta Tenuta** and **Mariarosaria Leporini**[*]

*Department of Pharmacy, Health and Nutritional Sciences, University of Calabria, Edificio Polifunzionale, Arcavacata di Rende (CS) 87036, Italy*

**Abstract:** Additives are added to food in order to stabilize or increase the nutritional quality and quality and/or safety of the food matrix. Moreover, additives have a technological function and could improve the sensory properties of food.

For a long time, synthetic food additives are largely applied in food industries. Since the last year, there has been a decrease in chemical additives which are less welcome by consumers who prefer the use of additives from a natural source. In this chapter, several groups of additives are described such as antimicrobials, antioxidants and antibrowning agents, with colouring and flavouring agents.

**Keywords:** Additives, Colorants, Flavouring, Health, Nutrition, Preservatives.

## INTRODUCTION

Food additives are defined by "The Food Protection Committee of the Food and Nutrition Committee", as: "one or more substances, other than the food itself, which are intentionally added to food products for technological purposes in the production, processing, preparation, treatment, packaging, transport or storage of food, becoming directly or indirectly components of such foods." Over the last decades, following technological evolution, the use of food additives has expanded considerably, about 2500 additives are added to foods in order to have a certain effect even if their use has a remote origin. The various benefits recognized for additives are a safer and nourishing diet, with a better choice of raw materials at a lower cost. Benefits generally fall into four categories:

1. Health benefits as they decrease health risks or offer health benefits. Two types of health benefits can be provided by food additives as they prevent and/or reduce

---

[*] **Corresponding author Mariarosaria Leporini:** Department of Pharmacy, Health and Nutritional Sciences, University of Calabria, Edificio Polifunzionale, Arcavacata di Rende (CS) 87036, Italy; E-mail: mariarosarialeporini@tiscali.it

the onset of diseases and other food components that improve nutrition.

2. They provide benefits in terms of abundance, economic availability and diversity. The use of additives such as preservatives prevents food spoilage and increases the shelf life of food products while reducing their costs. In addition, they have indirect health benefits as they protect nutrients, prevent microbial growth and offer a more nutritious supply of raw materials.

3. Benefits of hedonism sensory satisfaction: these include the best colour, flavour and texture to increase the sensory characteristics of food that attract consumers.

4. Benefits of improved convenience: additives are more important in affluent societies because they reduce the preparation time.

The health benefits observed from food additives are of primary importance, while the greater practicality is of less importance. With the increasing level of consumer information, for greater public awareness of their eating habits, the distrust toward synthesised and processed additives is growing steadily and is today considered to be one of the main threats to a healthy lifestyle. For this reason, the future of food additives seems to be more directed to natural products as they are harmless to health. They are able to protect the body especially with the action of natural antioxidants such as polyphenols, carotenoids, and tocopherols that fight against the oxidative stress caused by free radicals. In the socio-cultural reality of industrialized countries, conscious nutrition not only aims to protect citizens but is also a crucial factor in reducing healthcare costs caused annually by food-borne diseases; in fact, it is important to remember that in these countries, the re-education campaigns are now increasing, inculcating healthy and balanced eating habits in people. Considering the growing consumer demand on transparency, the future of additives will be increasingly linked to concepts of naturalness, genuineness and multifunctionality.

## NATURAL ANTIMICROBIALS

Antimicrobials, a class of preservatives labelled with E and INS numbers ranging from 200 to 290 are employed for the control of growth of microorganisms during the shelf-life [3]. Several studies have described the use of natural compounds for the preservation of both easily perishable foods such as fresh meat and fish products, as well as fermented foods such as cheeses [4 - 7]. The use of essential oils (EO) or natural extracts could be replaced by chemical additives that contribute to the so-called "*green label*" food, which consumers are particularly attracted to, as they are shown to be natural. Natural extracts derived from different vegetable matrices, consisting mainly of essential oils, hydroalcoholic extracts and other derivatives, contain a wide range of secondary metabolites which can slow down or stop the growth of microorganisms such as bacteria, molds and yeasts [8, 9]. Antimicrobial compounds of natural origin are usually contained in different parts of plants: leaves (sage, rosemary, basil, thyme, oregano, and marjoram), flowers and buds (cloves), seeds (cumin, fennel, nutmeg and parsley), bulbs (garlic and onion), and fruits (cardamom and pepper). Therefore, essential oils and their constituents, often in the form of spices, have always been in use to improve the aroma of foodstuffs and their extensive antimicrobial activity is known in terms of a spectrum of action [10, 11]. Such compounds can act directly on the microbial cell by inhibiting the growth or production of toxic secondary metabolites such as in the case of mycotoxins. Furthermore, the inhibitory activity of essential oils is greater for gram-positive bacteria than gram-negative bacteria [9, 11 - 13]. In nature, there are more than 1,300 plants characterized by the presence of compounds with acclaimed antimicrobial activity. Over 30,000 molecules have been identified and tested for potential applications in food systems, and most of them belong to phenolic compounds. Essential oils of cumin and coriander exhibited an antimicrobial effect against *Pseudomonas fluorescens, Staphylococcus aureus,* and *Aeromonas hydrophila* [14, 15]. The extracts of marjoram and basil are strongly active against *Bacillus cereus, Enterobacter aerogenes, Escherichia coli* and *Salmonella spp.,* whereas essential oils of sage and rosemary inhibited the development of *Listeria monocytogenes* and *Staphylococcus aureus* [11]. Different authors determined the minimum inhibitory concentration (MIC) and the spectrum of action for some essential oils. Gutierrez *et al.* [11] described that oregano and thymus extracts are strongly active against enterobacteria and that the MIC of oregano and thymus essential oils against *Enterobacter cloacae* is 190 and 440 ppm, respectively, against *Lactobacillus brevis,* at 55 and 440 ppm, and against *Bacillus cereus, being* 425 and 745 ppm, respectively. The inhibitory activity expressed by the natural substances can be attributed to a single molecule or to a set of these molecules that intervene at the cellular level in multiple sites by affecting the cell externally or the cytoplasm [4, 16, 17]. Possible mechanisms of action may affect the cell membrane since the hydrophobicity of some compounds allows them to penetrate and interfere with the membrane itself by altering its structure and functionality. This mechanism of action would explain the greater inhibitory activity of gram-positive microorganisms compared to gram-negative, in fact, in the latter, there is an outer capsule that wraps the cell wall and does not allow the entry of hydrophobic substances the inside the cell. Naturally-occurring compounds, in addition to altering the cell wall structure, may interfere with the cell wall protein functions involved in the transport processes of essential cellular components. The antimicrobial activity of thyme extract against *Salmonella typhimurium* and *S. aureus* is due to the ability of phenolic constituents to bind proteins by altering their normal functions [18]. In addition, Tassou *et al.* [5]

suggested that the antimicrobial effect of mint EO is basically linked to alteration of membrane permeability and destruction of the electron transport system. Certain compounds such as carvacrol, carvone, thymol and trans-cinnamaldehyde in *E. coli O157:H7* broth cultures cause an increase in the extracellular concentration of ATP, an event that indicates a destructive action of such molecules against the cytoplasmic membrane [19]. Moreover, carvacrol induces HSP60 protein synthesis and inhibits flagellin synthesis by depriving the bacterium of its pathogenicity [20]. Table **1** presents some antimicrobial activities and components of spices and herbs [21].

**Table 1. Antimicrobial activity and flavor components of different spices and herbs.**

| Species and herbs | Flavor components | Antimicrobial activity |
|---|---|---|
| *Cinnamonum zeylanicum* | Eugenol and Cinnamic aldehyde | 75–100 (%) |
| Mustard (*Brassica* ssp.) | Allyl isothiocyanate | 50–75 (%) |
| *Myristica fragrans* | Sabinene, α-piene and Myristicin | 50–75 (%) |
| *Ocimum basilicum* | Methyl chavicol and Linalool | <50 (%) |
| *Origanum vulgare* | Thymol and Carvacrol | 75-100 (%) |
| *Pimenta dioca* | Eugenol and β-caryophyllene | 75–100 (%) |
| *Rosmarinus offinicalis* | Camphor, 1,8cineole, borneol and camphor | 75-100 (%) |
| *Salvia officinalis* | Thujone, 1,8-cinole, borneol and camphor | 50-75 (%) |
| *Syzgium aromaticum* | Eugenol | 75–100 (%) |
| *Thymus vulgaris* | Thymol and carvacol | 75-100 (%) |

As shown in Table **2**, different studies reported the application of essential oils and their components in dietary studies of the last 10 years [21].

**Table 2. Application of essential oils and their components in food studies.**

| Food | EO and components | Bacterial species |
|---|---|---|
| Chicken | Oregano, pimento, oregano | *Escherichia coli O157:H7 and Pseudomonas spp.* |
| Cod fillets | Eugenol | *Listeria monocytogenes,* |
| Fried meat | Oregano, sage and thyme | *Listeria monocytogenes B. cereus, P. aeruginosa, and Escherichia coli O157:H7* |
| Lettuce and Carrots | Carvacrol | *Listeria monocytogenes* |
| Kiwi fruit and Honeydew melon | Clove, cardamom, cinnamon, peppermint oil | *Streptococcus thermophilus* |
| Mozzarella cheese | Clove oil | *Listeria monocytogenes* |

*(Table 2) cont.....*

| Food | EO and components | Bacterial species |
|---|---|---|
| Meat | Clove oil, coriander, eugenol, thyme oils,oregano, encapsulated rosemary EO | *Listeria monocytogenes, Escherichia coli O157:H7* and *Aeromonas hydrophila* |
| Salmon | Geraniol, carvacrol and citral | *Salmonella typhimurium* |
| Semi-skimmed milk | Oregano oil | *Photobacterium phosphoreum* |
| Yoghurt | Mint oil | *Salmonella enteritidis* |

Clove, oregano and thyme EO and compounds such as eugenol showed the ability to inhibit microbial growth of *L. monocytogenes, Aeromonas hydrophila* in meat products [22].

## NATURAL ANTIOXIDANTS

Antioxidants are a class of preservatives. Antioxidants labelled E300-E326, as food preservatives can be used in food products for preventing lipid and/or vitaminic oxidation; in fact, oxidation has a profound effect on the quality of food, all of the major food components are susceptible to oxidation. The consequence is manifested in the reduction of the shelf-life, compromising its appearance, structure, sensory properties and nutritional value and changes in aroma and savour, structure and function and loss of nutritional value. Furthermore, the oxidation of pigments causes a reduction in visual attractiveness due to colour alteration which is reflected in a decrease in food product marketing. Hence the role of antioxidants for the prevention of oxidative processes responsible for the rancidity and off-flavour in foods [3]. Among the antioxidant food additives, the most commonly used are: vitamins C and E, butylated hydroxyanisole, BHA and butylated hydroxytoluene, BHT) [3]. In the past, Native Americans used natural blueberries as antioxidants to prevent the oxidation of meat. In 1980, consumers' demand for natural antioxidant ingredients started increasing. Antioxidants are particularly useful for the preservation of dried and frozen foods [23]. The vegetable phenols inhibit the formation of radicals of lipids catalyzed by metals and radiations [24, 25] and also peroxides, hydroxides and individual oxygen radicals [25 - 27].

The tocopherols, most present in nuts, are recognized as powerful natural antioxidants and are used as preservatives in products based on meat, oils and dairy products given their resistance to high temperature and low volatility processing phases. Ascorbic acid, found in many species of the genus *Citrus*, is used as a preservative in cured meats, fruit juices, jams, and some canned foods. Carotenoids and phenolic compounds also have these properties. The Food and Drug Administration normalizes the application and concentrations allowed for the use of both natural and synthetic food additives. Several natural extracts are recognized as GRAS (*Generally Recognized As Safe*) [28]. Several studies proved the antioxidant effect of herbs and spices such as *Origanum vulgare, Rosmarinus, Thymus, Cinnamomum verum, Capsicum, Myristica and Ocimum basilicum* [29 - 31]. The main constituents of herbs and spices are represented by a) phenolic acids, most studied, such as rosmarinic, caffeic and gallic acids, b) phenolic diterpenes such as carnosol and carnosic acid c) flavonoids: quercetin, catechin, kaempferol, naringenin, apigenin and hesperetin, d) carotenoids, e) constituents of essential oils: carvacrol, eugenol, thymol and menthol [28]. *Rosmarinus* and *Origanum vulgare* extracts are recognized as potential antioxidants and are added as natural ingredients in meat processing. Carnosic and rosmarinic acids, as well as carnosol are mainly responsible for this protective activity [32]. Moreover, Zhang *et al.* [33], demonstrated the antioxidant action of liquorice extracts. Table **3** reports a collection of studies regarding the application of natural antioxidants in the food industry [34].

**Table 3. Application of natural antioxidants.**

| Natural Antioxidants | Active Compounds | Treated Meat Product |
|---|---|---|
| Essential oils | Terpenoids | Turkey meat patties and beef burgers |
| Fruits and leaves extracts | Flavonoids and water-soluble vitamins | Cooked burger patties, raw and cooked pork patties |
| Nuts and seeds extracts | Tocopherols, tocotrienols and polyphenols | Restructured steaks |
| Spices, herbs and extracts | Phenolic acids and terpenoids | Breakfast sausage and precooked pork |

The addition of antioxidants increases oxidative stability to improve organoleptic properties and nutritional value of meat products [35 - 39]. *Youdim et al.* [40] reported that dietary supplementation with thymus EO and thymol in aged rats showed a positive effect on superoxide dismutase and glutathione peroxidase enzyme. Furthermore, an antioxidant effect on muscle tissue was observed following dietary supplementation of oregano in a dose of 50-100 mg/kg to feeding chickens [40]. The results obtained in the study by Forte *et al.* [41] confirmed that the use of aqueous extracts of oregano in diets enriched with PUFA improved the oxidation resistance of meat and enhanced the taste of meat.

## ANTIBROWNING AGENTS

Another class of preservatives is represented by anti-browning agents used to prevent browning in food products. Many foods are subject to degradation reactions during manipulation, storage and processing [42, 43]. These reactions are divided into enzymatic browning and non-enzymatic browning. Enzymatic browning is determined by the oxidation of quinone polyphenols for the action of the polyphenol oxidase enzyme and followed by the quinone polymerization reaction. This effectively reduced the shelf life of fresh mushrooms, fresh fruit, potatoes, salads *etc*. [44]. Non-enzymatic browning reactions can originate, for example, from the Maillard reaction involving reducing sugars and amino acids [45]; this produces melanoidins in foods such as cereals, fruit, dairy, and vegetables products [46]. To reduce non-enzymatic browning, sulphites are added to the food matrix. However, adverse reactions such as allergic reaction, have been observed following the use of these compounds. As a result, the U.S. Food and Drug Administration has forbidden the use of sulphites in some raw fruit and vegetable products. Today ascorbic acid represents a valid alternative to sulphuring agents. The antibrowning action of ascorbic acid is related to its ability to reduce quinones and therefore avoid the additional reactions that lead to the formation of dark pigments. Therefore, the main effect of ascorbic acid is the inhibitor of the enzyme browning reaction, not as a PPO inhibitor. However, ascorbic acid has a direct inhibitory effect on PPO [47 - 49]. Currently, the main suppliers of ascorbic acid or burner inhibitors of eritorbic acid are Monsanto Chemical Company (Snow Fresh), EPL Technologies, Inc. (Fresh Potato) and Montrose-Haeuser Co., Inc. (NatureSeal). Many companies provide the ingredients from which these formulations can be made.

## NUTRITIONAL ADDITIVES

Another class of additives is nutritional additives. Their use has increased because the consumers are more interested in the safety of their "health". The category of nutritional additives includes the use of pure chemical compounds, minerals, vitamins, amino acids and fatty acids to improve and maintain the nutritional quality of food. With this purpose, folacin and ascorbic acids are used as fortificants in the soft drink. Carotenoids are added not only as food colorants but also as precursors of vitamin A. Vitamin E is used to prevent lipid peroxidation and to protect vitamin A from oxidation in the intestinal tract. Furthermore, at the cellular level, vitamin E, seems to protect the membranes by scavenging the free radicals containing oxygen. The main sources of vitamin E are vegetable oils, including soybeans, maize, cottonseed and safflower, products derived from these oils, as well as wheat germ, nuts and different cereals.

## FOOD COLORANTS

Since ancient times, the addition of colorants to foods has made them more appealing. Synthetic colorants are frequently used for their stability, availability, and low cost. However, several studies demonstrated the possible toxic effects of these compounds that limit their use. For this reason, the search for natural colorants is constantly increasing. Flavonoids (mainly anthocyanins), carotenoids, chlorophyll, betalains, and curcumin are the main food colorants from the plant kingdom.

Anthocyanins comprise a group of natural compounds responsible for the blue, purple, magenta, red, and violet colour of several plant species. Anthocyanins are anthocyanidins glycosides. The six most abundant anthocyanidins namely pelargonidin, delphinidin, malvidin, cyaniding, petunidin, and peonidin (Fig. **1**) are found in the skin of grape, plums and red apples, and in strawberries, blueberries, and shiso (*Perilla ocimoidis* var. *cripsa*) leaves. Anthocyanidins are, in general, less soluble and unstable in aqueous media than anthocyanins. Therefore, glycosylation is expected to confer a major solubility and stability to the pigment. The colour of anthocyanin solutions is significantly influenced by pH. Generally, below pH 3, anthocyanin solutions exhibit a red coloration. When the pH of such solutions is raised, their red colour normally fades to the point where they appear colourless (pH in the range 4-5). Further increases in pH give rise to blue and purple anthocyanins solutions. Upon storage or heat treatment, the colour of these solutions changes from blue to yellow. As reported by Timberlake [50], anthocyanins have not toxic and mutagenic effects, but only bring benefits both in the medical and in food sectors.

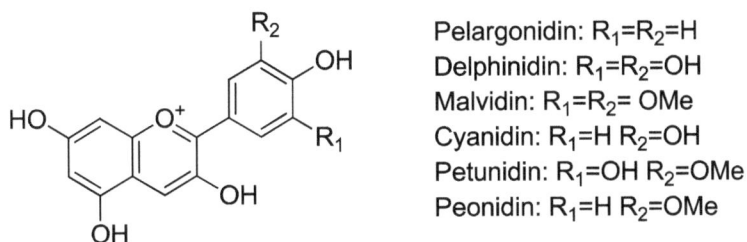

Pelargonidin: $R_1=R_2=H$
Delphinidin: $R_1=R_2=OH$
Malvidin: $R_1=R_2= OMe$
Cyanidin: $R_1=H$ $R_2=OH$
Petunidin: $R_1=OH$ $R_2=OMe$
Peonidin: $R_1=H$ $R_2=OMe$

**Fig. (1).** Structure of some major anthocyanins.

Carotenoids are commonly distributed in bacteria, fungi, animals, and algae but mainly in plants and, in particular, in carrots, peppers, and tomatoes [51]. The most abundant compound of this class is β-carotene (Fig. **2**). It is widely used in dairy products, cakes, soup, and confectionery. Moreover, it is added to several nutraceutical beverages and functional foods. Other carotenoids used for colouring food are annatto, saffron, and gardenia extracts [3].

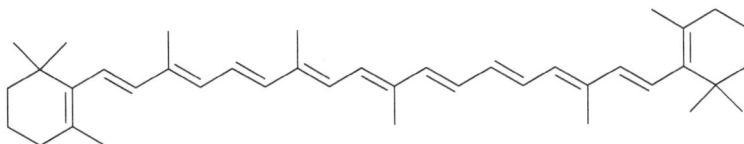

**Fig. (2).** Structure of β-carotene.

Annatto Fig. (**3**) is an orange-yellow pigment extracted from the pericarp of the seeds of *Bixa Orellana*. Generally, annatto contains 4.5-5.5% pigments that consist of 70-80% bixin. There are two forms of annatto obtained from different methods of extraction of seeds. The oil-soluble form is called bixin while the water-soluble form is called norbixin. Bixin is extracted by using non-polar solvents including vegetable oils. Norbixin is obtained in the presence of alkali leading to the hydrolysis of bixin.

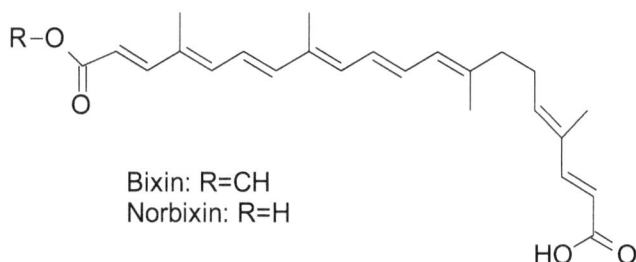

Bixin: R=CH
Norbixin: R=H

**Fig. (3).** Structure of annatto pigments.

The tinctorial value of bixin is equivalent to that of β-carotene. It is employed in dairy and fat-based food products, like cheese, margarine, bakery products and creams.

The fat-soluble bixin is also used, in addition to other food colorants, to have a different tonality of colour. Norbixin is added in cheese, smoked fish, snack foods, sugar confectionery, meat products (*e.g.*, frankfurter sausages) and bakery products [52].

Saffron is a water-soluble extract produced from the flower of *Crocus sativus*, *C. albiflouris*, *C. lutens*, *Cedrela toona*, *Nyctasthes arbortristes*, *Verbascum phlomoides*, and *Gardenia jasminoides*. Crocin, the digentiobioside ester of crocetin Fig. (**4**), is the dominant compound of saffron. Other constituents are β-carotene, zeaxanthin, and certain flavouring components (mainly picrocrocin and safranal).

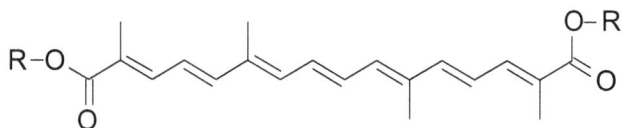

**Fig. (4).** Structure of saffron pigment.

Usually, saffron is added as an intensifier the yellow colour of food like in soups, certain confectionery goods and meat, where a spicy flavour is desirable [3]. New food colorant is lycopene, characterized by an intense red colour. The major source of lycopene is tomato, followed by watermelon and red grapefruit. The strong stability of this pigment for industrial production has brought to its use as a new commercial natural colorant [53]. Lycopene is used as a colorant in beverages, bread, confectionery, boiled sweets, and cakes.

Betalains occur in both yellow (vulgaxanthins) and red forms (betanins). These compounds are water-soluble and usually stable at moderately acid pH. Light, heat, and oxygen accelerate their decomposition. Although betalains showed a limited distribution, their importance is enhanced by their presence in some food crops, namely beetroot, chard, and amaranth.

Betanin represents one of the most common red pigments obtained from the red beetroot *Beta vulgaris* Fig. (**5**).

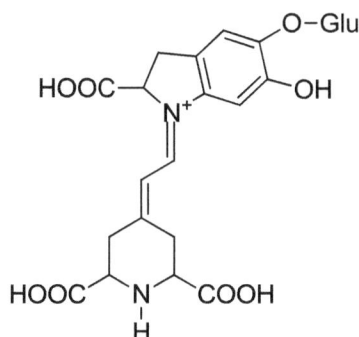

**Fig. (5).** Betanin

Vulgaxanthine I and II are the yellow principal compounds extracted from *B. vulgaris* var. *lutea* Fig. (**6**). Betanin and vulgaxanthine can exclusively be added in products with a short shelf-life and not subjected to heat treatments.

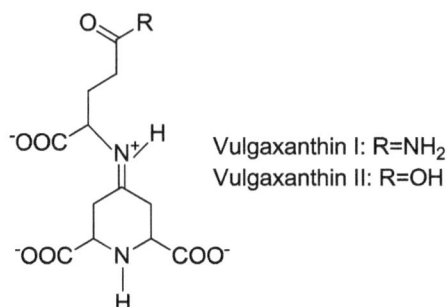

Vulgaxanthin I: R=NH$_2$
Vulgaxanthin II: R=OH

**Fig. (6).** Vulgaxanthin I and II, which is extracted from the yellow beet root.

Chlorophyll is the most extensively distributed natural pigment that occurs in the leaves and other parts of almost all plants. In nature, there are two main types of chlorophyll, chlorophylls a and chlorophyll b. The chlorophyll a is a bluish-green pigment, instead type b is yellowish-green in colour. The chlorophyll is a porphyrin pigment, consisting of four pyrrole rings combined along *via* methine linkages. There is also a magnesium atom inside the porphyrin structure, held in position by two covalent and two coordinate bonds. Principally, chlorophyll pigments are extracted from dried plant materials [54]. The most used plant materials are lucerne, alfalfa and nettles. In the food industry, chlorophyll is used for colouring sugar confectionery, chewing gum, soups, edible oil, and dairy products. Chlorophyll is used, also, in the pharmaceutical and cosmetic industries [3].

*Curcuma longa* is the main source of turmeric, obtained from the root and it is responsible for a fluorescent yellow colour. By grinding the tuber, a powder is obtained that comprises three pigments: bisdemethoxycurcumin, demethoxy-curcumin and curcumin. The curcumin is insoluble in water and represents the principal pigment [54]. Traditionally, it is added to the food as a spice rather than as a colouring agent, even if the uses of this extract are rather restricted for the characteristic odour and sharp taste and for its sensitivity to light and to alkaline conditions. After the deodorization process, the odourless extract is principally utilised in food products such as in mustard, soups, confectionery, pickles and canned products. It is also used in acidic food products and salad dressing for its strong stable pH.

## PIGMENTS FROM ANIMAL AND INSECT SOURCES

### Cochineal

Cochineal belongs to the quinonoid pigments, characterized by red colour. The very popular cochineal pigment industrially used is carminic acid, obtained from the female Dactylopius coccus Costa, a parasite of plants from *Opuntia* and *Nopale* genera. For a lot of time, it was used as a red dye, in particular for dyeing fabrics, while today, it is of great value as a colorant in food [3]. Other pigments are Armenian red, Kermes, Polish Cochineal, and Lac dyes. Carminic acid Fig. (**7**) is the principal cochineal pigment used in the industry, but it has little intrinsic colour that conglomerates with diverse metals, such as aluminium, imparting a bright red colour. The product obtained from this complex is known as carmine and it is utilised for jams, preserves, syrups, baked goods and confectionery. However, it has a range of colours, from pale "strawberry" to near "black currant" [55], corresponding to varying ratio of carminic acid to aluminium.

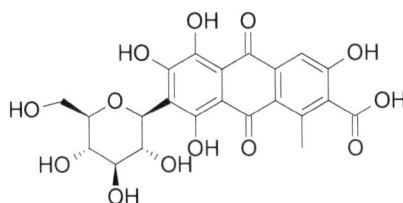

**Fig. (7).** Carminic acid.

## Heme Pigments

Heme possesses four pyrrolic rings such as chlorophyll, but the difference is the central iron atom instead of the magnesium atom. In the animal kingdom, heme is associated with complexes that form proteins such as haemoglobin in the blood and myoglobin in the muscle and its function is of a carrier of oxygen in the body. In the oxygenated blood, the complex is red because the central iron atom is oxidized, subjecting heat to the complex brownish in colour, characteristic of cooked meat because the oxygen atom bound will be lost. The heme pigments are not toxic as confirmed by several studies conducted on animals. However, the characteristic colour has limited their use only in the food where the colour of cooked meat is preferred for example, in sausages and meat analogues [3].

## FLAVOURING AGENTS

In 1969, the Society of Flavor Chemists [3] defined: "a flavour is a substance which may be a single chemical entity, or a mixture of chemicals of natural or synthetic provenance, whose primary purpose is to provide all or part of the unique effect to any food or other products taken in the mouth". Furthermore, the Council of Europe has defined: "flavouring is a substance which has prevalently odor-producing properties and which likely influences the taste".

Essential ingredients for adding flavour are spices and essential oils. People use spices specially to modify or improve the flavour of food. The most important spices came from the east, particularly from India, but now it is possible to grow these spices and herbs in diverse parts of the world. Both chemical and natural flavours are reported in Table **4**. The number of synthetic chemicals authorized for use in food flavours increases continuously, with approximately 1600 till date. Instead, the natural materials could be averaged to around 600.

**Table 4. Sources of materials used in flavour compounding.**

| | |
|---|---|
| Natural source | Botanical (Fruit and vegetable juice, extract and distillate, herbs, spices, nuts) Animal (drippings, seafood byproducts, enzyme- modified cheese, meat extract) |
| Chemical source | Benzaldehyde, Cinnamic alcohol |

Before the 1900, 90% of the materials used for flavours were of natural provenance, after this data, the majority of known chemical products were generated synthetically with an economic cost. For this reason, the industry prefers the use of artificial flavours [3].

The function of a flavour agent is to give pleasant sensation to tobacco, beverages or pharmaceuticals depending on its different uses. The functions of a flavour are different, however, in many ways of utilisation, one application is more prominent than the other. It is important to differentiate three principal classes of functions: economic, physiological and psychological. Most of the flavouring agents fulfil all of these functions; however, each of them will have a diverse contribution. It is necessary to modify the taste of many foods to make more palatable and desirable the food with undesirable tastes (*e.g.* vitamins and soya). A further example is the use of flavour to prevent the loss of flavour during the food manipulations or to prolong freshness during conservation. Different studies specify that the taste can modify the metabolic rejoinder to a fatty meal [56, 57].

Other studies demonstrate that oral stimulation affects intestinal absorption [58].

Flavours are used with different products in the pharmaceutical, food and oral hygiene sectors. Flavoured products are divided into two groups:

- Flavour-dependent. This term indicates foods and beverages that, without the application of flavours, cannot exist; for example gelatin desserts, chewing gum, powdered artificial beverages, carbonated and non-juice drinks and hard-boiled candy.

- Flavour-independent. This term defines the products for which flavours are legally banned or can be marketed, not having flavours. For example, the first type of products includes milk, butter and orange juice in which flavour consolidation is prohibited, except if a product is identified as a new product. While the second type consists of crackers, cereals and nuts.

## NATURAL RAW MATERIALS

Since ancient times, herbs and spices have been added to food for their nutritional value and properties, to enhance the sensory properties, and to act as preservatives. Herbs and spices are a good substitute for chemical additives because they are safe. Essential oils are blends of volatile compounds obtained, primarily by steam distillation, from aromatic and medicinal plants. In the Mediterranean region, there are many aromatic plants rich in essential oils, such as thyme, rosemary, and sage [59].

Considering the fact that flavour industry is principally interested in the sensory quality of materials, it is very unusual that a spice or any other natural food product is utilised in its natural form. The spice or food is elaborated to remove the chemical compounds (fiber, cellulose, pectin, *etc.*). The objective is to have the complete concentration of aromatic chemicals within the minimum totality of neutral compounds at the most desirable composition of flavour profile, cost, and stability. Practically, one factor usually has to be renounced to increase the other. It is important to see that flavours obtained by the industry in the late 19th century were approximatively 90% natural, ensued principally from essential oils and spices. In the 1950s, flavours change into circa being 90% artificial, due to the disponibility of synthetic chemicals. In the 1980s and 1990s, natural flavours comprised more or less 70% of the flavours [3].

The genus *Salvia* (Lamiaceae) is constituted around 900 species, distributed all over the world, several of which with a great economic advantage, because they are used as spices and flavouring agents by cosmetic and perfumery industries [60, 61]. Since the ancient times, *Salvia* sp. have been used for the treatment of rheumatism, fever, chronic bronchitis, and mental disorders [62, 63].

The most common *Salvia* species are *S. fruticosa* Mill., *S. officinalis* L., and *S. lavandulifolia* Vahl [63]. *S. officinalis* (garden sage, sage, or common sage) is a perennial, evergreen subshrub, with woody stems, grayish leaves and blue to purplish flowers. It is typical in the Mediterranean area [63, 64]. Essential oil or dried leaves of sage are used as a savoury food flavouring [65]. In all European countries, it is one of the most widely used spices in the kitchen to add flavour to meat, fish, soups and vegetables.

## CONCLUDING REMARKS

Interest in food additives, mainly in those of natural origin, has increased significantly over the past years. This increase is expected to continue because of interest of food industries, consumers, and the scientific communities. Consumers are more aware of the potential role of food in the prevention of several diseases in addition to their nutritional value. This determines a greater interest and a growing demand for natural additives in contrast to the use of synthetic additives. Synthetic additives are widely used in the past years due to their stability, availability, and low cost. However, the use of some of these food additives is not free from side effects to health that limited their use. For these reasons, the consumer seeks high-quality food in which natural additives are used.

## CONSENT FOR PUBLICATION

Not applicable.

## CONFLICT OF INTEREST

The authors declare that there are no conflicts of interest.

## ACKNOWLEDGEMENTS

This chapter is the outcome of an in-house financially non-supported study.

## REFERENCES

[1]    Darby WJ. Risk versus benefits: the future of food safety. The nature of benefits. Nutr Rev 1980;
       38(1): 37-44.
       [http://dx.doi.org/10.1111/j.1753-4887.1980.tb05840.x] [PMID: 6892654]

[2]    Food Safety Council, Social and Economic Committee. Principles and processes for making food
       safety decisions. Food Technol 1980; 34(3): 89-125.

[3]    Branen AL, Davidson PM, Salminen S, Thorngate JH III. Food Additives. 2nd ed. New York, Basel:
       Marcel Dekker Inc 2001; pp. 1-952.

[4]    Nychas GJE. Natural antimicrobials from plants.New methods of food preservation. Glasgow,
       Scotland: Blackie Academic & Professional 1995; pp. 58-89.
       [http://dx.doi.org/10.1007/978-1-4615-2105-1_4]

[5]    Tassou C, Koutsoumanis K, Nychas GJE. Inhibition of Salmonella enteritidis and Staphylococcus
       aureus in nutrient broth by mint essential oil. Food Res Int 2000; 33(3-4): 273-80.
       [http://dx.doi.org/10.1016/S0963-9969(00)00047-8]

[6]    González-Molina E, Domínguez-Perles R, Moreno DA, García-Viguera C. Natural bioactive
       compounds of Citrus limon for food and health. J Pharm Biomed Anal 2010; 51(2): 327-45.
       [http://dx.doi.org/10.1016/j.jpba.2009.07.027] [PMID: 19748198]

[7]    Zhou GH, Xu XL, Liu Y. Preservation technologies for fresh meat - a review. Meat Sci 2010; 86(1):
       119-28.
       [http://dx.doi.org/10.1016/j.meatsci.2010.04.033] [PMID: 20605688]

[8]    Burt SA, Reinders RD. Antibacterial activity of selected plant essential oils against Escherichia coli
       O157:H7. Lett Appl Microbiol 2003; 36(3): 162-7.
       [http://dx.doi.org/10.1046/j.1472-765X.2003.01285.x] [PMID: 12581376]

[9]    Chorianopoulos NG, Giaouris ED, Skandamis PN, Haroutounian SA, Nychas GJE. Disinfectant test
       against monoculture and mixed-culture biofilms composed of technological, spoilage and pathogenic
       bacteria: bactericidal effect of essential oil and hydrosol of Satureja thymbra and comparison with
       standard acid-base sanitizers. J Appl Microbiol 2008; 104(6): 1586-96.
       [http://dx.doi.org/10.1111/j.1365-2672.2007.03694.x] [PMID: 18217930]

[10]   Nychas GJE, Tassou CC, Skandamis P. Antimicrobials from herbs and spices.Natural antimicrobials
       for the minimal processing of foods. New York: CRC Press Woodhead Publishers 2003; pp. 176-200.
       [http://dx.doi.org/10.1533/9781855737037.176]

[11]   Gutierrez J, Rodriguez G, Barry-Ryan C, Bourke P. Efficacy of plant essential oils against foodborne
       pathogens and spoilage bacteria associated with ready-to-eat vegetables: antimicrobial and sensory
       screening. J Food Prot 2008; 71(9): 1846-54.
       [http://dx.doi.org/10.4315/0362-028X-71.9.1846] [PMID: 18810868]

[12]   Marino M, Bersani C, Comi G. Impedance measurements to study the antimicrobial activity of
       essential oils from Lamiaceae and Compositae. Int J Food Microbiol 2001; 67(3): 187-95.
       [http://dx.doi.org/10.1016/S0168-1605(01)00447-0] [PMID: 11518428]

[13]   Kim S, Fung DY. Antibacterial effect of water-soluble arrowroot (Puerariae radix) tea extracts on

foodborne pathogens in ground beef and mushroom soup. J Food Prot 2004; 67(9): 1953-6.
[http://dx.doi.org/10.4315/0362-028X-67.9.1953] [PMID: 15453588]

[14]   Wan J, Wilcock A, Coventry MJ. The effect of essential oils of basil on the growth of Aeromonas hydrophila and Pseudomonas fluorescens. J Appl Microbiol 1998; 84(2): 152-8.
[http://dx.doi.org/10.1046/j.1365-2672.1998.00338.x] [PMID: 9633630]

[15]   Fricke G, Hoyer H, Wermter R, Paulus H. Staphylococcus aureus as an example of the influence of lipophilic components on the microbiological activity of aromatic extracts. Arch Lebensmit- teltechn 1998; 49: 107-11.

[16]   Davidson PM. Chemical preservatives and naturally antimicrobial compounds.Food microbiology fundamentals and frontiers. 2nd ed. Washington: ASM Press 2001; pp. 593-628.

[17]   López-Malo A, Palou E. Storage stability of pineapple slices preserved by combined methods. Int J Food Sci Technol 2008; 43(2): 289-95.
[http://dx.doi.org/10.1111/j.1365-2621.2006.01433.x]

[18]   Juven BJ, Kanner J, Schved F, Weisslowicz H. Factors that interact with the antibacterial action of thyme essential oil and its active constituents. J Appl Bacteriol 1994; 76(6): 626-31.
[http://dx.doi.org/10.1111/j.1365-2672.1994.tb01661.x] [PMID: 8027009]

[19]   Helander IM, Alakomi HL, Latva-Kala K, *et al.* Characterisation of the action of selected essential oil components on Gram-negative bacteria. J Agric Food Chem 1998; 46(9): 3590-5.
[http://dx.doi.org/10.1021/jf980154m]

[20]   Burt SA, van der Zee R, Koets AP, *et al.* Carvacrol induces heat shock protein 60 and inhibits synthesis of flagellin in Escherichia coli O157:H7. Appl Environ Microbiol 2007; 73(14): 4484-90.
[http://dx.doi.org/10.1128/AEM.00340-07] [PMID: 17526792]

[21]   Tajkarimi MM, Ibrahim SA, Cliverb DO. Antimicrobial herb and spice compounds in food: A review. Food Control 2010; 21(9): 1199-218.
[http://dx.doi.org/10.1016/j.foodcont.2010.02.003]

[22]   Burt S. Essential oils: their antibacterial properties and potential applications in foods--a review. Int J Food Microbiol 2004; 94(3): 223-53.
[http://dx.doi.org/10.1016/j.ijfoodmicro.2004.03.022] [PMID: 15246235]

[23]   Mattill HA. Antioxidants. Annu Rev Biochem 1947; 16: 177-92.
[http://dx.doi.org/10.1146/annurev.bi.16.070147.001141] [PMID: 20259061]

[24]   Buettner GR. The pecking order of free radicals and antioxidants: lipid peroxidation, alpha-tocopherol, and ascorbate. Arch Biochem Biophys 1993; 300(2): 535-43.
[http://dx.doi.org/10.1006/abbi.1993.1074] [PMID: 8434935]

[25]   Hanasaki Y, Ogawa S, Fukui S. The correlation between active oxygens scavenging and antioxidative effects of flavonoids. Free Radic Biol Med 1994; 16(6): 845-50.
[http://dx.doi.org/10.1016/0891-5849(94)90202-X] [PMID: 8070690]

[26]   Laughton MJ, Evans PJ, Moroney MA, Hoult JR, Halliwell B. Inhibition of mammalian 5-lipoxygenase and cyclo-oxygenase by flavonoids and phenolic dietary additives. Relationship to antioxidant activity and to iron ion-reducing ability. Biochem Pharmacol 1991; 42(9): 1673-81.
[http://dx.doi.org/10.1016/0006-2952(91)90501-U] [PMID: 1656994]

[27]   Tournaire C, Croux S, Maurette MT, *et al.* Antioxidant activity of flavonoids: efficiency of singlet oxygen (1 delta g) quenching. J Photochem Photobiol B 1993; 19(3): 205-15.
[http://dx.doi.org/10.1016/1011-1344(93)87086-3] [PMID: 8229463]

[28]   Brewer MS. Natural antioxidants: sources, compounds, mechanisms of action, and potential applications. Compr Rev Food Sci Food Saf 2011; 10(4): 221-47.
[http://dx.doi.org/10.1111/j.1541-4337.2011.00156.x]

[29]   Kong B, Zhang H, Xiong YL. Antioxidant activity of spice extracts in a liposome system and in

cooked pork patties and the possible mode of action. Meat Sci 2010; 85(4): 772-8.
[http://dx.doi.org/10.1016/j.meatsci.2010.04.003] [PMID: 20430533]

[30]   Velioglu YS, Mazza G, Gao L, Oomah BD. Antioxidant activity and total phenolics in selected fruits, vegetables, and grain products. J Agric Food Chem 1998; 46(10): 4113-7.
[http://dx.doi.org/10.1021/jf9801973]

[31]   Yoo KM, Lee CH, Lee H, Moon B, Lee CY. Relative antioxidant and cytoprotective activities of common herbs. Food Chem 2008; 106(3): 929-36.
[http://dx.doi.org/10.1016/j.foodchem.2007.07.006]

[32]   Aruoma OI, Halliwell B, Aeschbach R, Löligers J. Antioxidant and pro-oxidant properties of active rosemary constituents: carnosol and carnosic acid. Xenobiotica 1992; 22(2): 257-68.
[http://dx.doi.org/10.3109/00498259209046624] [PMID: 1378672]

[33]   Zhang Q, Ye M. Chemical analysis of the Chinese herbal medicine Gan-Cao (licorice). J Chromatogr A 2009; 1216(11): 1954-69.
[http://dx.doi.org/10.1016/j.chroma.2008.07.072] [PMID: 18703197]

[34]   Jiang J, Xiong YL. Natural antioxidants as food and feed additives to promote health benefits and quality of meat products: A review. Meat Sci 2016; 120: 107-17.
[http://dx.doi.org/10.1016/j.meatsci.2016.04.005] [PMID: 27091079]

[35]   Kasapidou E, Wood JD, Richardson RI, Sinclair LA, Wilkinson RG, Enser M. Effect of vitamin E supplementation and diet on fatty acid composition and on meat colour and lipid oxidation of lamb leg steaks displayed in modified atmosphere packs. Meat Sci 2012; 90(4): 908-16.
[http://dx.doi.org/10.1016/j.meatsci.2011.11.031] [PMID: 22177553]

[36]   Lynch MP, Kerry JP, Buckley DJ, Faustman C, Morrissey PA. Effect of dietary vitamin E supplementation on the colour and lipid stability of fresh, frozen and vacuum-packaged beef. Meat Sci 1999; 52(1): 95-9.
[http://dx.doi.org/10.1016/S0309-1740(98)00153-3] [PMID: 22062148]

[37]   Phillips AL, Faustman C, Lynch MP, Govoni KE, Hoagland TA, Zinn SA. Effect of dietary α-tocopherol supplementation on color and lipid stability in pork. Meat Sci 2001; 58(4): 389-93.
[http://dx.doi.org/10.1016/S0309-1740(01)00039-0] [PMID: 22062429]

[38]   Franz C, Baser KHC, Windisch W. Essential oils and aromatic plants in animal feeding a European perspective: A review. Flavour Fragrance J 2010; 25(5): 327-40.
[http://dx.doi.org/10.1002/ffj.1967]

[39]   Delles RM, Xiong YL, True AD, Ao T, Dawson KA. Dietary antioxidant supplementation enhances lipid and protein oxidative stability of chicken broiler meat through promotion of antioxidant enzyme activity. Poult Sci 2014; 93(6): 1561-70.
[http://dx.doi.org/10.3382/ps.2013-03682] [PMID: 24879706]

[40]   Youdim KA, Deans SG. Effect of thyme oil and thymol dietary supplementation on the antioxidant status and fatty acid composition of the ageing rat brain. Br J Nutr 2000; 83(1): 87-93.
[http://dx.doi.org/10.1017/S000711450000012X] [PMID: 10703468]

[41]   Forte C, Branciari R, Pacetti D, *et al.* Dietary oregano (Origanum vulgare L.) aqueous extract improves oxidative stability and consumer acceptance of meat enriched with CLA and n-3 PUFA in broilers. Poult Sci 2018; 97(5): 1774-85.
[http://dx.doi.org/10.3382/ps/pex452] [PMID: 29462413]

[42]   Nichols R. Post-harvest physiology and storage.The biology and technology of the cultivated mushroom. New York: John Wiley & Sons 1985; pp. 195-210.

[43]   Feinberg B, Olson RL, Mullins WR. Prepeeled potatoes.Potato Processing. 4th ed. New York: AVI–Van Nostrand Reinhold 1987; pp. 697-726.

[44]   Huxsoll CC, Bolin HR, King AD Jr. Physicochemical changes and treatments for lightly processed fruits and vegetables. In: Jen JJ, Ed. Quality factors of fruits and vegetables: chemistry and

technology. American Chemical Society203-15.
[http://dx.doi.org/10.1021/bk-1989-0405.ch016]

[45]   Hodge JE. Dehydrated foods: chemistry of browning reactions in model system. J Agric Food Chem 1953; 1(15): 928-43.
[http://dx.doi.org/10.1021/jf60015a004]

[46]   Labuza TP, Schmidl MK. Advances in the control of browning reactions in foods.Role of chemistry in the quality of processed food. Westport, CT: Food & Nutrition Press 1986; pp. 65-95.

[47]   Tressler DK, DuBois C. No browning of cut fruit when treated by new process. Food Ind 1944; 16(9): 763-5.

[48]   Esselen WB Jr, Powers JJ, Woodward R. d-Isoascorbic acid as an antioxidant. Ind Eng Chem 1945; 37: 295-9.
[http://dx.doi.org/10.1021/ie50423a023]

[49]   Vámos-Vigyázó L. Polyphenol oxidase and peroxidase in fruits and vegetables. Crit Rev Food Sci Nutr 1981; 15(1): 49-127.
[http://dx.doi.org/10.1080/10408398109527312] [PMID: 6794984]

[50]   Timberlake CF. The biological properties of Anthocyanins. NATCOL. Quarterly Information Bulletin 1988; 1: 4-15.

[51]   Weedon BCL, Moss GP. Carotenoids, isolation and analysis.. Basel, Boston and Berlin: Carotenoids handbook. Birkhäuser 1995; 1: pp. 27-70.

[52]   Preston HD, Rickard MD. Extraction and chemistry of Annatto. Food Chem 1980; 5(1): 47-56.
[http://dx.doi.org/10.1016/0308-8146(80)90063-1]

[53]   Nir Z, Hartal D, Raveh Y. Lycopenes from tomatoes- a new commercial natural carotenoid. Intl Food Ingredients 1993; 6: 45-51.

[54]   Humphrey AM. Chlorophyll. Food Chem 1980; 5(1): 57-67.
[http://dx.doi.org/10.1016/0308-8146(80)90064-3]

[55]   Lloyd AG. Extraction and chemistry of cochineal. Food Chem 1980; 5(1): 91-107.
[http://dx.doi.org/10.1016/0308-8146(80)90067-9]

[56]   Michael N, Brand JG, Kare MR, Carpenter RG. Energy intake, weight gain, and fat deposition in rats fed flavoured, nutritionally controlled diets in a multichoice ("cafeteria") design. J Nutr 1985; 1447-58.

[57]   Ramirez I. Oral stimulation alters digestion of intragastric oil meals in rats. Am J Physiol 1985; 248(4 Pt 2): R459-63.
[PMID: 3985188]

[58]   Threatte RM, Giduck SA, Kling M. Oropharyngeal stimulation of glucose absorption from the small intestine in conscious, unrestrained rats. Fed Proc 1986; 45(3): 537-361.

[59]   Nieto G. Biological activities of three essential oils of the Lamiaceae family. Medicines (Basel) 2017; 4(3): 63-73.
[http://dx.doi.org/10.3390/medicines4030063] [PMID: 28930277]

[60]   Kamatou GPP, Van Zyl RL, VanVuuren SF, *et al.* Chemical composition, leaf trichome types and biological activities of the essential oils of four related *Salvia* species indigenous to Southern Africa. J Essent Oil Res 2006; 18(1): 72-9.
[http://dx.doi.org/10.1080/10412905.2006.12067125]

[61]   Longaray Delamare AP, Moschen-Pistorello IT, Artico L, Atti-Serafini L, Echeverrigaray S. Antibacterial activity of the essential oils of *Salvia officinalis* L. and *Salvia triloba* L. cultivated in South Brazil. Food Chem 2007; 100(2): 603-8.
[http://dx.doi.org/10.1016/j.foodchem.2005.09.078]

[62]   Kamatou GPP, Viljoen AM, Gono-Bwalya AB, *et al.* The *in vitro* pharmacological activities and a chemical investigation of three South African *Salvia* species. J Ethnopharmacol 2005; 102(3): 382-90.
[http://dx.doi.org/10.1016/j.jep.2005.06.034] [PMID: 16099614]

[63]   Raal A, Orav A, Arak E. Composition of the essential oil of *Salvia officinalis* L. from various European countries. Nat Prod Res 2007; 21(5): 406-11.
[http://dx.doi.org/10.1080/14786410500528478] [PMID: 17487611]

[64]   Mirjalili MH, Salehi P, Sonboli A, Vala MM. Essential oil variation of *Salvia officinalis* aerial parts during its phenological cycle. Chem Nat Compd 2006; 42(1): 19-23.
[http://dx.doi.org/10.1007/s10600-006-0027-4]

[65]   Perry NB, Anderson RE, Brennan NJ, *et al.* Essential oils from dalmatian sage (*Salvia officinalis* l.): variations among individuals, plant parts, seasons, and sites. J Agric Food Chem 1999; 47(5): 2048-54.
[http://dx.doi.org/10.1021/jf981170m] [PMID: 10552494]

# CHAPTER 3

# Anti-Browning Agents

**Faiza Mumtaz**[1,2], **Fazlullah Khan**[3,4] and **Kamal Niaz**[5,*]

[1] *Department of Pharmacology, School of Medicine, Tehran University of Medical Sciences, Tehran, Iran*

[2] *Experimental Medicine Research Center, Tehran University of Medical Sciences, Tehran, Iran*

[3] *International Campus, Tehran University of Medical Sciences (IC-TUMS), Tehran, Iran*

[4] *Department of Toxicology and Pharmacology, Faculty of Pharmacy, Tehran University of Medical Science, Tehran-1417614411, Iran*

[5] *Department of Pharmacology and Toxicology, Faculty of Bio-Sciences, Cholistan University of Veterinary and Animal Sciences (CUVAS), Bahawalpur-63100 Pakistan*

**Abstract:** Browning of food is a major concern in the food industry. The endogenous polyphenol oxidases (PPOs) are responsible for causing enzymatic browning of fresh-cut fruits and vegetables. The use of sulfites has been replaced by anti-browning agents due to the consumer awareness about potential adverse events and increased regulatory scrutiny associated with the use of sulfites. The objective of this study was to shed light on the potential role of different antibrowning agents to extend the shelf life and maintain the quality of fresh-cut fruits and vegetables. The antibrowning capacity is measured by calculating the reduced browning reaction of the cut surfaces and, retaining total visual quality. These agents can reduce cut surface browning through their potential mechanisms by acting as acidulants, chelating agents, complexing agents, enzyme inhibitors or reducing agents. Anti-browning agents can be used alone or in combination with either other agents or with other physical methods to control browning reaction.

**Keywords:** Anti-browning, Browning, Chelating agents, Food, Polyphenol oxidases.

## INTRODUCTION

It is well known that in the last few years society's awareness about the potential health benefits of consuming fruits and vegetables has increased.

* **Corresponding author Dr. Kamal Niaz:** DVM, PhD, Assistant Professor, Department of Pharmacology and Toxicology, Faculty of Bio-Sciences, Cholistan University of Veterinary and Animal Sciences (CUVAS), Bahawalpur-63100 Pakistan; Tel: +923129360054; E-mail: kamalniaz1989@gmail.com

The consumer demand for fresh minimally processed ready-to-use fruits and vegetables is increasing with every passing day. The minimally processed fruits and vegetables are generally more appealing to customers compared to the original raw materials. Therefore, the supply of fresh-cut fruits with high quality in a convenient form has risen in the market. The main advantage of minimally processed foods is the maintenance of their biological and physiological activities due to their live tissues [1]. For this reason, food industries have tried to develop advance techniques to process fruits and vegetables. The shelf life of fresh-cut products is the main concern to limit their use due to microbial contamination, browning and desiccation [2, 3]. Among the quality attributes of minimally processed food items especially fruits and vegetables, colour of products is one of the important quality attributes to assess quality and aesthetic value. Therefore, maintaining the colour and preventing the browning of the surface of minimally processed food are the major points of concern for food industries [4].

The food processing operations induce enhanced ethylene synthesis, enzymatic and non-enzymatic browning, microbial contamination, softening of fresh-cut fruits and exposure to oxygen, all resulting in compromised quality [5, 6].

Browning is the process of the development of brown colouration on the surface of fresh-cut fruits and it is a major phenomenon in industrial food processing which implicates the loss of product quality before supply to end-users. Food industry is facing main challenges regarding browning reactions which are enhanced by tissue damage during processing operations, such as peeling, cutting, pureeing, pitting, freezing, commenting or pulping and shredding of fresh fruits and vegetables. As discussed, the browning process causes low market value and shorter shelf-life of products due to the deleterious changes in the appearance and organoleptic properties of foods [7].

Enzymatic or non-enzymatic browning reactions are a major concern with regard to the aesthetic properties of products [8, 9]. It has been reported that the browning reactions adversely affect the quality, nutritional value and safety of foods. Polyphenol oxidases (PPOs) are present in all fruits and vegetables and are responsible for oxidative or enzymatic browning. Therefore, the PPO activity is enhanced in fruits and vegetables that are particularly sensitive to oxidative browning. These include potatoes, apples, mushrooms, bananas, peaches, fruit juices and wines [10].

Along with enzymatic browning, there is a series of non-enzymatic chemical reactions occuring such as polymerization of endogenous phenolic compounds which cause surface browning of fresh-cut fruits and vegetables. Although our main point of concern is enzymatic browning, non-enzymatic browning occurs majorly due to the Maillard reaction, which occurs when mixtures of reducing sugars and amino acids are heated together [11].

To stop the browning reaction, at least one component among oxygen, phenolic compounds and PPOs must be removed from the system by exclusion or removal of one or both of the substrates either the oxygen molecule or phenols. Furthermore, other factors that prevent the browning reactions are to lower the pH less than 3 or more units below the optimum level, reverse melanin formation or adding compounds that inhibit PPO [12]. Before 1986, these unwanted reactions were successfully controlled by the addition of sulphites however, after the ban by government agencies on the use of sulphites as food additives, food item manufacturers looked for rapid replacements [13]. Therefore, food experts and researchers started to use other agents like sulfur-containing amino acids, ascorbic acid and some other organic acids to control browning [14].

Moreover, for fresh-cut fruits, a number of chemicals and their compositions are described as anti-browning agents [15, 16]. The anti-browning agents are used in a very low concentration because the inhibition of anti-browning agents is independent of their concentration. In minimally processed fresh-cut fruits and vegetables, citric acid and ascorbic acid have been evaluated largely for their anti-browning activity [17]. The use of combined treatments to overcome browning reactions are thought to be more effective [18].

## MECHANISM OF ENZYMATIC BROWNING

A copper containing oxido-reductase responsible for browning is called PPO [19]. Browning is the main problem faced by fresh-cut products (food items), which occurs in the presence of oxygen when the enzyme PPO converts the phenolic compounds into dark coloured pigments. Browning process does not occur in intact plant cells since phenolic compounds are separated from the PPO in cell vacuoles which are present in cytoplasm [3]. Rapid browning occurs when the tissues are damaged after slicing or cutting and PPO mixed with phenolic compounds lead to fast browning reaction. To date, enzymatic browning is one of the primary causes of quality degradation in food industries. The food industries developed various physical and chemical methods, either alone or in combination, to overcome the browning reaction [20, 21].

As far as the mechanism of developing enzymatic browning is concerned, it occurs due to the formation of unstable product anions by the interaction of oxygen, phenolic compounds and PPOs. This happens because fruit peeling or cutting leads to the excretion of the substrate of fruit cell membranes, which contain PPOs that in the presence of oxygen dehydrogenate polyphenols are transformed in its unstable form. These unstable products are further involved in the reactions which are responsible for the development of dark coloured pigments in freshly cut fruits [22].

To elucidate the mechanism in detail, it has been demonstrated that PPO can catalyse two types of reactions, one is the o-hydroxylation of monophenols to o-diphenols and the other is oxidation of o-diphenols to o-quinones. In enzymatic browning, the oxidation of phenol compounds by PPO in the presence of oxygen cause browning of food items [23]. Various anti-browning agents along with mechanisms of action are mentioned in Table **1**. Furthermore, the quinones undergo subsequent reactions to form dark-coloured pigments responsible for causing browning [24]. Therefore, the PPO activity is measured to quantify the anti-browning activity of compounds on fresh cut fruits. As far as the role of oxygen is concerned, increased levels of oxygen are particularly effective in inhibiting enzymatic browning by causing substrate inhibition of PPO. Although the subsequent formation of high levels of colourless quinones, alternatively, may cause feedback inhibition of PPO [25].

Table 1. Classification of anti-browning agents according to their mechanism of action.

| Class | Members | Mechanism |
|---|---|---|
| Acidulants | Citric acid, Malic acid, Phosphoric acids | Irreversible inactivation of PPO by reducing pH below 3 |
| Reducing agents | Ascorbic acid and analogues, Sulfit agents, Sulphur-containing amino acids, Phenolic acids | Act by causing the chemical reduction of the pigment precursors |
| Chelating agents | Sorbic acid, Polycarboxylic acids, Phosphate, EDTA | Either chelate with copper in the active site of PPO enzyme in browning catalysed by PPO or reduce the amount of copper available for incorporation into holoenzyme |
| Complexing agents | Cyclodextrin, Chitosan | Entrapping or forming complex with PPO substrate |
| Enzyme treatments | Oxygenase, Protease, O-methyltransferase | Inhibit PPOs |
| Enzyme Inhibitors | Aliphatic alcohols, Aromatic carboxylic acids, Anions, Peptides, Resorcinols | Inhibit PPOs |

## ANTI-BROWNING AGENTS

Previously, sulfites were used as anti-browning agents in food industries because these agents were able to inhibit enzymatic and non-enzymatic browning reactions effectively. There are growing concerns in using these chemical agents as anti-browning agents due to their potential to cause deleterious health effects and there is an increased demand for regulatory scrutiny to develop and find some functional alternatives to sulfites to be used as anti-browning agents [26].

By definition, anti-browning agents are the chemicals which interact chemically with either enzymes or intermediates of pigment formation. Therefore, browning inhibitors avoid the formation of coloured compounds by reacting with enzymes or react with the substrates or products of enzymes. A variety of different anti-browning agents that function as preferred substrates belong to different chemical groups and are used by food industries to overcome browning reactions inhibiting enzyme activity, substituting or removing its substrates either oxygen molecules or phenolics [27].

Browning of food items can be stopped by the removal of oxygen from the surface of fresh-cut fruits and vegetables as browning is an oxidation reaction. Therefore, browning reaction can be stopped by the use of anti-browning agents, which interact with molecular oxygen in one way or the other. Several types of chemical substances are used in the food industry to control browning reaction by directly inhibiting PPO or by acting indirectly with PPO products. Other agents act by rendering the medium inadequate for initiation of the browning process. The agents which react indirectly with products of PPO and can stop the PPO activity before converting into dark pigments on the surface of fresh-cut fruits or vegetables [28, 29].

As demonstrated, anti-browning agents are the most feasible approach for the prevention of browning in the food industry. However, the use of anti-browning agents to control enzymatic browning is limited due to their toxicity, high cost, effect on taste, aroma and texture of the product [3, 30]. Browning process is influenced by various factors including the different types of reactants participating in processing, the temperature used, pH and variety of metal ions. Therefore, by controlling these factors using various physical methods, browning process can be avoided along with the use of anti-browning agents. The reduction of temperature and oxygen, use of edible coatings or treatment with gamma irradiation or high pressure are the most commonly used physical methods to control the browning process [25].

Reaction of browning is specifically sensitive to and influenced by temperature variation. As well as, the temperature variation is also crucial for the storage of food items. It has been noticed that storage at low temperature during the storage, handling and processing of fresh-cut fruits and vegetables is efficient enough to control browning reactions either enzymatic or non-enzymatic instead of the fact that browning process cannot stop completely by lowering temperature. The slow-down of PPO activity by lowering temperature (0-4 °C) is far from optimal for these enzymes [31].

The cost associated with keeping food items cold all the time to prevent browning is a noticeable issue for manufacturers. Therefore, manufacturers are looking for some cost effective and more efficient methods to inhibit browning of food items [32]. It has been studied that an efficient anti-browning agent maintains its anti-browning potential during all storage conditions even at room temperature for a long time. Commonly, the anti-browning agents alone or in combination are used in the form of solution, frequently in the form of formulation to inhibit browning reaction [33].

The impact of different anti-browning agents has been tested on different kinds of treatments. The anti-browning agents maintained the initial light colour of fresh-cut fruits to use in the food industry and maintained a high content of vitamin C, phenolic compounds and antioxidant activity (FRAP, DPPH) [34]. As shown in Table **2**, to prevent browning reactions different chemical additives could be used *i.e.* ascorbic acid, citric acid, calcium propionate, calcium lactate, calcium ascorbate, carboxylic acids, chelators, thiol containing compounds, cysteine, glutathione or specific enzyme inhibitors such as 4-hexylresorcinol [15, 35 - 37].

Table 2. Representative browning inhibitory agents according to their chemical groups.

| Anti-browning agents | Classification |
|---|---|
| Carboxylic acids | Acetic, Citric, Fumaric, Formic, Lactic, Malic, Melanoid pyruvic, Oxalic, Oxaloacetic, Succinic, Tartaric |
| Ascorbic acids | Erythorbic, Na-erythrobate, Ascorbic, Ascorbic-2-phosphate, Ca-ascorbate, Mg-ascorbate, Fe-ascorbate |
| Sulfur-containing amino acids | Cysteine, Glutathione, Histidine, Methionine, N-acetylcysteine |
| Phenolic acids | Gallic, Kojic, Caffeic, Chlorogenic, Cinnamic, Ferulic, Coumaric |
| Resorcinol | 4-Hexyl resorcinol |
| Others Agents | EDTA, Honey, Aliphatic alcohols, NaCl CaCl$_2$ |

## Organic Acids

Acidulants are the chemical compounds that lower the pH of the medium. Anti-browning agents acidulants have a widespread application in the food industry to control enzymatic browning. These agents are used in combination with other anti-browning agents to control browning effectively. Among the organic acids, the carboxylic acids are used effectively as anti-browning agents in minimally processed food items [38].

It has also been evaluated that the inhibitory mechanisms of organic acids exert their action through maintaining the pH well below the one required for optimal PPO activity (pH 5-7) because PPO activity varies with changes in pH and nature of the substrate. The enzyme PPO is inactive below pH 3 or 4 hence; the mechanism of action of acidulants is to maintain the pH well below that necessary for the optimal catalytic activity of PPO [39 - 41].

## *Citric Acid*

Citric acid is among the most widely used anti-browning agents in the food industry and belongs to the organic acids class. It inhibits PPO activity as well as chelates with copper in the active site of holoenzyme. Citric acid can be used alone or in combination with other agents to exert its anti-browning activity in the food industry [41, 42]. Citric acid reacts with PPOs by acting as an acidulant and chelating agent and therefore, inactivating the enzyme PPO through reducing pH and chelating copper in the active site of PPO [14, 43].

Other organic acids used as an alternative to citric acid to inhibit browning reaction are malic, tartaric and malonic acids. Inorganic agents including phosphoric and hydrochloric acids could be used as an alternative to citric acid. The risk is more in using other acids compared to citric acid due to their higher price, limited availability and negative impact on taste. By lowering the pH, the inhibitory effect of citric acid becomes double [34, 43]. It was evaluated that citric acid was a non-competitive inhibitor of PPO activity in lettuce [44]. The anti-browning activity of citric acid was accessed by its inhibitory action on the quality of banana smoothie [45], fresh-cut apples [46], fresh-cut potatoes [47], fresh-cut royal delicious apples [48] and green table olives [49].

## *Oxalic Acid*

Although oxalic acid is not an approved food additive yet it is present naturally as an essential component in a vast number of plants, such as asparagus, broccoli, Brussels sprout, carrot, garlic, lettuce, onion, parsley, pea, potato, radish, spinach, tomato and turnip. It exhibits its anti-browning activity through inhibition of PPO as well as its binding with the active sites of copper, to form an inactive complex not available for browning. Oxalic acid avoided the formation of catechol-quinone formation and quinone was not available for bleaching [41, 50]. The anti-browning effect of oxalic acid was checked for potatoes and apples [51, 52], baby spinach leaves [53], unripe grapes [40] and green table olives [49]. The inhibition potential of oxalic acid was influenced by concentration and pH. It has been reported that on mushroom PPO, oxalic acid shows competitive inhibition. In contrast, oxalic acid showed non-competitive inhibition to PPO activity of artichoke, as well as competitive inhibition to celery root PPO [54].

## *Acetic Acid*

It has been studied that phenylalanine ammonia lyase (PAL) activity is completely inhibited by acetic acid which is required in the biosynthesis of phenolic compounds. These also inhibited the production of wound-induced phenolics. Thus, the reversible inhibition of phenylalanine ammonia lyase activity by acetic acid is required to exert its activity as an anti-browning inhibitor [41, 55]. The anti-browning activity of acetic acid was accessed by its inhibitory action on okra [56] and dried banana [57].

## Phenolic Acids

The anti-browning capacity can be correlated to the strong antioxidant activity of compounds. The anti-browning activity of phenolic acids is attributed to the complex formation of metal ions with the phenolic acids. Phenolic acids are reducing agents, as a result, in the presence of phenolic acids the metal ions cannot influence browning, although metal ions usually increase browning. Phenolic acids such as chlorogenic acid and ferulic acid are categorized as antioxidants and widely distributed in the plant kingdom. These agents prevent enzymatic browning through scavenging free radicals, as well as by forming a complex with various metal ions [58, 59].

At the position of hydroxy groups of phenolics is the site where its copper–phenolic acid complex is formed with metal ions to exhibit its anti-browning activity. All other phenolics, such as protocatechuic acid or caffeic acid, with ortho-dihydroxy groups of phenols form copper–phenolic acid complexes to inhibit the browning process [31, 60].

## *Kojic acid*

Kojic acid is chemically 5-hydroxy-2-hydroxymethyl-y-pyrone and produced metabolically by various species of *Aspergillus* and *Penicillium* and found in many fermented Japanese foods. Although, kojic acid is very effective as an anti-browning agent yet its use in the food industry is limited due to its cost. It was evaluated that kojic acid acts as a reducing agent as well as an inhibitor to PPOs [61]. It was used as an anti-browning agent in mushrooms to inhibit PPO activity [62]. Another study showed the role of kojic acid to inhibit browning in shrimp either by direct inhibition of PPO or by chemical reduction of pigment precursor to a colourless compound [19, 63]. Its anti-browning effect was studied on mushroom, potato, apple, white shrimp, and spiny lobster [64]. Among many tested phenolic acids, kojic acid has the highest inhibitory activity on browning of apple slice [17]. The anti-browning effect of kojic acid was evaluated by using apple juice [65], litchi fruit [66], lotus seeds [67] and pistachio and mushroom [68].

## *Cinnamic Acid*

The pleasant flavour of cinnamic acid will be a useful synergist for inhibiting browning since its flavouring capacity allows direct addition to food items. Cinnamic acid which is an aromatic carboxylic acid, as well as its phenolic relatives which are present in many essential oils from plants such as ferulic acid, coumaric acid and caffeic acid effectively perform their preservative and flavouring actions [69]. The inhibition of browning was evaluated by using cloudy apple juice [70], fresh cut pears [71] and lotus seeds [67].

## **Ascorbic Acid and Its Derivatives**

Ascorbic acid is a widely used reducing agent and anti-browning agent which maintains the flavour and texture of food items. Therefore, consumers feel it near to unprocessed food because the effectiveness of this agent is temporary [72]. Ascorbic acid and its derivatives like erythorbic acid have frequently been used interchangeably as antioxidants by the food industry, acting as reducing agents and oxidizing irreversibly in reaction. They also reduce the pH to some extent. These agents are highly nonspecific and cause off-colour and off-flavour to materials with which they react. Another disadvantage of using these agents in the food industry is their low penetration and non-specificity for cellular matrix of the food to act effectively [12, 42].

Ascorbic acid is converted into dehydroascorbic acid derivatives by oxidation which is more stable compared to ascorbic acid. The ascorbyl-6 esters of fatty acids are another stable form of ascorbic acid; these are less effective compared to ascorbic acid as the onset of browning is achieved later. Enzymatic browning is believed to be prevented by ascorbic acid specifically through the reduction of quinone products to their original polyphenol compounds [43, 56, 73]. Ascorbic acid (1% solution) along with its derivatives was used effectively to reverse browning reactions in apple slices and potatoes [17, 74].

The efficacy of ascorbic acid on slices of pineapple was checked and researchers found ascorbic acid as an effective natural agent to control enzymatic browning [75]. The anti-browning effect of ascorbic acid was checked against lettuce and it was observed that phenolics content was protected from oxidation by ascorbic acid [44]. Furthermore, the anti-browning effect was evaluated in cloudy apple juice [70], green coconut water [76], apple juice [77], fresh cut apples [78], fresh-cut royal delicious apples [48] and green table olives [49].

## Sulfhydryl Compounds/Sulfur Containing Amino Acids

Enzymatic browning is an oxidation process therefore reducing agents are applied to prevent discoloration. Reducing agents are compounds that act as anti-browning agents by converting back o-quinone which is a colourless product resulting from PPO activity to its previous form called o-diphenol. Reducing agents react temporarily during the reaction to control browning as reactants are irreversibly oxidised during reaction [79]. Sulfhydryl compounds are recommended to be used as anti-browning agents and are more effective compared to other reducing agents *i.e.* ascorbic acid. Cysteine and glutathione are well-known for their anti-browning effects in the food industry. Therefore, enzymatic and non-enzymatic browning could effectively be inhibited by using particularly sulfites and sulfur-containing amino acids or peptides [80].

A number of thiol-containing agents including gluthatione, L-cysteine, mercaptoethanol, and thiourea have been evaluated as inhibitors of enzymatic browning. The primary anti-browning effect of sulfhydryl compounds is generated through their interaction with the o-quinones formed by enzymatic catalysis producing stable, colourless products. The low concentration of sulphur containing amino acids such as cysteine and glutathione mediate their anti-browning effect. However, limitation to the use of sulphur containing amino acids as anti-browning agents is due to the unpleasant odour and negative effect on food taste when these agents are used in higher concentrations [81].

Although, the exact mechanism of inhibition of sulphur containing amino acids on PPO is still unclear yet, it is believed that they exert their anti-browning activity by converting more reactive o-quinones to produce less reactive diphenols by blocking the enzymatic browning reactions. Secondly, it works as an anti-browning agent by acting as a chelating agent to complex with copper in PPO, which in turn, inhibits browning by restricting copper to participate in the browning reactions [74, 82]. These agents have been successfully used as anti-browning inhibitors for minimally processed fruits like potatoes [14], apples [83], lychee fruit [84], pears and other fruit beverages [39].

### *Cysteine*

Sulfhydryl-containing amino acids like L-cysteine act by a complex mechanism. These agents inhibit the formation of brown pigments by reacting with the quinone intermediates to form stable colourless compounds. Thereafter, PPO activity is inhibited by cysteine-quinone adducts. Along with this, the direct inhibitory effect of cysteine on PPO through the formation of stable complexes with copper has also been evaluated [43, 85].

Cysteine is a thiol containing compound and also a reducing agent that controls browning reaction. A direct and stable complex is formed when cysteine combines with copper after reacting with PPO. It was reported that in papaya extracts, cysteine was used to investigate its anti-browning activity. Cysteine also reacts with quinone products to form colourless conjugated compounds to act as an anti-browning agent [86]. Although cysteine is very effective as anti-browning agent, its use needs more financial resources as these agents are very expensive to be used commercially . Their cost effective alternatives may include sulfur-containing amino acids such as L-cysteine, cystine, L-methionine and N-acetylcysteine. The inhibition of browning by L-cysteine was studied in apple juice [65] and cloudy apple juice [70]. The anti-browning effect of cysteine was checked against lettuce and it was observed that phenolics content was protected from oxidation [44, 87].

## *Glutathione*

Glutathione markedly inhibited PPO activity *in vitro* as reported already in previous studies and its use in food industries as an anti-browning agent is safe for human health [88].

## Cyclodextrins and Chitosan

Both cyclodextrins and chitosan are classified under complex agents, used to inhibit enzymatic browning in the food industry. As far as the mechanism of action of cyclodextrins as an anti-browning agent is concerned, they inhibit browning either by the formation of inclusion complexes with phenolics or by entrapment of PPO products or substrates, ultimately depleted PPO substrate. They are also used in combination with other known anti-browning agents such as chelating agents, reducing agents or acidulants [89]. The soluble type of cyclodextrins can be used in the solution form and insoluble type of cyclodextrin is used as a packed form in a column. The beta-cyclodextrin is less water soluble and has more capacity to bind with PPO to inhibit its activity [90]. However, the diffusion of beta cyclodextrin is low as tested by using diced apples to inhibit browning reactions [91].

The anti-browning effect of beta cyclodextrin was also determined by using cloudy apple juice [70]. The main disadvantage of using cyclodextrin is its negative effect on the colour and flavour of industrial food items as it binds non-specifically to form inclusion complex. Another disadvantage is its high cost, specifically of insoluble cyclodextrin, to be used as a food additive. The binding capacity of cyclodextrins also varies with the type of phenolic compounds [92, 93].

Chitosan is also a complexing agent and often used as an anti-browning agent. Its anti-browning activity was determined on minimally processed apples [94]. The anti-browning capacity of oligo chitosan was also determined on apple juice [95].

## Resorcinols

Resorcinols are categorised under enzyme inhibitors, acting as anti-browning agents. Substituted resorcinols are a novel type of resorcinols, isolated from fig extracts initially. 4-substituted resorcinols are stable compounds and very specific to interact with PPO activity and more effective to inhibit browning reactions compared to sulphites in the food industry [96, 97].

### *4-hexyl Resorcinol*

4-hexyl resorcinol has high potential to be used as a safe anti-browning agent in the food industry. It is a synthetic 4-substituted resorcinol that is structurally related to phenolic substrates. Its mechanism of action to inhibit browning reaction is by PPO inhibition, which has high potential among 4-substituted resorcinols to act as browning inhibitor [39, 98]. It exists in two forms, water-soluble 4-hexylresorcinol is stable, nontoxic, non-mutagenic and non-carcinogenic compounds. The anti-browning capacity of this compound was initially checked in shrimp malanosis. 4-hexylresorcinol has also been used to avoid browning reactions in fresh and dried slices of apples, avocado, grape juices, Japanese quince fruit and potatoes [39, 99 - 101]. This agent has no toxicity and was proved to be safe for use in the food industry [65, 85, 102].

### Phosphate-based Compounds

As discussed previously, the PPO enzyme contains copper in its active site and in the browning reaction catalysed by PPO the chelating agents believed to either bind with copper at active site or reduce the level of copper which in turn bind with holoenzyme to cause browning. Phosphate-based compounds are chelating agents including metaphosphate, polyphosphate and sodium acid pyrophosphate which have low solubility in cold water. These agents have been used as anti-browning agents for fresh-cut fruits and vegetables. The solubility of these agents can be enhanced when used at low concentrations or already dissolved in water. These agents are usually used in combination with other anti-browning agents [103, 104].

## Other Miscellaneous Compounds

### EDTA

EDTA is known as ethylenediaminetetraacetic acid, is a metalloenzyme containing copper in its centre. In the food industry it is commonly used as a chelating agent for metals. In fresh cut fruits and vegetables it is used in combination with other anti-browning agents. It had been used in apple slices and apple juice as anti-browning agent in combination with other anti-browning agents or alone [91, 105].

### Amino Acids, Peptides and Protein

The anti-browning effect of bovine serum albumin which is a protein, casein hydrolysate (protein hydrolysate) and L-amino acids on PPO catalysis and inhibition was evaluated in mushroom, avocado and banana. The PPO activity of mushroom was avoided by using low concentrations of L-lysine, glycine, L-histidine and L-phenylalanine [106].

### Sodium Chloride

Sodium chloride classified under halides is used as an anti-browning agent. It is believed to inhibit PPO activity and leads to a decrease in pH. It exerts its effect in the food industry on minimally processed food items. It has been reported that chloride binding with sodium is a weak browning inhibitor and more quantity of chloride is required to inhibit PPO activity [107, 108].

### Calcium Chloride

Calcium can be used as an effective anti-browning agent either alone or in combination with other browning inhibitors. Basically, it was used to firm tissues of fresh-cut fruits and vegetables [109]. Calcium is used in combination with other anti-browning agents to inhibit browning reactions. It has been reported to enhance the anti-browning effect of ascorbic acid and citric acid on slices of pear when used in 1% concentration. It has been reported that its effects were not due to inhibition of PPO [48, 110].

### Aromatic Carboxylic Acids

These agents have structural similarity with phenolic substrates and like carboxylic acids these agents also inhibit PPO activity. Among aromatic carboxylic acids, benzoic acid and cinnamic acids are both PPO inhibitors and do not offer long lasting protection against browning reactions. It has been studied that both compounds underwent slow conversion to PPO substrate during the progress of their anti-browning activity [39, 91, 111].

## *Other Anions*

A number of anions including halides, sulphate and nitrate are using in the food industry. As far as their mechanism of action is concerned, halides inhibit PPO activity. It has been reported that sulphate and nitrate have no effect on the PPOs activity possibly due to their large ionic radii [112].

## ANTI-BROWNING AGENTS FROM NATURAL SOURCES

Consumers are more conscious not only about the shelf-life and appearance of fresh-cut fruits but also are aware of the use of synthetic additives used to improve, for instance, the colour and consistency retention [113]. Consumers want to use minimally processed food items containing natural anti-browning agents which resemble to natural, unprocessed food products. Therefore, the food industries focus on the use of natural anti-browning agents and additives instead of artificial ones against fruit browning. The research is focused on natural sources to overcome the browning reactions. Grapefruit seed extract [114], onion extract [115], rice bran extract [116], rosemary extract [117], honey for fresh-cut apples [118], natural juice of cranberries (*Vaccinium macrocarpon Ait*) [119], pineapple juice [120], rhubarb juice [121], for fresh cut pears slices treatment, Japanese quince (*Chaenomeles japonica)* juices [119] and kiwifruit puree [122], were used to evaluate their potential as anti-browning agents in food industries.

### Honey

It has been reported that honey inhibits PPO enzyme to exert anti-browning activity and catalysed browning reaction by direct inhibition of the enzyme. It has been evaluated that honey also acts by its reaction with quinonoid which is a product of PPO catalysis [109, 123]. The anti-browning activity of honey was also confirmed by dipping slices of peeled apples and ginger in a honey solution [81, 124].

### Aliphatic Alcohols

The inhibition provided by natural methods is very fascinating for researchers [10]. It has been reported that alcoholic compounds including ethanol weakly inhibit PPO activity. Other aliphatic alcohols also inhibit PPO enzyme and the inhibitory effect of aliphatic alcohols is directly related to the increased number of carbon atoms. The anti-browning effects of natural aliphatic alcohols have been studied on PPO enzymes of grapes and apples [91, 125].

## COMBINED USE OF ANTI-BROWNING AGENTS

It has been studied that the most relevant anti-browning effect could be achieved by using different anti-browning agents. Previously various anti-browning agents had been used in combination to exert their inhibitory effect on the browning process in minimally processed fruits and vegetables [38]. In sliced potatoes, the combination of citric acid and ascorbic acid reversed the browning process [126]. The combinations of ascorbic acid, erythorbic acid and citric acid prevented the browning of sliced apples [127]. The browning reaction in sliced apples reversed by using a combination of ascorbic acid and calcium chloride [128]. The combined anti-browning effect of ascorbic acid, $CaCl_2$, citric acid was studied on potato slices to inhibit browning [129]. In litchi fruit, the combination of glutathione and citric acid was used to prevent browning reaction [84]. A combination of ascorbic acid and kojic acid has been used to inhibit browning reactions in food industry [130]. The combination of ascorbic acid, citric acid, carbon dioxide and nitrogen was used to study browning inhibition on banana smoothie [45]. To study browning inhibition on potatoes combination of citric acid, ascorbic acid and sodium metabisulfite was used [131], whereas the combination of ascorbic acid along with ethanol was also used as browning inhibitor [132].

## CONCLUSION

In the field of research, the efficiency of anti-browning is being checked by treating food items especially fruits with different anti-browning agents. These agents are the most effective alternative to sulphites in the food industry to control browning reactions on the surface of fresh-cut fruits and vegetables. Suitable treatments should give better visual results to control browning reactions. The present study sheds light on the best effective use of anti-browning agents on fresh-cut fruits. To choose a suitable browning inhibitory agent is a difficult task and depends on a number of factors including cost, method of treatment, efficacy and their effects on taste, texture, flavour, or colour of products in particular.

## CONSENT FOR PUBLICATION

Not applicable.

## CONFLICT OF INTEREST

The author confirms that this chapter contents have no conflict of interest.

## ACKNOWLEDGEMENTS

All the authors of the manuscript thank and acknowledge their respective universities and institutes.

## REFERENCES

[1]   Manolopoulou E, Varzakas T. Application of antibrowning agents in minimally processed cabbage J Food Nutr Disor 3 2014; 1:2

[2]   Kim D, Smith N, Lee C. Apple cultivar variations in response to heat treatment and minimal processing. J Food Sci 1993; 58(5): 1111-4.
      [http://dx.doi.org/10.1111/j.1365-2621.1993.tb06126.x]

[3]   Alzamora S, Tapia MS, López-Malo A. Minimally processed fruits and vegetables: Boom Koninklijke Uitgevers. 2000.

[4]   Lamikanra O. Fresh-cut fruits and vegetables: science, technology, and market. CRC press 2002.
      [http://dx.doi.org/10.1201/9781420031874]

[5]   Ahvenainen R. New approaches in improving the shelf life of minimally processed fruit and vegetables. Trends Food Sci Technol 1996; 7(6): 179-87.
      [http://dx.doi.org/10.1016/0924-2244(96)10022-4]

[6]   Tochi B, Wang Z, Xu SY, Zhang W. Effect of stem bromelain on the browning of apple juice. Am J Food Technol 2009; 4: 146-53.
      [http://dx.doi.org/10.3923/ajft.2009.146.153]

[7]   De Rigal D, Cerny M, Richard-Forget F, Varoquaux P. Inhibition of endive (Cichorium endivia L.) polyphenoloxidase by a Carica papaya latex preparation. Int J Food Sci Technol 2001; 36(6): 677-84.
      [http://dx.doi.org/10.1046/j.1365-2621.2001.00498.x]

[8]   He Q, Luo Y. Enzymatic browning and its control in fresh-cut produce. Stewart Postharvest Rev 2007; 3(6): 1-7.
      [http://dx.doi.org/10.2212/spr.2007.6.16]

[9]   Billaud C, Roux E, Brun-Merimee S, Maraschin C, Nicolas J. Inhibitory effect of unheated and heated D-glucose, D-fructose and L-cysteine solutions and Maillard reaction product model systems on polyphenoloxidase from apple. I. Enzymatic browning and enzyme activity inhibition using spectrophotometric and polarographic methods. Food Chem 2003; 81(1): 35-50.
      [http://dx.doi.org/10.1016/S0308-8146(02)00376-X]

[10]  Laurila E, Ahvenainen R. Minimal processing of fresh fruits and vegetables. 2002.
      [http://dx.doi.org/10.1533/9781855736641.3.288]

[11]  Leiva-Valenzuela GA, Quilaqueo M, Lagos D, Estay D, Pedreschi F. Effect of formulation and baking conditions on the structure and development of non-enzymatic browning in biscuit models using images. J Food Sci Technol 2018; 55(4): 1234-43.
      [http://dx.doi.org/10.1007/s13197-017-3008-7] [PMID: 29606738]

[12]  Whitaker JR, Lee CY. Recent advances in chemistry of enzymatic browning. Enzymatic Browning Prev 1995; 600: 2-7.
      [http://dx.doi.org/10.1021/bk-1995-0600.ch001]

[13]  Duxbury D, Ed. Stabilizer blend extends shelf life of fresh fruit, vegetables. Food Proc 1988.

[14]  Gunes G, Lee CY. Color of minimally processed potatoes as affected by modified atmosphere packaging and antibrowning agents. J Food Sci 1997; 62(3): 572-5.
      [http://dx.doi.org/10.1111/j.1365-2621.1997.tb04433.x]

[15]  Rojas-Graü MA, Sobrino-López A, Soledad Tapia M, Martín-Belloso O. Browning inhibition in fresh-cut 'Fuji' apple slices by natural antibrowning agents. J Food Sci 2006; 71(1): S59-65.

[http://dx.doi.org/10.1111/j.1365-2621.2006.tb12407.x]

[16] Suttirak W, Manurakchinakorn S. Potential application of ascorbic acid, citric acid and oxalic acid for browning inhibition in fresh-cut fruits and vegetables. Walailak J Sci Technol 2011; 7(1): 5-14.

[17] Son S, Moon K, Lee C. Inhibitory effects of various antibrowning agents on apple slices. Food Chem 2001; 73(1): 23-30.
[http://dx.doi.org/10.1016/S0308-8146(00)00274-0]

[18] González-Aguilar GA, Ayala-Zavala J, Olivas G, De la Rosa L, Álvarez-Parrilla E. Preserving quality of fresh-cut products using safe technologies. J Verbraucherschutz Lebensmsicherh 2010; 5(1): 65-72.
[http://dx.doi.org/10.1007/s00003-009-0315-6]

[19] Jukanti A. Polyphenol Oxidase (s): Importance in Food Industry Polyphenol Oxidases (PPOs) in Plants. Springer 2017; pp. 93-106.
[http://dx.doi.org/10.1007/978-981-10-5747-2_6]

[20] Rojas-Graü MA, Grasa-Guillem R, Martín-Belloso O. Quality changes in fresh-cut Fuji apple as affected by ripeness stage, antibrowning agents, and storage atmosphere. J Food Sci 2007; 72(1): S036-43.
[http://dx.doi.org/10.1111/j.1750-3841.2006.00232.x] [PMID: 17995895]

[21] Underhill S, Critchley C. Lychee pericarp browning caused by heat injury. HortScience 1993; 28(7): 721-2.
[http://dx.doi.org/10.21273/HORTSCI.28.7.721]

[22] Arias E, López-Buesa P, Oria R. Extension of fresh-cut "Blanquilla" pear (Pyrus communis L.) shelf-life by 1-MCP treatment after harvest. Postharvest Biol Technol 2009; 54(1): 53-8.
[http://dx.doi.org/10.1016/j.postharvbio.2009.04.009]

[23] Kavrayan D, Aydemir T. Partial purification and characterization of polyphenoloxidase from peppermint (Mentha piperita). Food Chem 2001; 74(2): 147-54.
[http://dx.doi.org/10.1016/S0308-8146(01)00106-6]

[24] Ni Eidhin DM, Murphy E, O'Beirne D. Polyphenol oxidase from apple (Malus domestica Borkh. cv Bramley's Seedling): purification strategies and characterization. J Food Sci 2006; 71(1): C51-8.
[http://dx.doi.org/10.1111/j.1365-2621.2006.tb12388.x]

[25] James JB, Ngarmsak T, Rolle R. Processing of fresh-cut tropical fruits and vegetables: A technical guide. RAP Publication (FAO) eng no 2010/16. 2010.

[26] Ramalingam C, Srinath R, Islam NN. Isolation and characterization of bromelain from pineapple (Ananas comosus) and comparing its anti-browning activity apple juice with commercial antibrowning agents. Elixir Food Sci 2012; 45: 7822-6.

[27] Soliva-Fortuny RC, Martín-Belloso O. New advances in extending the shelf-life of fresh-cut fruits: a review. Trends Food Sci Technol 2003; 14(9): 341-53.
[http://dx.doi.org/10.1016/S0924-2244(03)00054-2]

[28] Persic M, Mikulic-Petkovsek M, Slatnar A, Veberic R. Chemical composition of apple fruit, juice and pomace and the correlation between phenolic content, enzymatic activity and browning. Lebensm Wiss Technol 2017; 82: 23-31.
[http://dx.doi.org/10.1016/j.lwt.2017.04.017]

[29] Toledo L, Aguirre C. Enzymatic browning in avocado (Persea americana) revisited: History, advances, and future perspectives. Crit Rev Food Sci Nutr 2017; 57(18): 3860-72.
[http://dx.doi.org/10.1080/10408398.2016.1175416] [PMID: 27172067]

[30] Biegańska-Marecik R, Czapski J. The effect of selected compounds as inhibitors of enzymatic browning and softening of minimally processed apples. Acta Sci Pol Technol Aliment 2007; 6(3): 37-49.

[31] Tomás-Barberán FA, Espín JC. Phenolic compounds and related enzymes as determinants of quality in

fruits and vegetables. J Sci Food Agric 2001; 81(9): 853-76.
[http://dx.doi.org/10.1002/jsfa.885]

[32] Kwak EJ, Lim SI. Inhibition of browning by antibrowning agents and phenolic acids or cinnamic acid in the glucose–lysine model. J Sci Food Agric 2005; 85(8): 1337-42.
[http://dx.doi.org/10.1002/jsfa.1994]

[33] Chaisakdanugull C, Theerakulkait C, Wrolstad RE. Pineapple juice and its fractions in enzymatic browning inhibition of banana [Musa (AAA group) Gros Michel]. J Agric Food Chem 2007; 55(10): 4252-7. [Musa (AAA Group) Gros Michel].
[http://dx.doi.org/10.1021/jf0705724] [PMID: 17439237]

[34] Ibrahim R, Osman A, Saari N, Rahman RA. Effects of anti-browning treatments on the storage quality of minimally processed shredded cabbage. J Food Agric Environ 2004; 2: 54-8.

[35] Gomes MH, Fundo JF, Santos S, Amaro AL, Almeida DP. Hydrogen ion concentration affects quality retention and modifies the effect of calcium additives on fresh-cut 'Rocha'pear. Postharvest Biol Technol 2010; 58(3): 239-46.
[http://dx.doi.org/10.1016/j.postharvbio.2010.07.004]

[36] Oms-Oliu G, Rojas-Graü MA, González LA, Varela P, Soliva-Fortuny R, Hernando MIH, *et al.* Recent approaches using chemical treatments to preserve quality of fresh-cut fruit: A review. Postharvest Biol Technol 2010; 57(3): 139-48.
[http://dx.doi.org/10.1016/j.postharvbio.2010.04.001]

[37] Chiabrando V, Giacalone G. Maintaining quality of fresh-cut apple slices using calcium ascorbate and stored under modified atmosphere. Acta Aliment 2013; 42(2): 245-55.
[http://dx.doi.org/10.1556/AAlim.42.2013.2.12]

[38] Yousuf B, Qadri OS, Srivastava AK. Recent developments in shelf-life extension of fresh-cut fruits and vegetables by application of different edible coatings: A review. Lebensm Wiss Technol 2017; 89: 198-209.
[http://dx.doi.org/10.1016/j.lwt.2017.10.051]

[39] McEvily AJ, Iyengar R, Otwell WS. Inhibition of enzymatic browning in foods and beverages. Crit Rev Food Sci Nutr 1992; 32(3): 253-73.
[http://dx.doi.org/10.1080/10408399209527599] [PMID: 1418602]

[40] Tinello F, Lante A. Evaluation of antibrowning and antioxidant activities in unripe grapes recovered during bunch thinning. Aust J Grape Wine Res 2017; 23(1): 33-41.
[http://dx.doi.org/10.1111/ajgw.12256]

[41] Singh B, Suri K, Shevkani K, Kaur A, Kaur A, Singh N. Enzymatic Browning of Fruit and Vegetables: A Review. Enzymes Food Technol Springer 2018; pp. 63-78.

[42] da Silva JDF, Correa APF, Kechinski CP, Brandelli A. Buffalo cheese whey hydrolyzed with Alcalase as an antibrowning agent in minimally processed apple. J Food Sci Technol 2018; 55(9): 3731-8.
[http://dx.doi.org/10.1007/s13197-018-3303-y] [PMID: 30150833]

[43] Ali HM, El-Gizawy AM, El-Bassiouny RE, Saleh MA. Browning inhibition mechanisms by cysteine, ascorbic acid and citric acid, and identifying PPO-catechol-cysteine reaction products. J Food Sci Technol 2015; 52(6): 3651-9.
[PMID: 26028748]

[44] Altunkaya A, Gökmen V. Effect of various inhibitors on enzymatic browning, antioxidant activity and total phenol content of fresh lettuce (Lactuca sativa). Food Chem 2008; 107(3): 1173-9.
[http://dx.doi.org/10.1016/j.foodchem.2007.09.046]

[45] Wang S, Lin T, Man G, Li H, Zhao L, Wu J, *et al.* Effects of anti-browning combinations of ascorbic acid, citric acid, nitrogen and carbon dioxide on the quality of banana smoothies. Food Bioprocess Technol 2014; 7(1): 161-73.
[http://dx.doi.org/10.1007/s11947-013-1107-7]

[46] Chen C, Hu W, He Y, Jiang A, Zhang R. Effect of citric acid combined with UV-C on the quality of fresh-cut apples. Postharvest Biol Technol 2016; 111: 126-31.
[http://dx.doi.org/10.1016/j.postharvbio.2015.08.005]

[47] Tsouvaltzis P, Brecht JK. Inhibition of Enzymatic Browning of Fresh-Cut Potato by Immersion in Citric Acid is Not Solely Due to pH Reduction of the Solution. J Food Process Preserv 2017; 41(2)e12829
[http://dx.doi.org/10.1111/jfpp.12829]

[48] Kumar P, Sethi S, Sharma RR, Singh S, Varghese E. Improving the shelf life of fresh-cut 'Royal Delicious' apple with edible coatings and anti-browning agents. J Food Sci Technol 2018; 55(9): 3767-78.
[http://dx.doi.org/10.1007/s13197-018-3308-6] [PMID: 30150837]

[49] Mohsenabadi M, Ghasemnezhad M, Hashempour A, Sajedi RH. Inhibition of Polyphenol Oxidases and Peroxidase Activities in Green Table Olives by some Anti-browning Agents. ACS Agric Conspec Sci 2018; 82(4): 375-81.

[50] Prenen JA, Boer P, Dorhout Mees EJ. Absorption kinetics of oxalate from oxalate-rich food in man. Am J Clin Nutr 1984; 40(5): 1007-10.
[http://dx.doi.org/10.1093/ajcn/40.5.1007] [PMID: 6496379]

[51] Yoruk R, Yoruk S, Balaban M, Marshall M. Machine vision analysis of antibrowning potency for oxalic acid: A comparative investigation on banana and apple. J Food Sci 2004; 69(6): E281-9.
[http://dx.doi.org/10.1111/j.1365-2621.2004.tb10999.x]

[52] Zheng X, Brecht JK. Oxalic Acid Treatments. Novel Postharvest Treatments of Fresh Produce. CRC Press Taylor & Francis Group 2017; pp. 35-702.

[53] Cefola M, Pace B. Application of oxalic acid to preserve the overall quality of rocket and baby spinach leaves during storage. J Food Process Preserv 2015; 39(6): 2523-32.
[http://dx.doi.org/10.1111/jfpp.12502]

[54] Aydemir T, Akkanlı G. Partial purification and characterisation of polyphenol oxidase from celery root (Apium graveolens L.) and the investigation of the effects on the enzyme activity of some inhibitors. Int J Food Sci Technol 2006; 41(9): 1090-8.
[http://dx.doi.org/10.1111/j.1365-2621.2006.01191.x]

[55] Tomás-Barberán FA, Gil MI, Castaner M, Artés F, Saltveit ME. Effect of selected browning inhibitors on phenolic metabolism in stem tissue of harvested lettuce. J Agric Food Chem 1997; 45(3): 583-9.
[http://dx.doi.org/10.1021/jf960478f]

[56] Irshad M, Rizwan HM, Debnath B, Anwar M, Li M, Liu S, *et al.* Ascorbic Acid Controls Lethal Browning and Pluronic F-68 Promotes High-frequency Multiple Shoot Regeneration from Cotyldonary Node Explant of Okra (Abelmoschus esculentus L.). HortScience 2018; 53(2): 183-90.
[http://dx.doi.org/10.21273/HORTSCI12315-17]

[57] Sarpong F, Yu X, Zhou C, Hongpeng Y, Uzoejinwa BB, Bai J, *et al.* Influence of anti-browning agent pretreatment on drying kinetics, enzymes inactivation and other qualities of dried banana (Musa ssp.) under relative humidity-convective air dryer. J Food Meas Charact 2018; 12(2): 1229-41.
[http://dx.doi.org/10.1007/s11694-018-9737-0]

[58] Kweon M-H, Hwang H-J, Sung H-C. Identification and antioxidant activity of novel chlorogenic acid derivatives from bamboo (*Phyllostachys edulis*). J Agric Food Chem 2001; 49(10): 4646-55.
[http://dx.doi.org/10.1021/jf010514x] [PMID: 11600002]

[59] Sukhonthara S, Kaewka K, Theerakulkait C. Inhibitory effect of rice bran extracts and its phenolic compounds on polyphenol oxidase activity and browning in potato and apple puree. Food Chem 2016; 190: 922-7.
[http://dx.doi.org/10.1016/j.foodchem.2015.06.016] [PMID: 26213057]

[60] Natella F, Nardini M, Di Felice M, Scaccini C. Benzoic and cinnamic acid derivatives as antioxidants:

structure-activity relation. J Agric Food Chem 1999; 47(4): 1453-9.
[http://dx.doi.org/10.1021/jf980737w] [PMID: 10563998]

[61]   Dong X, Zhang Y, He J-L, *et al.* Preparation of tyrosinase inhibitors and antibrowning agents using green technology. Food Chem 2016; 197(Pt A): 589-96.
[http://dx.doi.org/10.1016/j.foodchem.2015.11.007] [PMID: 26616992]

[62]   Cabanes J, Chazarra S, Garcia-Carmona F. Kojic acid, a cosmetic skin whitening agent, is a slow-binding inhibitor of catecholase activity of tyrosinase. J Pharm Pharmacol 1994; 46(12): 982-5.
[http://dx.doi.org/10.1111/j.2042-7158.1994.tb03253.x] [PMID: 7714722]

[63]   Mills EC, Alcocer MJ, Morgan MR. Biochemical interactions of food-derived peptides. Trends Food Sci Technol 1992; 3: 64-8.
[http://dx.doi.org/10.1016/0924-2244(92)90132-G]

[64]   Chen JS, Wei C-i, Rolle RS, Otwell WS, Balaban MO, Marshall MR. Inhibitory effect of kojic acid on some plant and crustacean polyphenol oxidases. J Agric Food Chem 1991; 39(8): 1396-401.
[http://dx.doi.org/10.1021/jf00008a008]

[65]   İyidoğan N, Bayındırlı A. Effect of L-cysteine, kojic acid and 4-hexylresorcinol combination on inhibition of enzymatic browning in Amasya apple juice. J Food Eng 2004; 62(3): 299-304.
[http://dx.doi.org/10.1016/S0260-8774(03)00243-7]

[66]   Shah HMS, Khan AS, Ali S. Pre-storage kojic acid application delays pericarp browning and maintains antioxidant activities of litchi fruit. Postharvest Biol Technol 2017; 132: 154-61.
[http://dx.doi.org/10.1016/j.postharvbio.2017.06.004]

[67]   Chen SN, Xie RP, Li J, Fan YW, Liu XR, Zhang B, *et al.* Alteration on phenolic acids and the appearance of lotus (*Nelumbo nucifera Gaertn*) seeds dealt with antistaling agents during storage. Int J Food Prop 2018; 21(1): 1481-94.
[http://dx.doi.org/10.1080/10942912.2018.1489834]

[68]   Fattahifar E, Barzegar M, Gavlighi HA, Sahari M. Evaluation of the inhibitory effect of pistachio (*Pistacia vera* L.) green hull aqueous extract on mushroom tyrosinase activity and its application as a button mushroom postharvest anti-browning agent. Postharvest Biol Technol 2018; 145: 157-65.
[http://dx.doi.org/10.1016/j.postharvbio.2018.07.005]

[69]   Said S, Neves F, Griffiths A. Cinnamic acid inhibits the growth of the fungus Neurospora crassa, but is eliminated as acetophenone. Int Biodeterior Biodegradation 2004; 54(1): 1-6.
[http://dx.doi.org/10.1016/j.ibiod.2003.11.002]

[70]   Özoğlu H, Bayındırlı A. Inhibition of enzymic browning in cloudy apple juice with selected antibrowning agents. Food Control 2002; 13(4-5): 213-21.
[http://dx.doi.org/10.1016/S0956-7135(02)00011-7]

[71]   Sharma S, Rao TR. Xanthan gum based edible coating enriched with cinnamic acid prevents browning and extends the shelf-life of fresh-cut pears. Lebensm Wiss Technol 2015; 62(1): 791-800.
[http://dx.doi.org/10.1016/j.lwt.2014.11.050]

[72]   Komthong P, Igura N, Shimoda M. Effect of ascorbic acid on the odours of cloudy apple juice. Food Chem 2007; 100(4): 1342-9.
[http://dx.doi.org/10.1016/j.foodchem.2005.10.070]

[73]   Molnar-Perl I, Friedman M. Inhibition of browning by sulfur amino acids. 3. Apples and potatoes. J Agric Food Chem 1990; 38(8): 1652-6.
[http://dx.doi.org/10.1021/jf00098a006]

[74]   Sapers G, Miller R. Enzymatic browning control in potato with ascorbic acid-2-phosphates. J Food Sci 1992; 57(5): 1132-5.
[http://dx.doi.org/10.1111/j.1365-2621.1992.tb11281.x]

[75]   Lozano-De-Gonzalez PG, Barrett DM, Wrolstad RE, Durst RW. Enzymatic browning inhibited in fresh and dried apple rings by pineapple juice. J Food Sci 1993; 58(2): 399-404.

[http://dx.doi.org/10.1111/j.1365-2621.1993.tb04284.x]

[76]  Tan T, Cheng L, Bhat R, Rusul G, Easa A. Effectiveness of ascorbic acid and sodium metabisulfite as anti-browning agent and antioxidant on green coconut water (Cocos nucifera) subjected to elevated thermal processing. Int Food Res J 2015; 22(2): 631.

[77]  Dong X, Zhu Q, Dai Y, *et al.* Encapsulation artocarpanone and ascorbic acid in O/W microemulsions: Preparation, characterization, and antibrowning effects in apple juice. Food Chem 2016; 192: 1033-40.
[http://dx.doi.org/10.1016/j.foodchem.2015.07.124] [PMID: 26304444]

[78]  Saba MK, Sogvar OB. Combination of carboxymethyl cellulose-based coatings with calcium and ascorbic acid impacts in browning and quality of fresh-cut apples. Lebensm Wiss Technol 2016; 66: 165-71.
[http://dx.doi.org/10.1016/j.lwt.2015.10.022]

[79]  Iyengar R, McEvily AJ. Anti-browning agents: alternatives to the use of sulfites in foods. Trends Food Sci Technol 1992; 3: 60-4.
[http://dx.doi.org/10.1016/0924-2244(92)90131-F]

[80]  Friedman M. Chemistry, biochemistry, and dietary role of potato polyphenols. A review. J Agric Food Chem 1997; 45(5): 1523-40.
[http://dx.doi.org/10.1021/jf960900s]

[81]  Lim WY, Wong CW. Inhibitory effect of chemical and natural anti-browning agents on polyphenol oxidase from ginger (*Zingiber officinale* Roscoe). J Food Sci Technol 2018; 55(8): 3001-7.
[http://dx.doi.org/10.1007/s13197-018-3218-7] [PMID: 30065409]

[82]  Nirmal NP, Benjakul S, Ahmad M, Arfat YA, Panichayupakaranant P. Undesirable enzymatic browning in crustaceans: causative effects and its inhibition by phenolic compounds. Crit Rev Food Sci Nutr 2015; 55(14): 1992-2003.
[http://dx.doi.org/10.1080/10408398.2012.755148] [PMID: 25584522]

[83]  Buta JG, Moline HE, Spaulding DW, Wang CY. Extending storage life of fresh-cut apples using natural products and their derivatives. J Agric Food Chem 1999; 47(1): 1-6.
[http://dx.doi.org/10.1021/jf980712x] [PMID: 10563838]

[84]  Jiang Y, Fu J. Inhibition of polyphenol oxidase and the browning control of litchi fruit by glutathione and citric acid. Food Chem 1998; 62(1): 49-52.
[http://dx.doi.org/10.1016/S0308-8146(97)00144-1]

[85]  Nicolas JJ, Richard-Forget FC, Goupy PM, Amiot MJ, Aubert SY. Enzymatic browning reactions in apple and apple products. Crit Rev Food Sci Nutr 1994; 34(2): 109-57.
[http://dx.doi.org/10.1080/10408399409527653] [PMID: 8011143]

[86]  Richard-Forget FC, Goupy PM, Nicolas JJ. Cysteine as an inhibitor of enzymic browning. 2. Kinetic studies. J Agric Food Chem 1992; 40(11): 2108-13.
[http://dx.doi.org/10.1021/jf00023a014]

[87]  Pace B, Capotorto I, Ventura M, Cefola M. Evaluation of L-cysteine as anti-browning agent in fresh-cut lettuce processing. J Food Process Preserv 2015; 39(6): 985-93.
[http://dx.doi.org/10.1111/jfpp.12312]

[88]  Fan X, Sokorai K, Phillips J. Development of antibrowning and antimicrobial formulations to minimize *Listeria monocytogenes* contamination and inhibit browning of fresh-cut "Granny Smith" apples. Postharvest Biol Technol 2018; 143: 43-9.
[http://dx.doi.org/10.1016/j.postharvbio.2018.04.009]

[89]  Favre LC, Dos Santos C, López-Fernández MP, Mazzobre MF, Buera MDP. Optimization of β-cyclodextrin-based extraction of antioxidant and anti-browning activities from thyme leaves by response surface methodology. Food Chem 2018; 265: 86-95.
[http://dx.doi.org/10.1016/j.foodchem.2018.05.078] [PMID: 29884399]

[90]  Billaud C, Regaudie E, Fayad N, Richard-Forget F, Nicolas J. Effect of cyclodextrins on polyphenol

oxidation catalyzed by apple polyphenol oxidase 1995.
[http://dx.doi.org/10.1021/bk-1995-0600.ch023]

[91] Sapers G, El-Atawy Y, Hicks K, Garzarella L. Effect of emulsifying agents on inhibition of enzymatic browning in apple juice by ascorbyl palmitate, laurate and decanoate. J Food Sci 1989; 54(4): 1096-7.
[http://dx.doi.org/10.1111/j.1365-2621.1989.tb07958.x]

[92] He J, Guo F, Lin L, Chen H, Chen J, Cheng Y, *et al.* Investigating the oxyresveratrol β-cyclodextrin and 2-hydroxypropyl-β-cyclodextrin complexes: The effects on oxyresveratrol solution, stability, and antibrowning ability on fresh grape juice. LWT 2019; 100: 263-70.
[http://dx.doi.org/10.1016/j.lwt.2018.10.067]

[93] Singh V, Jadhav SB, Singhal RS. Interaction of polyphenol oxidase of Solanum tuberosum with β-cyclodextrin: Process details and applications. Int J Biol Macromol 2015; 80: 469-74.
[http://dx.doi.org/10.1016/j.ijbiomac.2015.07.010] [PMID: 26187193]

[94] Volpe S, Torrieri E, Cavella S. Use of chitosan and chitosan-caseinate coating to prolong shelf life of minimally processed apples. Ital J Food Sci 2018; •••: 30-5.

[95] Zhang J, Zhao P, Liu B, Meng X. Use of Oligochitosan as an Inhibiting Agent of Apple Juice Enzymatic Browning. J Food Process Preserv 2017; 41(4)e13062
[http://dx.doi.org/10.1111/jfpp.13062]

[96] Lee SY, Baek N, Nam TG. Natural, semisynthetic and synthetic tyrosinase inhibitors. J Enzyme Inhib Med Chem 2016; 31(1): 1-13.
[http://dx.doi.org/10.3109/14756366.2015.1004058] [PMID: 25683082]

[97] Brown JW, Green JK. Antibrowning compositions. Google Patents 2015.

[98] Ortiz-Ruiz CV, Berna J, Rodriguez-Lopez JN, Tomas V, Garcia-Canovas F. Tyrosinase-catalyzed hydroxylation of 4-hexylresorcinol, an antibrowning and depigmenting agent: a kinetic study. J Agric Food Chem 2015; 63(31): 7032-40.
[http://dx.doi.org/10.1021/acs.jafc.5b02523] [PMID: 26176355]

[99] McEvily AJ, Iyengar R, Otwell S. Sulfite alternative prevents shrimp melanosis. Food Technol 1991.

[100] Krasnova I, Seglina D, Pole V. The effect of pre-treatment methods on the quality of dehydrated candied Japanese quince fruits during storage. J Food Sci Technol 2018; 55(11): 4468-76.
[http://dx.doi.org/10.1007/s13197-018-3375-8] [PMID: 30333643]

[101] Singh D, Ahmed N, Pal A, Kumar R, Mirza A. Effect of anti browning agents and slice thickness on drying and quality of apple slices var. Red Chief. J Appl Hortic 2015; 17(1)

[102] Vamos-Vigyazo L. Prevention of enzymatic browning in fruits and vegetables: Rev Principles Practice. 1995.

[103] Gardner J, Manohar S, Borisenok WS. Method and composition for preserving fresh peeled fruits and vegetables. Google Patents 1991.

[104] Dodd J. Method for the prevention of the discoloration of fruit. Google Patents 2014.

[105] Moon KM, Lee B, Cho WK, Lee BS, Kim CY, Ma JY. Swertiajaponin as an anti-browning and antioxidant flavonoid. Food Chem 2018; 252: 207-14.
[http://dx.doi.org/10.1016/j.foodchem.2018.01.053] [PMID: 29478533]

[106] Liu X, Lu Y, Yang Q, Yang H, Li Y, Zhou B, *et al.* Cod peptides inhibit browning in fresh-cut potato slices: A potential anti-browning agent of random peptides for regulating food properties. Postharvest Biol Technol 2018; 146: 36-42.
[http://dx.doi.org/10.1016/j.postharvbio.2018.08.001]

[107] Mayer A, Harel E. Phenoloxidases and their significance in fruit and vegetables. Food Enzymol 1991; 1: 373-98.

[108] Yi L, Van Boekel M, Lakemond C. Extracting Tenebrio molitor protein while preventing browning:

effect of pH and NaCl on protein yield. J Insects Food Feed 2017; 3(1): 21-31.
[http://dx.doi.org/10.3920/JIFF2016.0015]

[109]  Wen B, Wu X, Boon-Ek Y, Xu L, Pan H, Xu P, *et al.* Effect of honey and calcium dips on quality of fresh-cut nectarine (*Prunus persica L. Batsch*). Agric Nat Resour (Bangk) 2018; 52(2): 140-5.
[http://dx.doi.org/10.1016/j.anres.2018.06.015]

[110]  Rosen JC, Kader AA. Postharvest physiology and quality maintenance of sliced pear and strawberry fruits. J Food Sci 1989; 54(3): 656-9.
[http://dx.doi.org/10.1111/j.1365-2621.1989.tb04675.x]

[111]  Gonçalves S, Moreira E, Grosso C, Andrade PB, Valentão P, Romano A. Phenolic profile, antioxidant activity and enzyme inhibitory activities of extracts from aromatic plants used in Mediterranean diet. J Food Sci Technol 2017; 54(1): 219-27.
[http://dx.doi.org/10.1007/s13197-016-2453-z] [PMID: 28242919]

[112]  Nooshkam M, Varidi M, Bashash M. The Maillard reaction products as food-born antioxidant and antibrowning agents in model and real food systems. Food Chem 2019; 275: 644-60.
[http://dx.doi.org/10.1016/j.foodchem.2018.09.083] [PMID: 30724245]

[113]  Corbo MR, Bevilacqua A, Campaniello D, D'Amato D, Speranza B, Sinigaglia M. Prolonging microbial shelf life of foods through the use of natural compounds and non-thermal approaches–a review. Int J Food Sci Technol 2009; 44(2): 223-41.
[http://dx.doi.org/10.1111/j.1365-2621.2008.01883.x]

[114]  Park W, Lee D, Cho S, Eds. Effect of grapefruit seed extract and antibrowning agents on the keeping quality of minimally processed vegetables. Int Symposium Vegetable Quality Fresh Fermented Vegetables. 483.

[115]  Kim M-J, Kim CY, Park I. Prevention of enzymatic browning of pear by onion extract. Food Chem 2005; 89(2): 181-4.
[http://dx.doi.org/10.1016/j.foodchem.2004.02.018]

[116]  Theerakulkait C, Boonsiripiphat K. Effect of rice bran extract on browning and polyphenol oxidase activity in vegetable and fruit. Kasetsart J 2007; 41: 272-8. [Nat Sci].

[117]  Xiao C, Zhu L, Luo W, Song X, Deng Y. Combined action of pure oxygen pretreatment and chitosan coating incorporated with rosemary extracts on the quality of fresh-cut pears. Food Chem 2010; 121(4): 1003-9.
[http://dx.doi.org/10.1016/j.foodchem.2010.01.038]

[118]  Jeon M, Zhao Y. Honey in combination with vacuum impregnation to prevent enzymatic browning of fresh-cut apples. Int J Food Sci Nutr 2005; 56(3): 165-76.
[http://dx.doi.org/10.1080/09637480500131053] [PMID: 16009631]

[119]  Krasnova I, Dukaļska L, Segliņa D, Mišina I, Kārkliņa D. Influence of anti-browning inhibitors and biodegradable packaging on the quality of fresh-cut pears.
[http://dx.doi.org/10.2478/prolas-2013-0026]

[120]  Perera N, Gamage T, Wakeling L, Gamlath G, Versteeg C. Colour and texture of apples high pressure processed in pineapple juice. Innov Food Sci Emerg Technol 2010; 11(1): 39-46.
[http://dx.doi.org/10.1016/j.ifset.2009.08.003]

[121]  Son S, Moon K, Lee C. Rhubarb juice as a natural antibrowning agent. J Food Sci 2000; 65(8): 1288-9.
[http://dx.doi.org/10.1111/j.1365-2621.2000.tb10598.x]

[122]  Yi J, Kebede B, Kristiani K, Grauwet T, Van Loey A, Hendrickx M. Minimizing quality changes of cloudy apple juice: The use of kiwifruit puree and high pressure homogenization. Food Chem 2018; 249: 202-12.
[http://dx.doi.org/10.1016/j.foodchem.2017.12.088] [PMID: 29407925]

[123]  Chen L, Mehta A, Berenbaum M, Zangerl AR, Engeseth NJ. Honeys from different floral sources as

inhibitors of enzymatic browning in fruit and vegetable homogenates. J Agric Food Chem 2000; 48(10): 4997-5000.
[http://dx.doi.org/10.1021/jf000373j] [PMID: 11052768]

[124]   Oszmianski J, Lee CY. Inhibition of polyphenol oxidase activity and browning by honey. J Agric Food Chem 1990; 38(10): 1892-5.
[http://dx.doi.org/10.1021/jf00100a002]

[125]   Inam-ur-Raheem M, Saeed M, Aslam HKW, Shakeel A, Raza MS, Afzal F. Effect of various minimal processing treatments on quality characteristics and nutritional value of spinach. National Institute of Food Science and Technology University of Agriculture Faisalabad 2015; 3(2-3): 76-83.

[126]   Langdon T. Preventing of browning in fresh prepared potatoes without the use of sulfiting agents. Food Technol 1987.

[127]   Santerre CR, Cash J, Vannorman D. Ascorbic acid/citric acid combinations in the processing of frozen apple slices. J Food Sci 1988; 53(6): 1713-6.
[http://dx.doi.org/10.1111/j.1365-2621.1988.tb07823.x]

[128]   Pizzocaro F, Torreggiani D, Gilardi G. Inhibition of apple polyphenoloxidase (PPO) by ascorbic acid, citric acid and sodium chloride. J Food Process Preserv 1993; 17(1): 21-30.
[http://dx.doi.org/10.1111/j.1745-4549.1993.tb00223.x]

[129]   Mattila M, Ahvenainen R, Hurme E. Prevention of browning of pre-peeled potato.

[130]   Fukusawa R, Wakabayashi H, Natori T. Inhibitor of tyrosinases in foods 1982. Japanese Patent.57-40875

[131]   Ierna A, Rizzarelli P, Malvuccio A, Rapisarda M. Effect of different anti-browning agents on quality of minimally processed early potatoes packaged on a compostable film. Lebensm Wiss Technol 2017; 85: 434-9.
[http://dx.doi.org/10.1016/j.lwt.2017.03.043]

[132]   Gao J, Luo Y, Turner E, Zhu Y. Mild concentration of ethanol in combination with ascorbic acid inhibits browning and maintains quality of fresh-cut lotus root. Postharvest Biol Technol 2017; 128: 169-77.
[http://dx.doi.org/10.1016/j.postharvbio.2016.12.002]

# CHAPTER 4

# Antioxidant Food Additives

**Ilias Marmouzi**[1,*], **Shahira M. Ezzat**[2,3], **Mourad Kharbach**[1,4] **and Abdelhakim Bouyahya**[5]

[1] *Biopharmaceutical and Toxicological Analysis Research Team, Laboratory of Pharmacology and Toxicology, Faculty of Medicine and Pharmacy, University Mohammed V-Rabat, Morocco*

[2] *Pharmacognosy Department, Faculty of Pharmacy, Cairo University, Kasr El-Ainy Street, Cairo11562, Egypt*

[3] *Department of Pharmacognosy, Faculty of Pharmacy, October University for Modern Science and Arts (MSA), 6thOctober, 12566 Egypt*

[4] *Department of Analytical Chemistry, Applied Chemometrics and Molecular Modelling, CePhaR, Vrije Universiteit Brussel (VUB), Laarbeeklaan 103, B-1090Brussels, Belgium*

[5] *Laboratory of Human Pathology Biology, Faculty of Sciences, Department of Biology, Genomic Center of Human Pathology, Mohammed V University in Rabat, Morocco*

**Abstract:** Food additives, especially antioxidant preservatives, are key elements in the food industry and production. Food antioxidants can be natural products such as extracts and purified natural metabolites, or synthetic compounds. They act as radical scavengers, chelators, quenchers, or antioxidant regenerators. Generally, food antioxidants target the preservation of food without altering its taste and colour. Synthetic antioxidants are cheap, easy to use and efficient as preservative agents; however, consumers tend to seek natural antioxidants. This chapter focuses on the different functional antioxidants such as polyphenols, tocopherols that can be used as food additives. These compounds are characterized by different chemical structures and different mechanisms of actions.

**Keywords:** Food additives, Natural antioxidants, Oxidation, Preservatives, Synthetic antioxidants.

## INTRODUCTION

The use of food additives is an ancestral practice. For instance, improving the taste by using smoked meat and submerging it into saltwater is an old preservative knowledge. Adding spices for flavoring and the role of sugar in storage is a significant advancement in the field of food additives. Food additives are defined

---

* **Corresponding author Ilias Marmouzi:** Biopharmaceutical and Toxicological Analysis Research Team, Laboratory of Pharmacology and Toxicology, Faculty of Medicine and Pharmacy, University Mohammed V-Rabat, Morocco

**Seyed Mohammad Nabavi** *et al.* **(Eds.)**

as any substance intended to affect or may reasonably be expected to affect the characteristics of any food [1]. According to the FDA, they include substances used in the production, processing, treatment, packaging, transportation or storage [2]. They are acquainted with foodstuff to perform particular technologic functions that can vary from preserving the food, color modifying, increasing taste sweetness and performing texture changes. Antioxidants are universally recognized as dietary supplements for their potential to prevent or inhibit the peroxidation or oxidation deterioration process in food matrices. The natural antioxidant additives are widely added in many food matrices for conserving freshness and prolonging shelf-life (fishes, meats, oils, cereals, salads, sauces, cooked and fried foods and dairy products). The utilization of such compounds during the manufacturing of foodstuffs is strictly controlled [3]. The legislation, law enforcement for regulating and supervision of food additives is mainly organized by the European Food Safety Authority (EFSA), the European Union (EU), and the Food and Drug Administration of the United States of America (FDA). In addition, the JECFA (Joint Food and Agriculture Organization (FAO)/World Health Organization (WHO)) Expert Committee on Food Additives, and the Codex Alimentarius are also important foundations that are concerned with safety risks, perform testing, and issue statements regarding food additives [3 - 6]. According to the EFSA, food additives could be classified into 6 groups, depending on the function they have in foodstuff. The groups are preservatives, nutritional additives, colouring agents, flavouring agents, texturizing agents, and miscellaneous agents. Each food additive is given a number, which indicates the group it belongs to, preceded by the letter "E", representing Europe. The added quantity of each additive is strictly calculated for each foodstuff, so the overall daily consumption by an individual does not exceed the Admissible Daily Intake (ADI), which is the cumulative amount of a specific additive consumed everyday does not have any hazardous effect on health [7 - 9]. Preservatives are one of the most important groups of additives, their E numbers range from E200 to E399. They could be divided into three functional sub-groups, which are: antimicrobials, antioxidants and anti-browning agents [3]. In fact, the antioxidant food additives protect the foodstuff from being rancid, losing color, developing odours, losing texture, or any other processes that may occur in foodstuffs. The reactions that protect the food are the same ones that protect cells in biological organisms, and have a specific aim, to avoid oxidation, allowing the food to be in good condition for a longer time [7, 8]. The trend of replacing synthetic antioxidants by safer natural mixtures has been imposed by the worldwide preference of the food industry and stimulated by consumer choices regarding side effects; some of the natural antioxidants are present inherently in foods or are artificially added during processing [10]. This chapter reviews and summarizes the natural and functional antioxidant food additives approved by the international regulations.

## FOOD RANCIDITY AND AUTO-OXIDATION

Oxidation, free radical formation and scavenging reactions virtually occur in all living organisms and biological systems not only in the human body. Food does not differ from other living systems, thus it is liable to autoxidation, lipid peroxidation and other forms of oxidation. Food antioxidants have the same function as the endogenous antioxidants of the human body; they protect the food from free radicals attack, preserving its organoleptic properties, texture, nutritional value and safety. Unsaturated fatty acids, cholesterol and phospholipids are responsible for autoxidation of fats through lipid peroxidation which can either be mediated by the lipoxidase enzyme or spontaneously [11 - 13]. This process adversely affects the organoleptic properties producing the rancid taste in food, reducing colour, changing food texture, thus decreasing the nutritional value and forming toxic end products, alkynes, epoxides, ketones and malondialdehydes [14 - 16]. Fish usually has a high content of unsaturated fatty acids and metals in their flesh and skin; absorbed from the surrounding aquatic systems thus it is highly susceptible to autoxidation of its fats. Regarding vegetables, dried fruits and vegetable oils are the most liable to destruction by homolytic removal of β carbon-carbon bonds, or the formation of alkanes or alcohols. Cysteine, methionine, lysine, arginine, histidine, tryptophan, valine, serine and proline are the most susceptible amino acids to damages coming from metal-ion interactions, photochemical reactions and carbonyl groups causing protein autoxidation [17, 18].

Lipid oxidation is a major concern for the food industry because as it produces rancid taste and odors, decreases the shelf life, alters texture and colour and decreases the nutritional values of high-lipid content foods [19]. Lipid oxidation is a matter of many factors such as temperature, oxygen, metal catalysts however it can be delayed or even prevented by the action of antioxidant compounds [20]. Generally, food emulsions are excellent models of food products that deteriorate rapidly by lipid oxidation reactions. There is a growing interest these days in oil-in-water emulsions as they constitute the basis of many innovative food products and their properties determine the quality of the obtained final product [21]. Therefore, it is necessary to understand the endogenous and exogenous factors which regulate the oxidative degradation of oil-in-water food emulsion and control lipid oxidation mechanisms during the formulation, production and storage of relevant products [22].

## MECHANISMS OF ANTIOXIDANT ACTIVITY

Natural antioxidants isolated from herbs, spices and vegetables are used to hinder the rancidity caused by the oxidation of unsaturated fats [23]. Natural antioxidants could be grouped as vitamins (ascorbic acid and tocopherols), carotenoids (xanthophylls and carotenes), flavonoids and phenolic acids. Antioxidant molecules exert their activity by various mechanisms [24]: (*i*) Free radical quencher; (*ii*) Singlet oxygen scavengers; (*iii*) Chelation of metal ions that catalyze the oxidative reactions. Tocopherols, are among the first identified antioxidants, which were used to prevent lipid oxidation as well as the oxidative destruction of carotenes due to their chain breaking activity. They scavenge peroxyl radical and hinder the fatty acid oxidation chain reactions [25]. Carotenoids (xanthophylls and carotenes) are $C_{40}$-terpenoids and act as fat-soluble antioxidants formed by isoprene as the building unit. Moreover, they inhibit lipid oxidation by quenching singlet oxygen ($^1O_2$) or reacting with free radicals [26].

Ascorbic acid (vitamin C) is one of the most important antioxidants [27]. Ascorbic acid acts as a radical chain terminator through the transformation of non-toxic and non-radical products [28]. Being a mildly electronegative compound, ascorbic acid has the ability to donate electrons to a wide variety of substrates such as superoxide radical anion, hydrogen peroxide, hydroxyl radical, singlet oxygen and reactive nitrogen oxide [11, 28]. Chelators function as antioxidants through the obstruction of the activity of catalytic metals, accordingly they prevent the initial oxidation step which is the production of reactive species such as oxygen, lipid, or protein radicals. Metal chelators used in food are selected on the basis of their ability to maintain minerals in a bioavailable form and to eliminate any chance for internal or external metals to participate in redox reactions. This second function is of primary concern from the antioxidant point of view [29]. The most important character of the food chelators is the presence of *O*-containing ligands, which tend to stabilize iron and copper in their oxidized or noncatalytic form [30]. While the N-containing ligands tend to stabilize them in their more active reduced state [30]. Reducing systems usually exist in association with many of these biomolecules, assuring that the metal centres can be returned to their reduced state, thus maintaining their biological function [31]. Ethylenediaminetetraacetic acid (EDTA) is an amino-carboxylic acid-type chelator. Calcium disodium EDTA is allowed as a food additive by the European Union (EU), United States (US), and World Health Organization (WHO); the sodium salt, disodium EDTA, is allowed by the US and WHO but cannot be used in the EU [32, 33].

## NATURAL AND SYNTHETIC ANTIOXIDANTS

Natural antioxidants are extracted from plants, spices and food and can mainly be classified into five groups (radical scavengers, chelators, quenchers, oxygen scavengers, and antioxidant regenerators). Generally, natural and synthetic antioxidants used as food additives are classified into different functional groups Fig. (**1**); the most important classes are ascorbates, tocopherols, gallates, erythorbates, butylates, lactates, citrates and tartrates, tartrates, phosphates, malates, adipates, succinic acid, ethylene diamine tetra-acetic acid (EDTA) and rosemary extracts. Table **1** shows a list of authorized and official natural antioxidant food additives [34].

## PLANT EXTRACTS AND POLYPHENOLIC COMPOUNDS

The phenolic natural extracts have been used and incorporated as natural preservatives in many food matrices such as dairy, fish and meat products to avoid rancidity, spoilage, and bacterial infection [7, 35]. The most important used extracts are those from rosemary (*Rosmarinus officinalis L.*), salvia (*Salvia officinalis L.*), oregano (*Origanum vulgare L.*) and green tea. The rosemary phenolic extracts are rich in carnosic and rosmarinic acids and carnosol. They are approved as food antioxidants and are included in the European list of food additives, with the code number (E392) following specific criteria described in the European Union directives 2010/67/EU and 2010/69/EU repealed in 2013 by EU regulation 231/2012 and 1333/2008 [3, 36, 37]. Rosemary and also its active metabolites are mainly used for oils, fats, sauces, bakery wares, meat and fish among others [3, 38, 39]. Especially to avoid lipid oxidation in meat products [40], cooked turkey products [41], chicken frankfurters [42], sausage [43] and others [44]. In addition to that, salvia extract, which is rich in carnosic acid, carnosol and rosmarinic acid, presents a higher antioxidant power compared to rosemary phenolic extract; and can be used as an additive in vegetable oils, meat, chicken fat, and fried foods [16, 36]. On the other hand, oregano extract is relatively similar to rosemary and sage chemical composition, with rosmarinic and carnosic acids and carnosol as main compounds. Oregano possesses lower antioxidant capacity compared to salvia and rosemary extracts, however it is rich in apigenin and dihydroquercetin [3, 16, 36]. Oregano is an effective food additive in meat products [36]. Additionally, green tea antioxidants are applied to protect and improve the shelf-life of various food products such as pork sausage [45], sausages and fish [46, 47], extra virgin olive oil [48], apple products [49], rice starch products, and biscuits [50]. In fact, green tea catechins demonstrated higher antioxidant properties in diverse food products such as bread [51], meat, poultry and fish [52, 53]. Also, grape seed extracts have shown a considerable antioxidant and antimicrobial potential [52]. It has the ability to protect the raw or cooked meat and poultry products from the rancidity and undesirable flavours [44, 52]. Other extracts of interest include plums, cranberries, pomegranate and bearberry fruits [44, 54]. Among those extracts, only the rosemary extract is approved by EU legislation.

Polyphenolic compounds are one of the major groups of natural antioxidants. They are plant's secondary metabolites and can be divided into: flavonoids and non-flavonoids molecules. The flavonoids group is constituted by six subclasses: flavones, flavonols, chalcones, flavanones, isoflavones, flavanonols, flavanols and anthocyanins. The non-flavonoids group is divided as follows: isoflavonoids, lignans, stilbenoids, tannins, curcuminoids, coumarins, phenolic acids and hydroxycinnamic acids [55]. The use of polyphenolics as natural preservatives aims to extend food shelf life, organoleptic and nutritional characteristics respecting the consumer's prospects [55, 56]. Phenolics can be added to food as plant extract (mixture) or purified individual compounds. Natural polyphenolic that are used as antioxidants food additives, include phenolic acids (*e.g.* rosmarinic and carnosic acid), hydroxycinnamic acids (*e.g.* ferulic and chlorogenic acids), hydroxybenzoic acids (*e.g.* vanillic acid), flavonoids (*e.g.* quercetin, catechin and rutin), tannins (*e.g.* procyanidin, ellagic and tannic acids), coumarins (*e.g.* o-coumarine), anthocyanins (E163) (*e.g.* delphinidin), lignans (*e.g.* sesaminol), and stilbenes (*e.g.* resveratrol) [36, 55, 57 - 59].

Table 1. List of some natural food antioxidants. For some of these EFSA emitted a scientific opinion.

| Name | Molecular Formula | Source | Official Document |
|---|---|---|---|
| Rosmarinic acid | $C_{18}H_{16}O_8$ | *Ocimum basilicum, Rosmarinus officinalis* | [60] |
| Carnosic acid | $C_{20}H_{28}O_4$ | *Salvia officinalis, Rosmarinus officinalis* | |
| Ferulic acid | $C_{10}H_{10}O_4$ | *Angelica sinensis, Cimicifuga heracleifolia* | |
| Chlorogenic acid | $C_{16}H_{18}O_9$ | *Hibiscus sabdariffa* | |
| Vanillic acid | $C_8H_8O_4$ | *Angelica sinensis, Euterpe oleracea* | |
| Anthocyanins | - | Vaccinium species (Grape skin extract) | [61] |
| Quercetin | $C_{15}H_{10}O_7$ | *Capparis spinosa* | |
| Catechin | $C_{15}H_{14}O_6$ | Green tea, *Uncaria rhynchophylla* | |
| Rutin | $C_{27}H_{30}O_{16}$ | *Carpobrotus edulis*, citrus fruits, berries and apples | [62] |
| Procyanidin | $C_{30}H_{26}O_{13}$ | *Vitis vinifera, Euterpe oleracea* | |
| Tannic acid | $C_{76}H_{52}O_{46}$ | *Caesalpinia spinosa, Rhus semialata* | [63] |
| Tocopherol mixed | - | Vegetable oils (soybean and corn) | [64] |
| α-tocopherol | $C_{29}H_{50}O_2$ | | |
| γ-tocopherol | $C_{29}H_{50}O_2$ | | |
| δ-tocopherol | $C_{27}H_{50}O_2$ | | |
| Ascorbic acid | $C_6H_8O_6$ | Citrus fruits, broccoli | [65] |
| Carotenoids mixed | - | | |

*(Table 1) cont.....*

| Name | Molecular Formula | Source | Official Document |
|------|-------------------|--------|-------------------|
| α-carotene | $C_{40}H_{56}$ | Carrots, sweet potatoes, pumpkin | |
| β-carotene | $C_{40}H_{56}$ | Cantaloupe, carrots, mangoes, pumpkin, | |
| Lycopene | $C_{40}H_{56}$ | Tomatoes, carrots, watermelons, gac fruit | [66] |
| Annatto | $C_{24}H_{28}O_4$ | *Bixa orellana* | [67] |
| Lutein | $C_{40}H_{56}O_2$ | Spinach, kale and yellow carrots | [68] |
| Astaxanthin | $C_{40}H_{52}O_4$ | *Haematococcus pluvialis* | [69] |

## Tocopherols

Tocopherols (tocopherols and tocotrienols) (or vitamins E) are natural compounds formed from a series of benzopyranols. From a biochemical point of view, the two groups of molecules are formed of 20 carbon atoms attached to a benzene ring. However, the C16 side chain of tocopherols is saturated, while that of tocotrienols contains three trans double bonds [3, 64]. The four main constituents of both classes are called α-5,7,8-trimethyl (α-tocopherol or E3017), β-5,8-dimethyl (β-tocopherol), γ-7,8-dimethyl (γ-tocopherol or E308) and δ-8-methyl (δ-tocopherol or E309) (Table **1**). They are massively present in oils and plant tissues. This group occurs naturally in many foods (vegetable fats and nuts); α-tocopherol is mainly present in almonds, canola oil, sunflower seeds, and safflower oil, whereas γ -tocopherol is mainly found in some vegetable oils such as argan, canola, soybean, peanuts, walnuts, and pecans. Vitamin E or tocopherols extracted from deodorized vegetable oils are largely added as mixed adjuncts in foods. Tocopherols have potent antioxidant activity especially lipophilic antioxidant effects [64]. This antioxidant activity of tocopherols can be potentiated in the case of synergies with other compounds such as ascorbic acid and carotenoids [70]. However, some studies have shown that the use of tocopherols in the presence of rosmarinic acid or caffeic acid can have an antagonist effect that can lower their activities [8, 39, 71, 72]. The *in vitro* and *in vivo* antioxidant activity of tocopherols in various biological systems such as foods, cosmetics and pharmaceutical preparations are certainly due to their lipophilic nature. Indeed, these compounds by their ability to be located in membranes, they can interact rapidly with lipid hydroperoxides [64]. This reaction proceeds non-enzymatically to trap lipid peroxide radicals (radical species that propagate lipid peroxidation) [70].

## Ascorbates

Ascorbates are a group of natural antioxidants widely used in the food industry. This group is essentially composed of four main molecules: ascorbic acid (E300), sodium ascorbates (E301), calcium ascorbates (E302) and ascorbyl palmitate (E304) (Table 1). Among these four molecules, the plant products are very rich in ascorbic acid compared to ascorbates [3]. From a structural point of view, ascorbic acid (vitamin C) is an organic molecule whose structure is a cyclic ester with the presence of a ketone in the α-position. This molecule is known for its powerful antioxidant properties *in vivo* and *in vitro*. The antioxidant effect generated by ascorbic acid is due to the ability of this molecule to give two electrons to the molecules that surround it; in this case, the molecule becomes in an oxidized form called dehydro-ascorbic acid [65]. Ascorbic acid currently used as a standard antioxidant in humans to neutralize the free radicals and prevent oxidation at both cellular and molecular levels. However, this molecule is also widely used as a food additive registered under the code E300. Indeed, it has been shown for a long time to protect the oxidation of the food and therefore prevent their deterioration [38]. In addition, the use of ascorbic acid is often combined with other synthetic antioxidants such as butylated hydroxytoluene (BHT) and butylated hydroxyanisole (BHA) to increase their antioxidant capacity [65]. In addition, a combination of ascorbic acid and other natural compounds such as tocopherols has now shown some interesting results [16].

Sodium ascorbate (E301) is the sodium salt of vitamin C, known by its formulation 3-oxo-L-gulofuranolactone sodium enolate (Table 2). It is a molecule chemically synthesized from vitamin C, which has important antioxidant properties. In the food industry, sodium ascorbate is used in dry fermented products to prevent proteins and lipids oxidation. However, this molecule has recently shown to be implicated in pro-oxidant effects that have limited their use in food preservation [73]. Calcium ascorbate (E302) or the salt of ascorbic acid and calcium is a chemically synthesized molecule belonging to the ascorbate family. Thanks to its antioxidant properties, this molecule is used as an antioxidant in dairy and cooked products. Moreover, this additive has an important application against the browning of some food products essentially apples [74]. Fatty acid esters of ascorbic acid (ascorbyl palmitate or ascorbyl stearate) constitute ascorbate E334 (formula $C_{22}H_{38}O_7$). Despite being not widely used in comparison with other ascorbates, the E334 additive has potent antioxidant activity. In the food industry, this fat-soluble compound is applied to some products such as dairy products, cereals, meats, salads and sauces [75].

## Gallates

Gallic acid or hydroxybenzoic acid is a phenolic compound that is highly reactive in medicinal plants. This molecule is endowed with remarkable biological properties essentially its powerful antioxidant abilities. There are three other molecules derived from gallic acid (propyl ester, octyl ester and dodecyl ester of gallic acid). These compounds are food additives identified as propyl gallate (E310), octyl gallate (E3111) and dodecyl gallate (E312) (Table **2**). The most well-known additive is propyl gallate, which is an ester of gallic acid with propanol. In the food industry, propyl gallate plays a very important role in lipo-peroxidation inhibition [3]. On the other hand, it can also have other effects such as the maintenance of the organoleptic properties, the aroma and the color of the food. The activity of propyl gallate can be increased if its industrial application is carried out in combination with other additives such as BHT and BHA and citric acid. However, the other two compounds (octyl gallate and dodecyl gallate) are not widely used in the food industry [76, 77]. Their major effects seem to be related to the antioxidant properties they possess [78, 79]. Indeed, octyl gallate is a powerful antioxidant and antimicrobial agent. It specifically targets Gram positive (+) bacteria. The potential application of octyl gallate in the food industry is in dehydrated milk, fats, oils, potato products and cereals [80]. Regarding dodecyl gallate, which is present mainly in green tea, it has an important antioxidant activity due to the presence of hydroxyl and carboxyl groups in its structure. It also has antibacterial effects, but they remain less important [76].

## Butylates

From butyric acid, three main food additives were derived. These are tertbutylhydroquinone (TBHQ), butylated hydroxyanisole (BHA) and butylated hydroxytoluene (BHT) (Table **2**). The TBHQ molecule (E319) has powerful antioxidant properties, which encourages their industrial use in oils, cereals and meats. In some cases, this molecule is used in combination with other additives such as citric acid, propyl gallate and BHT [81]. BHA (E320) is a synthetic phenol compound. Despite its low solubility in water, BHA is used in the industry to control the rancidity of fats especially animal ones [39, 82]. BHT (E321) is the third additive derived from butyric acid. It has a potent antioxidant effect [83] on the peroxyl radicals present in foods; transforming them into phenoxy radicals of BHA. However, butylates have showed several side effects, such as genotoxic and carcinogenesis.

**Table 2. Functional antioxidant groups.**

| Additive group | Name | E number |
|---|---|---|
| Ascorbates | Ascorbic acid | 300 |
| | Sodium ascorbate | 301 |
| | Calcium ascorbate | 302 |
| | Fatty acid esters of ascorbic acid | 304 |

*(Table 2) cont.....*

| Additive group | Name | E number |
|---|---|---|
| Tocopherols | α-Tocopherol | 307 |
| | γ-Tocopherol | 308 |
| | δ-Tocopherol | 309 |
| Gallates | Propyl gallate | 310 |
| | Octyl gallate | 311 |
| | Dodecyl gallate | 312 |
| Butylates | Tertbutyl Hydroquinone | 319 |
| | Butylated hydroxyanisole | 320 |
| | Butylated hydroxytoluene | 321 |
| Erythrobates | Erythorbic acid | 315 |
| | Sodium erythrobate | 316 |
| Citrates | Citric acid | 330 |
| | Sodium citrate | 331 |
| | Potassium citrate | 332 |
| | Calcium citrate | 333 |
| | Triammonium citrate | 380 |
| Lactates | Lactic acid | 270 |
| | Sodium lactate | 325 |
| | Potassium lactate | 326 |
| | Calcium lactate | 327 |
| Rosemary extracts | Carnosol | 392 |
| | Carnosic | |
| EDTA | Calcium-dinatrium-EDTA | 385 |
| Succinic acid | Succinic acid | 363 |
| Adipates | Adipic acid | 355 |
| | Sodium adipate | 356 |
| | Potassium adipate | 357 |
| Malates | Sodium malate | 350 |
| | Potassium malate | 351 |
| | Calcium malate | 352 |

*(Table 2) cont.....*

| Additive group | Name | E number |
|---|---|---|
| Phosphates | Phosphoric acid | 338 |
| | Sodium phosphate | 339 |
| | Potassium phosphate | 340 |
| | Calcium phosphate | 341 |
| | Ammonium phosphate | 342 |
| | Magnesium phosphate | 343 |
| Tartrates | Tartrate acid | 334 |
| | Sodium tartrate | 335 |
| | Potassium tartrate | 336 |
| | Sodium-potassium tartrate | 337 |
| | Metatartaric acid | 353 |
| | Calcium tartrate | 354 |

## Other Functional Groups

The erythorbic acid or isoascorbic acid does not exist in nature; however, it is easily synthesized [85]. It is an organic molecule of the formula C6H8O6, and a stereoisomer of ascorbic acid. The erythorbate subgroup consists of two compounds, erythorbic acid (E315) and sodium erythorbate (E316) (Table **2**). The use of erythorbic acid in the food industry is often done in another form called sodium erythorbate (E316) [86]. The latter is used especially in frozen fruits, dried meat, vegetable oils and fats [85]. The industrial application of sodium erythorbate lies in its important antioxidant properties [67]. Another group is the lactates; which include organic molecules derived from lactic acid (E270). Among them, three are widely used in the food industry namely sodium lactate (E325), potassium lactate (E326) and lactate of calcium (E327) (Table **2**). Lactic acid is used in the preservation of vegetables, meat and dairy products. It acts as an antimicrobial, antioxidant and regulator of acidity. Sodium lactate and potassium lactate have a strong antioxidant activity [87]. They are applied mainly in the conservation of meat patties and fish [3]. Furthermore, Sodium lactate is sometimes used in synergy with other molecules such as ascorbic acid and thymol [88, 89]. While potassium lactate is combined with other compounds such as sodium diacetate and calcium ascorbate [90, 91]. Finally, calcium lactate is used mainly in fruits. Their main action is antibacterial which allows the inhibition of browning of food. It is sometimes combined with phosphate to increase antioxidant capacity in processed products [84, 92, 93]. Another tonic acidizing but also chelating agent is the citric acid (E330). The inhibition of citric acid inhibit browning of food and increases the time of food preservation [3]. Its positive action is potentiating when combined with other compounds such as ascorbic acid [94, 95]. Thus, from this acid, several food additives are synthesized like sodium citrate (E331), potassium citrate (E332) and calcium citrate (E333) and tri-ammonium citrate (E380) (Table **2**). Although these additives have common effects, each compound itself has a specific application property. For example, sodium citrate can chelate ions, adjust the acidity, and reduce the microbial load in certain food products such as meat and skim milk [3]. These effects can be enhanced by the synergistic combination of sodium citrate with other organic acids such as tartaric acid, malic acid and lactic acid [96]. However, potassium citrate and calcium citrate are considered powerful emulsifying, sequestering and antioxidant agents. They are used mainly in gelatin and cheese [97].

The Tartaric acid (2,3-dihydroxybutanedioic acid) is naturally present in several plants [3]. Tartaric acid is authorized as a food additive (E334) and from which other food additives called sodium tartrate salts (E335), tartrate potassium salts (E336), sodium-potassium tartrate salts (E334), metatartaric acid (E353) and calcium tartrate salts (E354) were synthesized and authorized (Table **2**). Tartaric acid and tartrate salts are used in the food industry primarily to regulate acidity and for their antioxidant powers. They were particularly applied in chocolate, preserves, cheese, fresh pasta, fats, oils and meat [3]. Moreover, despite its use as an additive (E338), the phosphoric acid plays a major role in the genesis of kidney disease; it has been associated with urinary changes that promote kidney stones [98]. In addition, several phosphoric acid salts such as sodium phosphate (E339), potassium phosphate (E340), calcium phosphate (E341), ammonium phosphate (E342) and magnesium phosphate (E343) are present in the food industry as powerful food additives (Table **2**). These additives are mainly used as pH buffers, chelating agents, antioxidants and acidifying agents. Indeed, these molecules can have synergies with citric acid and gallates to prevent oxidation. The major food applications of these molecules are labeled with fruit gelatin, cheese and powdered yeasts [99]. However, each additive in this group has its own effect on food preservation. Indeed, sodium phosphate (E339) is particularly used in foods such as meat, milk powder, fruit and cheese for its antioxidant, antimicrobial and sequestering properties. In addition, it may have also synergistic initiation with nisin, which increases its chelating and antimicrobial effects [100]. An example of preservatives used for bread dough and powdered juices is potassium phosphate (E340). This compound is able to establish a synergistic action with sodium acetate [101]. While, calcium phosphate (E241), which is considered an acidifying, antioxidant and anti-caking agent, is used in the baking industry, in canned fruit, powdered juices and cheese [100]. However, the two food additives (ammonium phosphate: E342 and magnesium phosphate: E343) do not have important applications in the food industry; they are only occasionally applied in bread, pasta, biscuits and pancakes [102]. Malic acid which is naturally present in several plant tissues, presents different derivatives whose malic acid salts such as sodium malate (E350), potassium malate (E351) and calcium malate (E350) are food additives (Table **2**). These additives are mainly used to regulate the acidity, flavor the product and adjust the pH. In addition, they also have antimicrobial and antioxidant effects [3]. The food additive adipic acid (1,6-hexanedioic acid) is an aliphatic carboxylic diacid widely used in the synthesis of polyamides. The compound (E355) is used mainly in the food industry to acidify non-alcoholic drinks or control the acidity of cosmetics. It can also be used for its antimicrobial and antioxidant properties, as well as a pH buffer and gelling factor agent [3]. Adipic acid can bind chemically with certain mineral salts such as sodium and potassium to give adipate sodium (E356) and adipate potassium (E357) (Table **2**). The main difference between these three compounds is their solubility in water as a function of temperature. The two salts of adipic acid are used also in the preservation of certain foods such as cheese and canned fruits [97, 99].

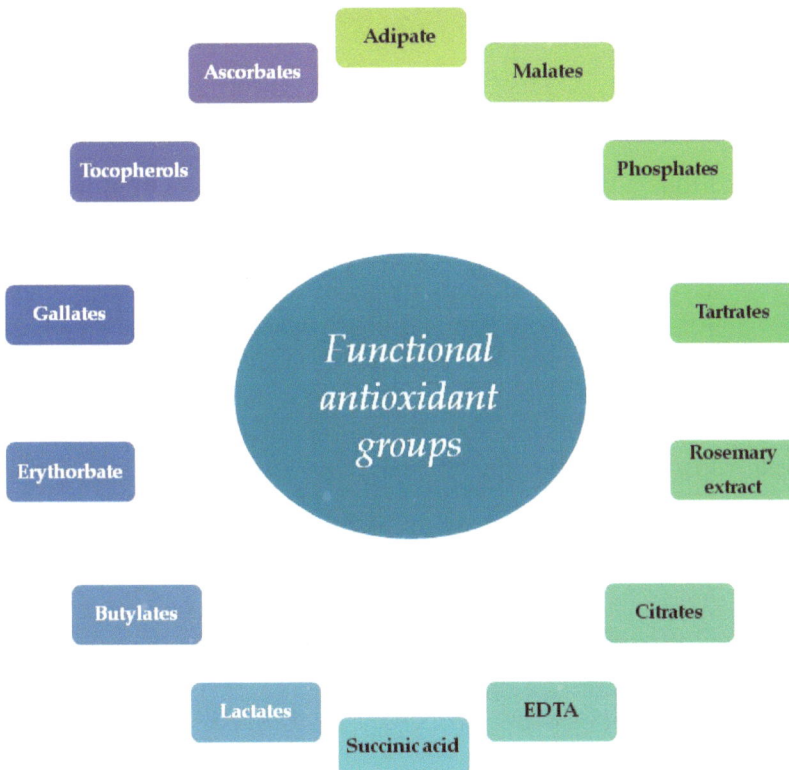

**Fig. (1).** Functional antioxidant groups.

Present in almost all living organisms, the succinic acid plays a crucial role in metabolism, essentially energy catabolism. Its synthesis is essentially from the malic or fumaric acid by the hydrogenation reaction [99]. Furthermore, this molecule has been produced as a fermentation product by biotechnology using *E. coli* as a producing strain. Succinic acid is considered a food additive (E363) because it has shown powerful antioxidant and antimicrobial properties. Its applications in foods are particularly carried out for the preservation of chicken meat, dairy products and baked goods [97, 99, 102]. Finally, the synthetic Calcium-dinatrium-EDTA is qualified as the food additive of code E385 (Table **2**). This molecule is particularly used as a sequestering and chelating of metal compounds as well as a powerful antioxidant [33]. The property of Calcium-dinatrium-EDTA can be potentiated by its combination with other compounds such as potassium ascorbate and lysosomes. This synergistic action essentially increases the antimicrobial potency of these compounds in certain food applications such as chicken meat, processed meat and fruits [16]. Moreover, the combination of calcium-dinatrium-EDTA and other antioxidants such as ascorbic acid and citric acid, BHA and BHT considerably increases the antioxidant activity of these substances especially in fresh and processed meat, fish, sauces, grains and seafood [33, 97, 102].

## CONCLUSION

Fresh consumed foods are generally free of preservatives and unprocessed. However, to prevent food deterioration between production and consumption, the vast majority of food products need necessary processing and additives. Fortunately, the large chemical variety of antioxidants, the diversity of their mechanisms of action and physicochemical characteristics are the key factors for a rationale design of food products with extended shelf life. Still one of the major issues of food additives is safety, generally related to natural based molecules or extracts. Although this perception can be erroneous, natural antioxidants are gaining interest and their application in modern formulations is increasing.

## CONSENT FOR PUBLICATION

Not applicable.

## CONFLICT OF INTEREST

The author confirms that this chapter contents have no conflict of interest.

## ACKNOWLEDGEMENTS

Declared none.

# REFERENCES

[1]   Furia TE. CRC handbook of food additives. CRC press 1973; Vol. 1.

[2]   Administration USF and D. Overview of food ingredients, additives & colors Retrieved March 2013; 21: 2013

[3]   Carocho M, Morales P, Ferreira IC F R. Antioxidants: Reviewing the chemistry, food applications, legislation and role as preservatives. Trends Food Sci Technol 2018; 71: 107-20.
[http://dx.doi.org/10.1016/j.tifs.2017.11.008]

[4]   FDA. Food additive status list. Food and Drug Admi 2006.

[5]   Meeting JFEC on FA. Organization WH Compendium of Food Additive Specifications: Addendum 8. Food & Agriculture Org 2000; Vol. 52.

[6]   (FEEDAP) EP on A and P or S used in AF. Guidance for the preparation of dossiers for technological additives. EFSA J 2012; 10(1): 2528.
[http://dx.doi.org/10.2903/j.efsa.2012.2528]

[7]   Carocho M, Barreiro MF, Morales P, Ferreira IC F R. Adding molecules to food, pros and cons: A review on synthetic and natural food additives. Compr Rev Food Sci Food Saf 2014; 13(4): 377-999.
[http://dx.doi.org/10.1111/1541-4337.12065]

[8]   Carocho M, Morales P, Ferreira IC F R. Natural food additives: Quo vadis? Trends Food Sci Technol 2015; 45(2): 284-95.
[http://dx.doi.org/10.1016/j.tifs.2015.06.007]

[9]   Carocho M, Morales P, Ferreira ICFR. Sweeteners as food additives in the XXI century: A review of what is known, and what is to come. Food Chem Toxicol 2017; 107(Pt A): 302-17.
[http://dx.doi.org/10.1016/j.fct.2017.06.046] [PMID: 28689062]

[10]  Kiokias S, Dimakou C, Oreopoulou V. Activity of natural carotenoid preparations against the autoxidative deterioration of sunflower oil-in-water emulsions. Food Chem 2009; 114(4): 1278-84.
[http://dx.doi.org/10.1016/j.foodchem.2008.10.087]

[11]  Carocho M, Ferreira IC F R. A review on antioxidants, prooxidants and related controversy: natural and synthetic compounds, screening and analysis methodologies and future perspectives. Food Chem Toxicol 2013; 51: 15-25.
[http://dx.doi.org/10.1016/j.fct.2012.09.021] [PMID: 23017782]

[12]  Liu Z. Kinetic study on the prooxidative effect of vitamin C on the autoxidation of glycerol trioleate in micelles. J Phys Org Chem 2006; 19(2): 136-42.
[http://dx.doi.org/10.1002/poc.1011]

[13]  Noguchi N, Yamashita H, Hamahara J, Nakamura A, Kühn H, Niki E. The specificity of lipoxygenase-catalyzed lipid peroxidation and the effects of radical-scavenging antioxidants. Biol Chem 2002; 383(3-4): 619-26.
[http://dx.doi.org/10.1515/BC.2002.064] [PMID: 12033451]

[14]  Ayala A, Muñoz MF, Argüelles S. Lipid peroxidation: production, metabolism, and signaling mechanisms of malondialdehyde and 4-hydroxy-2-nonenal. Oxid Med Cell Longev 2014; 2014360438
[http://dx.doi.org/10.1155/2014/360438] [PMID: 24999379]

[15]  Chen HJ, Gonzalez FJ, Shou M, Chung F-L. 2,3-epoxy-4-hydroxynonanal, a potential lipid peroxidation product for etheno adduct formation, is not a substrate of human epoxide hydrolase. Carcinogenesis 1998; 19(5): 939-43.
[http://dx.doi.org/10.1093/carcin/19.5.939] [PMID: 9635886]

[16]  Baines D, Seal R. Natural food additives, ingredients and flavourings. Elsevier 2012.
[http://dx.doi.org/10.1533/9780857095725]

[17]  Dean RT, Fu S, Stocker R, Davies MJ. Biochemistry and pathology of radical-mediated protein oxidation. Biochem J 1997; 324(Pt 1): 1-18.

[http://dx.doi.org/10.1042/bj3240001] [PMID: 9164834]

[18] Decker EA, Elias RJ, McClements DJ. Oxidation in foods and beverages and antioxidant applications: management in different industry sectors. Elsevier 2010.

[19] Alamed J, Chaiyasit W, McClements DJ, Decker EA. Relationships between free radical scavenging and antioxidant activity in foods. J Agric Food Chem 2009; 57(7): 2969-76.
[http://dx.doi.org/10.1021/jf803436c] [PMID: 19265447]

[20] Beker BY, Bakır T, Sönmezoğlu I, İmer F, Apak R. Antioxidant protective effect of flavonoids on linoleic acid peroxidation induced by copper(II)/ascorbic acid system. Chem Phys Lipids 2011; 164(8): 732-9.
[http://dx.doi.org/10.1016/j.chemphyslip.2011.09.001] [PMID: 21925488]

[21] Nikovska K. Oxidative stability and rheological properties of oil-in-water emulsions with walnut oil. Adv J Food Sci Technol 2010; 2(3): 172-7.

[22] Kiokias S, Oreopoulou V. Antioxidant properties of natural carotenoid extracts against the AAPH-initiated oxidation of food emulsions. Innov Food Sci Emerg Technol 2006; 7(1–2): 132-9.
[http://dx.doi.org/10.1016/j.ifset.2005.12.004]

[23] Anglin C, Mahon JH, Chapman RA. Antioxidant analysis, determination of antioxidants in edible fats. J Agric Food Chem 1956; 4(12): 1018-22.
[http://dx.doi.org/10.1021/jf60070a003]

[24] Shahidi F, Wanasundara PK, Wanasundara PD. Phenolic antioxidants. Crit Rev Food Sci Nutr 1992; 32(1): 67-103.
[http://dx.doi.org/10.1080/10408399209527581] [PMID: 1290586]

[25] Farhoosh R, Khodaparast MHH, Sharif A, Rafiee SA. Olive oil oxidation: rejection points in terms of polar, conjugated diene, and carbonyl values. Food Chem 2012; 131(4): 1385-90.
[http://dx.doi.org/10.1016/j.foodchem.2011.10.004]

[26] Burton GH, Ingold KU. Autoxidation of biological molecules. 1. The antioxidant activity of vitamin E and related chain reaction of unsaturated lipids. Food Chem 1981; 9: 21-5.

[27] Bielski BHJ, Richter HW, Chan PC. Some properties of the ascorbate free radical. Ann N Y Acad Sci 1975; 258(1): 231-7.
[http://dx.doi.org/10.1111/j.1749-6632.1975.tb29283.x] [PMID: 942]

[28] Davey M W. Plant L-ascorbic acid: chemistry, function, metabolism, bioavailability and effects of processing. J Sci Food Agric 2000; 80(7): 825-60.
[http://dx.doi.org/10.1002/(SICI)1097-0010(20000515)80:7<825::AID-JSFA598>3.0.CO;2-6]

[29] Decker EA. Strategies for manipulating the prooxidative/antioxidative balance of foods to maximize oxidative stability. Trends Food Sci Technol 1998; 9(6): 241-8.
[http://dx.doi.org/10.1016/S0924-2244(98)00045-4]

[30] Miller DM, Buettner GR, Aust SD. Transition metals as catalysts of "autoxidation" reactions. Free Radic Biol Med 1990; 8(1): 95-108.
[http://dx.doi.org/10.1016/0891-5849(90)90148-C] [PMID: 2182396]

[31] Page CC, Moser CC, Chen X, Dutton PL. Natural engineering principles of electron tunnelling in biological oxidation-reduction. Nature 1999; 402(6757): 47-52.
[http://dx.doi.org/10.1038/46972] [PMID: 10573417]

[32] Commission EU. Commission Regulation (EU) No 1129/2011 of 11 November 2011 amending Annex II to Regulation (EC) No 1333/2008 of the European Parliament and of the Council by establishing a Union list of food additives. Off J Eur Union L 2011; 295(4): 11-2.

[33] Shahidi F, Chandrasekara A. The use of antioxidants in the preservation of cereals and low-moisture foods.Handbook of Antioxidants for Food Preservation. Elsevier 2015; pp. 413-32.
[http://dx.doi.org/10.1016/B978-1-78242-089-7.00017-8]

[34]   EFSA Panel on Dietetic Products N and A (NDA). Scientific Opinion on the substantiation of health claims related to various food (s)/food constituent (s) and protection of cells from premature aging, antioxidant activity, antioxidant content and antioxidant properties, and protection of DNA, proteins. EFSA J 2010; 8(2): 1489.

[35]   Maqsood S, Benjakul S, Abushelaibi A, Alam A. Phenolic compounds and plant phenolic extracts as natural antioxidants in prevention of lipid oxidation in seafood: a detailed review. Compr Rev Food Sci Food Saf 2014; 13(6): 1125-40.
[http://dx.doi.org/10.1111/1541-4337.12106]

[36]   Embuscado M, Shahidi F. 2015.

[37]   Commission E. Commission Regulation (EU) No. 231/2012 of 9 March 2012 laying down specifications for food additives listed in Annexes II and III to Regulation (EC) No. 1333/2008 of the European Parliament and of the Council. Off J. Eur Union 2012; 83: 1-295.

[38]   Tai A, Iomori A, Ito H. Structural evidence for the DPPH radical-scavenging mechanism of 2-O--d-glucopyranosyl-l-ascorbic acid. Bioorg Med Chem 2017; 25(20): 5303-10.
[http://dx.doi.org/10.1016/j.bmc.2017.07.044] [PMID: 28789909]

[39]   Wang Y, Li F, Zhuang H, Chen X, Li L, Qiao W, *et al.* Effects of plant polyphenols and α-tocopherol on lipid oxidation, residual nitrites, biogenic amines, and N-nitrosamines formation during ripening and storage of dry-cured bacon. Lebensm Wiss Technol 2015; 60(1): 199-206.
[http://dx.doi.org/10.1016/j.lwt.2014.09.022]

[40]   McBride NTM, Hogan SA, Kerry JP. Comparative addition of rosemary extract and additives on sensory and antioxidant properties of retail packaged beef. Int J Food Sci Technol 2007; 42(10): 1201-7.
[http://dx.doi.org/10.1111/j.1365-2621.2006.01342.x]

[41]   Yu L, Scanlin L, Wilson J, Schmidt G. Rosemary extracts as inhibitors of lipid oxidation and color change in cooked turkey products during refrigerated storage. J Food Sci 2002; 67(2): 582-5.
[http://dx.doi.org/10.1111/j.1365-2621.2002.tb10642.x]

[42]   Rižnar K. Čelan Št, Knez Že, ŠKerget M, Bauman D, Glaser R. Antioxidant and antimicrobial activity of rosemary extract in chicken frankfurters. J Food Sci 2006; 71(7): C425-9.
[http://dx.doi.org/10.1111/j.1750-3841.2006.00130.x]

[43]   Sebranek JG, Sewalt VJH, Robbins KL, Houser TA. Comparison of a natural rosemary extract and BHA/BHT for relative antioxidant effectiveness in pork sausage. Meat Sci 2005; 69(2): 289-96.
[http://dx.doi.org/10.1016/j.meatsci.2004.07.010] [PMID: 22062821]

[44]   Karre L, Lopez K, Getty KJK. Natural antioxidants in meat and poultry products. Meat Sci 2013; 94(2): 220-7.
[http://dx.doi.org/10.1016/j.meatsci.2013.01.007] [PMID: 23501254]

[45]   Martínez L, Cilla I, Beltrán JA, Roncalés P. Antioxidant effect of rosemary, borage, green tea, pu-erh tea and ascorbic acid on fresh pork sausages packaged in a modified atmosphere: influence of the presence of sodium chloride. J Sci Food Agric 2006; 86(9): 1298-307.
[http://dx.doi.org/10.1002/jsfa.2492]

[46]   Alghazeer R, Saeed S, Howell NK. Aldehyde formation in frozen mackerel (Scomber scombrus) in the presence and absence of instant green tea. Food Chem 2008; 108(3): 801-10.
[http://dx.doi.org/10.1016/j.foodchem.2007.08.067] [PMID: 26065738]

[47]   Bozkurt H. Utilization of natural antioxidants: Green tea extract and Thymbra spicata oil in Turkish dry-fermented sausage. Meat Sci 2006; 73(3): 442-50.
[http://dx.doi.org/10.1016/j.meatsci.2006.01.005] [PMID: 22062482]

[48]   Rosenblat M, Volkova N, Coleman R, Almagor Y, Aviram M. Antiatherogenicity of extra virgin olive oil and its enrichment with green tea polyphenols in the atherosclerotic apolipoprotein-E-deficient mice: enhanced macrophage cholesterol efflux. J Nutr Biochem 2008; 19(8): 514-23.

[http://dx.doi.org/10.1016/j.jnutbio.2007.06.007] [PMID: 17904345]

[49]  Lavelli V, Vantaggi C, Corey M, Kerr W. Formulation of a dry green tea-apple product: study on antioxidant and color stability. J Food Sci 2010; 75(2): C184-90.
[http://dx.doi.org/10.1111/j.1750-3841.2009.01489.x] [PMID: 20492224]

[50]  Mildner-Szkudlarz S, Zawirska-Wojtasiak R, Obuchowski W, Gośliński M. Evaluation of antioxidant activity of green tea extract and its effect on the biscuits lipid fraction oxidative stability. J Food Sci 2009; 74(8): S362-70.
[http://dx.doi.org/10.1111/j.1750-3841.2009.01313.x] [PMID: 19799681]

[51]  Wang R, Zhou W. Stability of tea catechins in the breadmaking process. J Agric Food Chem 2004; 52(26): 8224-9.
[http://dx.doi.org/10.1021/jf048655x] [PMID: 15612821]

[52]  Perumalla AVS, Hettiarachchy NS. Green tea and grape seed extracts-Potential applications in food safety and quality. Food Res Int 2011; 44(4): 827-39.
[http://dx.doi.org/10.1016/j.foodres.2011.01.022]

[53]  O'sullivan CM, Lynch A-M, Lynch PB, Buckley DJ, Kerry JP. Assessment of the antioxidant potential of food ingredients in fresh, previously frozen and cooked chicken patties. Int J Poult Sci 2004; 3(5): 337-44.
[http://dx.doi.org/10.3923/ijps.2004.337.344]

[54]  Negi PS. Plant extracts for the control of bacterial growth: efficacy, stability and safety issues for food application. Int J Food Microbiol 2012; 156(1): 7-17.
[http://dx.doi.org/10.1016/j.ijfoodmicro.2012.03.006] [PMID: 22459761]

[55]  Galanakis CM. Polyphenols: Properties, Recovery, and Applications. Woodhead Publishing 2018.

[56]  Jongberg S, Terkelsen LS, Miklos R, Lund MN. Green tea extract impairs meat emulsion properties by disturbing protein disulfide cross-linking. Meat Sci 2015; 100: 2-9.
[http://dx.doi.org/10.1016/j.meatsci.2014.09.003] [PMID: 25282040]

[57]  Pokorny J. Antioxidants in food preservation. Handb food Preserv 2007; 2: 259-86.
[http://dx.doi.org/10.1201/9781420017373.ch11]

[58]  Kumar N, Pruthi V. Potential applications of ferulic acid from natural sources. Biotechnol Rep (Amst) 2014; 4: 86-93.
[http://dx.doi.org/10.1016/j.btre.2014.09.002] [PMID: 28626667]

[59]  Kaewprachu P, Osako K, Benjakul S, Rawdkuen S. Quality attributes of minced pork wrapped with catechin–lysozyme incorporated gelatin film. Food Packag Shelf Life 2015; 3: 88-96.
[http://dx.doi.org/10.1016/j.fpsl.2014.11.002]

[60]  (EFSA) EFSA. Use of rosemary extracts as a food additive-Scientific Opinion of the Panel on Food Additives, Flavourings, Processing Aids and Materials in Contact with Food. EFSA J 2008; 6(6): 721.
[http://dx.doi.org/10.2903/j.efsa.2008.721]

[61]  (ANS) EP on FA and NS added to F. Scientific Opinion on the re-evaluation of anthocyanins (E 163) as a food additive. EFSA J 2013; 11(4): 3145.
[http://dx.doi.org/10.2903/j.efsa.2013.3145]

[62]  EFSA Panel on Dietetic Products N and A (NDA). Scientific Opinion on the substantiation of health claims related to rutin and improvement of endothelium-dependent vasodilation (ID 1649, 1783) and protection of DNA, proteins and lipids from oxidative damage (ID 1784) pursuant to Article 13 (1) of Regul. EFSA J 2010; 8(10): 1751.
[http://dx.doi.org/10.2903/j.efsa.2010.1751]

[63]  (FEEDAP) EP on A and P or S used in AF. Scientific Opinion on the safety and efficacy of tannic acid when used as feed flavouring for all animal species. EFSA J 2014; 12(10): 3828.
[http://dx.doi.org/10.2903/j.efsa.2014.3828]

[64]   (ANS) EP on F additives and NS added to F. Scientific Opinion on the re-evaluation of tocopherol-rich extract (E 306), α-tocopherol (E 307), γ-tocopherol (E 308) and δ-tocopherol (E 309) as food additives. EFSA J 2015; 13(9): 4247.

[65]   (ANS) EP on F additives and NS added to F. Scientific Opinion on the re-evaluation of ascorbic acid (E 300), sodium ascorbate (E 301) and calcium ascorbate (E 302) as food additives. EFSA J 2015; 13(5): 4087.

[66]   Authority EFS. Revised exposure assessment for lycopene as a food colour. EFSA J 2010; 8(1): 1444. [http://dx.doi.org/10.2903/j.efsa.2010.1444]

[67]   Figueirêdo BC, Trad IJ, Mariutti LRB, Bragagnolo N. Effect of annatto powder and sodium erythorbate on lipid oxidation in pork loin during frozen storage. Food Res Int 2014; 65: 137-43. [http://dx.doi.org/10.1016/j.foodres.2014.07.016]

[68]   Ree E. Opinion of the Scientific Panel on Food Additives, Flavourings, Processing Aids and Materials in Contact with Food on a request from the Commission related to Lutein for use in foods for particular nutritional uses. EFSA J 2006; 315.

[69]   (EFSA) EFSA. Opinion of the Scientific Panel on additives and products or substances used in animal feed (FEEDAP) on the safety of use of colouring agents in animal nutrition-PART I. General Principles and Astaxanthin EFSA J 2005; 3(12): 291.

[70]   Seppanen CM, Song Q, Saari Csallany A. The antioxidant functions of tocopherol and tocotrienol homologues in oils, fats, and food systems. J Am Oil Chem Soc 2010; 87(5): 469-81. [http://dx.doi.org/10.1007/s11746-009-1526-9]

[71]   Barbosa-Pereira L, Cruz JM, Sendón R, de Quirós ARB, Ares A, Castro-López M, *et al.* Development of antioxidant active films containing tocopherols to extend the shelf life of fish. Food Control 2013; 31(1): 236-43. [http://dx.doi.org/10.1016/j.foodcont.2012.09.036]

[72]   Marcos B, Sárraga C, Castellari M, Kappen F, Schennink G, Arnau J. Development of biodegradable films with antioxidant properties based on polyesters containing α-tocopherol and olive leaf extract for food packaging applications. Food Packag Shelf Life 2014; 1(2): 140-50. [http://dx.doi.org/10.1016/j.fpsl.2014.04.002]

[73]   Berardo A, De Maere H, Stavropoulou DA, Rysman T, Leroy F, De Smet S. Effect of sodium ascorbate and sodium nitrite on protein and lipid oxidation in dry fermented sausages. Meat Sci 2016; 121: 359-64. [http://dx.doi.org/10.1016/j.meatsci.2016.07.003] [PMID: 27424306]

[74]   Wang H, Feng H, Luo Y. Control of browning and microbial growth on fresh-cut apples by sequential treatment of sanitizers and calcium ascorbate. J Food Sci 2007; 72(1): M001-7. [http://dx.doi.org/10.1111/j.1750-3841.2006.00210.x] [PMID: 17995885]

[75]   (ANS) EP on FA and NS added to F. Scientific Opinion on the re-evaluation of ascorbyl palmitate (E 304 (i)) and ascorbyl stearate (E 304 (ii)) as food additives. EFSA J 2015; 13(11): 4289.

[76]   (ANS) EP on F additives and NS added to F. Scientific Opinion on the re-evaluation of dodecyl gallate (E 312) as a food additive. EFSA J 2015; 13(5): 4086.

[77]   Food A. Scientific opinion on the re-evaluation of octyl gallate (E 311) as a food additive. EFSA J 2015; 13(10)

[78]   (ANS) EP on F additives and NS added to F. Scientific Opinion on the re-evaluation of propyl gallate (E 310) as a food additive. EFSA J 2014; 12(4): 3642.

[79]   Gálico DA, Nova CV, Guerra RB, Bannach G. Thermal and spectroscopic studies of the antioxidant food additive propyl gallate. Food Chem 2015; 182: 89-94. [http://dx.doi.org/10.1016/j.foodchem.2015.02.129] [PMID: 25842313]

[80]   Hsu F-L, Chang H-T, Chang S-T. Evaluation of antifungal properties of octyl gallate and its synergy

with cinnamaldehyde. Bioresour Technol 2007; 98(4): 734-8.
[http://dx.doi.org/10.1016/j.biortech.2006.04.002] [PMID: 16750625]

[81]     Gharavi N, El-Kadi AOS. tert-Butylhydroquinone is a novel aryl hydrocarbon receptor ligand. Drug
         Metab Dispos 2004.
         [PMID: 15608132]

[82]     Roushani M, Sarabaegi M. Electrochemical detection of butylated hydroxyanisole based on glassy
         carbon electrode modified by iridium oxide nanoparticles. J Electroanal Chem (Lausanne Switz) 2014;
         717: 147-52.
         [http://dx.doi.org/10.1016/j.jelechem.2014.01.013]

[83]     Ma Y, Pan J, Zhang G, Zhang Y. Binding properties of butylated hydroxytoluene with calf thymus
         DNA in vitro. J Photochem Photobiol B 2013; 126: 112-8.
         [http://dx.doi.org/10.1016/j.jphotobiol.2013.07.011] [PMID: 23911863]

[84]     Akoh CC. Food lipids: chemistry, nutrition, and biotechnology. CRC press 2017.
         [http://dx.doi.org/10.1201/9781315151854]

[85]     (ANS) EP on FA and NS added to food. Scientific Opinion on the re-evaluation of erythorbic acid (E
         315) and sodium erythorbate (E 316) as food additives. EFSA J 2016; 14(1): 4360.
         [http://dx.doi.org/10.2903/j.efsa.2016.4360]

[86]     Fidler MC, Davidsson L, Zeder C, Hurrell RF. Erythorbic acid is a potent enhancer of nonheme-iron
         absorption. Am J Clin Nutr 2004; 79(1): 99-102.
         [http://dx.doi.org/10.1093/ajcn/79.1.99] [PMID: 14684404]

[87]     Kwaw E, Ma Y, Tchabo W, *et al.* Effect of lactobacillus strains on phenolic profile, color attributes
         and antioxidant activities of lactic-acid-fermented mulberry juice. Food Chem 2018; 250: 148-54.
         [http://dx.doi.org/10.1016/j.foodchem.2018.01.009] [PMID: 29412905]

[88]     Brewer MS, Mckeith F, Martin SE, Dallmier AW, Meyer J. Sodium lactate effects on shelf-life,
         sensory, and physical characteristics of fresh pork sausage. J Food Sci 1991; 56(5): 1176-8.
         [http://dx.doi.org/10.1111/j.1365-2621.1991.tb04727.x]

[89]     Ilhak OI, Guran HS. Combined Antimicrobial Effect of Thymol and Sodium Lactate against L isteria
         monocytogenes and Salmonella Typhimurium in Fish Patty. J Food Saf 2014; 34(3): 211-7.
         [http://dx.doi.org/10.1111/jfs.12115]

[90]     Kim YH, Keeton JT, Smith SB, Maxim JE, Yang HS, Savell JW. Evaluation of antioxidant capacity
         and colour stability of calcium lactate enhancement on fresh beef under highly oxidising conditions.
         Food Chem 2009; 115(1): 272-8.
         [http://dx.doi.org/10.1016/j.foodchem.2008.12.008]

[91]     Kim YH, Keeton JT, Yang HS, Smith SB, Sawyer JE, Savell JW. Color stability and biochemical
         characteristics of bovine muscles when enhanced with L- or D-potassium lactate in high-oxygen
         modified atmospheres. Meat Sci 2009; 82(2): 234-40.
         [http://dx.doi.org/10.1016/j.meatsci.2009.01.016] [PMID: 20416750]

[92]     Kim YHB, Huff-Lonergan E, Lonergan SM. Effect of calcium lactate on m-calpain activity and
         protein degradation under oxidising conditions. Food Chem 2012; 131(1): 73-8.
         [http://dx.doi.org/10.1016/j.foodchem.2011.08.033]

[93]     Cruzen SM, Kim YHB, Lonergan SM, Grubbs JK, Fritchen AN, Huff-Lonergan E. Effect of early
         postmortem enhancement of calcium lactate/phosphate on quality attributes of beef round muscles
         under different packaging systems. Meat Sci 2015; 101: 63-72.
         [http://dx.doi.org/10.1016/j.meatsci.2014.11.004] [PMID: 25437452]

[94]     De'Nobili MD, Soria M, Martinefski MR, Tripodi VP, Fissore EN, Rojas AM. Stability of l-(+-
         -ascorbic acid in alginate edible films loaded with citric acid for antioxidant food preservation. J Food
         Eng 2016; 175: 1-7.
         [http://dx.doi.org/10.1016/j.jfoodeng.2015.11.015]

[95]    Liu K, Liu J, Li H, Yuan C, Zhong J, Chen Y. Influence of postharvest citric acid and chitosan coating treatment on ripening attributes and expression of cell wall related genes in cherimoya (Annona cherimola Mill.) fruit. Sci Hortic (Amsterdam) 2016; 198: 1-11.
[http://dx.doi.org/10.1016/j.scienta.2015.11.008]

[96]    Banipal TS, Kaur H, Kaur A, Banipal PK. Effect of tartarate and citrate based food additives on the micellar properties of sodium dodecylsulfate for prospective use as food emulsifier. Food Chem 2016; 190: 599-606.
[http://dx.doi.org/10.1016/j.foodchem.2015.05.130] [PMID: 26213016]

[97]    Jim S, Hong-Shum L. Antioxidant. Food Addit Data B. 2003; pp. 75-118.

[98]    Ritz E, Hahn K, Ketteler M, Kuhlmann MK, Mann J. Phosphate additives in food--a health risk. Dtsch Arztebl Int 2012; 109(4): 49-55.
[PMID: 22334826]

[99]    Belitz H-D, Grosch W, Schieberle P. Food additives. Food Chem 2009; 429-66.

[100]   Msagati T A M. The chemistry of food additives and preservatives. John Wiley & Sons 2012.
[http://dx.doi.org/10.1002/9781118274132]

[101]   Vickers PJ, Braybrook J, Lawrence P, Gray K. Detecting tartrate additives in foods: Evaluating the use of capillary electrophoresis. J Food Compos Anal 2007; 20(3–4): 252-6.
[http://dx.doi.org/10.1016/j.jfca.2006.05.002]

[102]   Davidson PM, Branen AL, Thorngate J, Salminen S. Food additives. CRC Press 2001.

# CHAPTER 5

# Antimicrobial Agents

**Ovais Sideeq**[1,2], **Fazlullah Khan**[2,3] and **Kamal Niaz**[4,*]

[1] *School of Medicine, Tehran University of Medical Sciences (TUMS), Tehran, Iran*

[2] *International Campus, Tehran University of Medical Sciences (IC-TUMS), Tehran, Iran*

[3] *Department of Toxicology and Pharmacology, Faculty of Pharmacy, Tehran University of Medical Science, Tehran-1417614411, Iran*

[4] *Department of Pharmacology and Toxicology, Faculty of Bio-Sciences, Cholistan University of Veterinary and Animal Sciences CUVAS), Bahawalpur-63100 Pakistan*

**Abstract:** Antimicrobial agents have been the target of numerous research studies for a long period of history and they still attract great research interest namely in what regards to the discovery of newer molecules or the search for newer sources of natural antimicrobials. Antimicrobial agents include drugs, supplements, and ointments which particularly act on bacteria, fungi, comprising molds and yeasts, viruses as well as parasites. Phytochemicals, essential oils, antimicrobial peptides, metal oxides like silver and gold, namely those found as nanoparticles, are being used to treat microbial infections. Antimicrobial pesticides, some of which are isolated from the bacteria themselves, are being studied to help eradicate pathogens in the clinic as well as being used by agricultural companies. There are also various food derivatives that are used as antimicrobial agents. In this chapter, antibacterial, antifungal, antiviral, and antiparasitic antimicrobial agents, which include natural and synthesized molecules used as food additives, are addressed. An outlook of recent advances in drugs and other procedures of treating microbial infections is also given. This chapter also focuses on antimicrobial essential oils and antimicrobial pesticides with a closer look at the effects of heat and radiation as antimicrobial therapies.

**Keywords:** Antimicrobial Peptides, Antibacterial, Antifungal, Antiviral, Food, Physical agents.

## INTRODUCTION

A naturally occurring or synthesized material that has killing or inhibitory effect on the growth of microbes, including bacteria, fungi, viruses, algae, or parasites,

\* **Corresponding author Dr. Kamal Niaz:** DVM, PhD, Assistant Professor, Department of Pharmacology and Toxicology, Faculty of Bio-Sciences, Cholistan University of Veterinary and Animal Sciences (CUVAS), Bahawalpur-63100 Pakistan; Tel: +923129360054; E-mail: kamalniaz1989@gmail.com

**Seyed Mohammad Nabavi *et al*. (Eds.)**

is known as an antimicrobial agent [1]. For decades, antimicrobial therapies have been developed to treat various infections caused by microorganisms [1]. Drugs and dietary supplements which are isolated from plants and other alternative forms are being used in medicine as antimicrobials [2]. In this chapter, antimicrobial agents that are used to inhibit and kill microbes are addressed in what regards to their classification and sources. Special attention is given to antimicrobials used in foods.

## CLASSIFICATION OF ANTIMICROBIAL AGENTS

### Antibacterial Agents

Antimicrobial peptides (AMPs), sometimes also called host defense peptides (HDPs), have been studied for their stimulation of the immune system and anti-inflammatory properties. Naturally occurring AMPs are broad-spectrum antimicrobials against many bacterial species which include both Gram-positive and Gram-negative bacteria. The effectiveness of AMPs against multidrug-resistant (MDR) bacteria with less resistance inclination is very interesting. Many AMPs are becoming a part of clinical use. Some of them include polymyxins (colistin and polymyxin B), daptomycin, vancomycin, and gramicidin. Licheniformis group of *Bacillus subtilis* var Tracy produces polypeptide bacitracin. The polypeptide bacitracin is active against a variety of Gram-positive bacteria such as Staphylococci, Streptococci, and Clostridia. This polypeptide was approved by the FDA back in 1948. Polymyxins (colistin and polymyxin B) are a product of the non-ribosomal synthetase system in Gram-positive bacteria like *Paenibacillus polymyxa*. For Gram-negative bacteria, polymyxins are lipopolysaccharide (LPS) specific thus they show selective toxicity. Colistin has two commercial forms: colistimethane sodium and colistin sulfate. Both forms are used to treat acute infections of *Pseudomonas aeruginosa* and are also used against different Gram-negative bacteria. Daptomycin, a lipopeptide antibiotic, disrupts membrane potential and eradicates susceptible Gram-positive bacteria. Glycopeptide antibiotics such as vancomycin act against methicillin-resistant *Staphylococcus aureus* (*S. aureus*) and *Streptococci*. Gramicidin has bactericidal activity against *Streptococcus pneumonia* (*S. pneumoniae*), *Streptococcus pyogenes*, *Staphylococcus aureus*, *Diphtheria bacilli*, and *Anaerobic bacilli*. Many peptides are currently being clinically investigated such as POL7080, a synthetic cyclo-peptide selective against *Pseudomonas bacteria*. HLF-11 shows antimicrobial activity against MDR gram-positive and Gram-negative bacteria. A cationic antimicrobial peptide, omiganan pentahydrochloride (CLS001) interacts with the cytoplasmic membranes of Gram-positive and Gram-negative bacteria and it is effective against *S. aureus* [3]. B-(arylsulfonyl) and B-(arylsulfinyl) are low molecular weight hydroxamic acid derivatives that displayed potent antibacterial activity against many pathogens like *Chlamydia pneumonia, Mycoplasma pneumonia, Haemophilus influenza,* and *Moraxella catarrhalis* [4]. A novel bacterial topoisomerase inhibitor (NBTI), GSK299423, displays strong inhibition of DNAgyrase lead supercoiling from *S. aureus* and *Escherichia coli* (*E. coli*) [5]. Phage lysins which are phage-encoded peptidoglycan hydrolases have been used against particular bacteria causing no effect on commensal microflora. They are genus or species selective and specific. It has also been studied that lysins have the ability to target multiple genes. When applied as purified recombinant proteins, they cause sudden lysis and death of Gram-positive bacterial cells. During pre-clinical trials in eliminating antibiotic-resistant *S. pneumoniae,* which causes pneumonia, acute otitis media (AOM), septicemia, bronchitis, and meningitis, the use of pneumococcal lysins Cp1-1 and Pal has been successful. Staphylococcal phage K produces LysK lysin which has been demonstrated active against nine species of staphylococcus including MRSA and VRSA. Among the recombinant lysins, PlyG and PlyPH are reported to act on *B. anthracis.* Different strains of *C. difficile* are lysed by CD27L, a lysin extracted from *C. difficile* phage CD27 [6]. The bacteria which are found on mucosal surfaces and tissues with infection are also controlled by using lysins. The lysin enzymes *in vitro* as well as *in vivo* are remarkably potent in lysing bacteria. Lysins act rapidly to cause a therapeutic effect [7]. A natural isoquinoline, berberine, is found in medicinal plants like *Coptis chinensis, Hydrastis canadensis, Berberis aristata, Coptis japonica,* and *Phellondendron amurense.* To date, berberine is active against diarrhea, gastroenteritis, and abdominal pain. Aminothiazolyl berberine derivatives and their precursor compounds are active against Gram-positive and Gram-negative bacteria. *A. baumanii,* which is Gram-negative drug-resistant, is inhibited by hexyl aminothiazolyl berberine derivative 9c and 2,4-dichlorobenzoyl [8]. Nanoparticles (NPs) demonstrate high efficacy against bacteria, for instance, Ag nanoparticles prevent the development of biofilms and also inhibit new bacterial colonies on biofilms. $MgF_2$ NPs prevent biofilm formation in pathogens like *E. coli* and *S. aureus.* ZnO NPs coated glass surfaces produce reactive oxygen species (ROS) that act against biofilm formation in *E. coli* and *S. aureus.* Regarding NPs, superparamagnetic iron oxide NPs (SPIONs) are known to be highly active against bacteria and biofilms. In *Salmonella typhimurium,* $TiO_2$ and ZnO NPs have the weak potential to cause frameshift mutation. $TiO_2$ NPs under UV illumination kill *Pseudomonas aeruginosa (-), Enterococcus hire (+), E. coli (-),* and *Bacteroides fragilis (-).* Silver Carbon Complexes (SCCs) with NPs are efficiently toxic against *P. aeruginosa (-), Burkholderia cepacia (-), methicillin-resistant S. aureus, multidrug resistant Acinetobacter baumanii (A. baumanii) (-),* and *Klebsiella pneumonia (-).* The growth of bacteria such as *B. subtilis* and *Yersinia pestis (-)* is inhibited by SCCs [9]. The edible mushroom *Lentinus edodes* is valued for its medical and food applications. Lenthionine, its bioactive component, is rich in sulfur showing antibacterial activity. The derivative of lenthionine, bis-(methylsulfi=only)-methyl] disulfide inhibits *S. aureus, Bacillus subtilis,* and *E. coli*. Chloroform and ethyl acetate extracts from dry mushrooms act against *Streptococcus mutans* and *Prevotella intermedia* [10]. The nanomaterial using bismuth presents as a potent inhibitor of bacteria. More concisely, bismuth oxide ($Bi_2O_3$) has shown efficient antibacterial activity and is low cytotoxic. The synergistic relation between Ag and $Bi_2O_3$ is due to the high concentration of $H_2O_2$ produced on the surface of $Ag/Bi_2O_3$ nanocomposites (ABNPs), which results in an increase of antibacterial activities against Gram-negative and Gram-positive bacteria as well as clinically drug-resistant bacteria. The effect is well seen in *E. coli, S. aureus, S. typhimurium,* and *P. vulgaris* [11]. The essential oil of *Thymus daenensis* when prepared to obtain a nanoencapsulated oil or nanoemulsion shows novel activity against biofilm formation against multi-drug resistant (MDR) *A. baumanii* [12]. The derivatives of the organometallics of penicillin, quinolone, and platensimycin have been studied and shown to suppress the resistance mechanisms of bacteria [13]. A variety of cobalt complexes have shown antibacterial activity against many Gram-negative bacteria as well as Gram-positive bacteria such as *S. aureus, B. subtilis*, *E. coli*, *P. aeruginosa*, *Shigella*, and *Klebsiella* [14]. Cefazolin antibiotic, when loaded with polycaprolactone (PCL), has shown improved effects in inhibiting bacterial growth such as on *S. aureus* [15]. Growth of *Bacillus subtilis* and *Streptococcus epidermidis* is inhibited by an aqueous extract from *Cordyceps sinensis*. Similarly, the extract from *P. australis* has an inhibitory effect on the growth of *S. epidermidis* [16]. Synthetic pis1, a piscidin family paralogue which is found in Atlantic cod, is effective against Gram-(+) and Gram-(-) bacteria which includes pathogens from fish like *Vibrio anguillarum* and *Yersinia ruckeri* [17]. The bacteriophage KARL-1 which is an aqueous extract, when combined with other antibiotics has shown improved effect against multi-drug resistant *A. baumannii* [18].

## Antifungal Agents

There are two compounds, piliformic acid and cytochalasin D, isolated from endophytic *Xylaria* species and they have been studied due to show fungistatic activities against anthracnose caused by *Colletotrichum gloeosporoides* [19]. A chitin-binding lectin (PgTeL) is present in pomegranate (*Punica granatum)* sarcotesta and it has antifungal actions against *Candida albicans* and *Candida krusei*. In *C. krusei*, the lectin has been shown to damage the cell wall while in *C. albicans* biofilm inhibitory action has been reported [20]. Derivatives of imidazole like butoconazole nitrate (BN) are considered antifungal drugs of choice against vaginal infections. BN has been studied to be effective against

*Candida* species [21]. Opportunistic and endemic fungal pathogens cause different types of disseminated infections. Ketoconazole, fluconazole, and itraconazole have been used as a treatment for such fungal pathogens. The treatment of choice in the initial therapy regarding invasive aspergillosis is amphotericin B. The beneficial alternative has been reported to be itraconazole. Irrespective of the degree of neutropenia present in cancer patients with candidemia, the treatment with fluconazole and amphotericin B showed equal effectiveness. The combination of fluconazole-terbinafine has been shown effective against isolates of *C. albicans* and *C. glabrata.* For the prevention of recurring infections of *Cryptococcus,* fluconazole is very efficient. For meningitis caused by *Histoplasma capsulatum,* amphotericin B is the drug of choice. Itraconazole has been effective against infections of *Blastomyces dermatitidis.* In HIV infected patients, ketoconazole oral tablets and itraconazole oral capsules show a potent effect in treating oral and esophageal candidiasis. But if HIV related infection is more advanced, their use is limited owing to the absorption of the drug. Recently, fluconazole has been standardized for treating infections in oropharyngeal candidiasis (OPC) and esophageal candidiasis. In vulvo-vaginal candidiasis, intravaginal therapy consisting of intravaginal regimens like clotrimazole vaginal tablet and tioconazole ointment in combination with an antifungal agent is more clinically effective in comparison to topical nystatin. By the use of topical antifungal agents, the spread of nail infections caused by dermatophytes like *Trichophyton* species and *Epidermophyton floccosum* which are usually followed by infectious yeasts like *Candida albicans* can be prevented. A new triazole derivative of fluconazole, voriconazole has been tested and reported to show wide-spectrum effect against fungal pathogens which are clinically important, such as *Candida* species, *Aspergillus* species, *Cryptococcus neoformans, B. dermatitidis, Coccidioides immitis, H. capsulatum, Fusarium,* and *Penicillium marneffei.* Similarly, SCH 56592, a triazole derivative of itraconazole, is effective against *Candida* species, *Aspergillus,* and *Cryptococcus neoformans* [22]. Some compounds extracted from plants like dimethyl pyrrole, hydroxydihydrocornin-aglycones, indole derivatives, *etc.* have been studied to show activities against fungi. Extracts of *Gaullher procumbens, Rhammus purshiand,* and *Anacardum pulsatilla* containing tannins and salicylic acid have antifungal properties. Potent antifungal activities have been reported for geranylated biphenyl derivative from Green fruits (Garcinia malvgostana/purple mangostana). Antifungal activities have also been noted from polyisoprenylated benzophenone which is derived from an ethanol extract of *Cuban propolis.* Amentoflavone, a flavone derivative of *Selaginella tamariscina* exhibits strong antifungal activity. Calusendine, dentatin, nor-dentatin, and derivatives of carbazole and clauszoline isolates of *Clausena excavata* which act as coumarin phenolic substances have antimycotic properties. Quinone derivatives such as naphthoquinones, kigelinone, isopinnatal, dihydro-a-lapachone, and lapachol which are isolated from *Kigelia pinnata* show antifungal properties. Various spirostanol steroidal saponins extracted from *Smilax medica* roots exhibit antifungal properties against many types of yeast like *C. albicans, C. glabrata,* and *C. tropicalis.* Dichloromethane isolate of *Securidaca longepedunculata,* yields a xanthone product, 1,7-dihydroxy-4-methoxy xanthone, which is antifungal for pathogens such as *A. niger, A. fumigatus,* and *Penicillium* species. Some alkaloids isolated from plant *Datura metel* are antifungal *in vitro* as well as *in vivo* against *Aspergillus* and *Candida* species [23]. Ciclopirox olamine, an antifungal drug has been studied to show a reduction in the acute and latent infections of the peripheral nervous system caused by HSV-1 [24]. *Mitracarpus frigidus* methanolic extract (MFM) *in vitro* as well as *in vivo* demonstrated favorable activity against *C. albicans* [25]. The echinocandins have strong fungicidal properties against *Candida* species, as well as those pathogens which are resistant to azoles [26]. Microcrystal of silver tungstate (α-Ag2WO4) has been studied to show a wide spectrum of antifungal activities [27]. Silver nanoparticles (Ag-NPs) are active against *Candida albicans* and *Saccharomyces cerevisiae* [28]. Chitosan and chitosan derivatives act as biopolymers which are orally safe to administer and have antifungal activities. Pyridine chitosan showed extreme antifungal properties against *Botrytis cinerea (B. cinerea)* and *Fulvia fulva (F. fulva)* [29]. Tacrolimus which is an isolate of *Streptomyces tsukubaensis* has a pivotal role in immunosuppression. The protein phosphatase affects fungal cells and has a role in pathogenesis and growth of some major species of fungi including *Cryptococcus neoformans, C. albicans,* and *Aspergillus fumigans* [30]. NPs of selenium enriched with cells and supernatant of *Lactobacillus plantarum* and *Lactobacillus johnsonii* demonstrated antifungal properties against *C. albicans* [31]. The use of probiotics shows a reduction of colonization of *Candida* on mucosal surfaces, relief from signs and symptoms of infection caused by fungi, and effective enhancement of conventional antifungal therapy [31]. A broad-spectrum triazole, Iiavuconazole is effective against all *Candida, Aspergillus,* and some dimorphic fungi like *Histoplasma capsulatum* and *Coccidiodes* species [32]. The naturally occurring herbs which include *Withania somnifera, Curcuma longa, Euphorbia hirta, Echinophora platybola, Zingiber officinale, Lawsonia inermis, Adenocalymma alliacum, Pogostemon parviflorus,* and *Swertia chirata* have been studied to show antifungal activities against *Candida albicans,* a causative agent of oral infection [33]. Pyrrolozinone and indolizinone derivatives have shown inhibitory effects on many fungi such as *Phomopsis adianticola, Magnaporthe oryzae,* and *Gloeosporium theae-sinensis* [34]. Recently, a synthetic antimycotic agent, Flucytosine in combination with amphotericin B has been studied to show potent effects against fungal pathogens like *Candida albicans, Candidia tropical,* and *Cryptococcus neoformans* [35]. Luliconazole has strong antifungal effects on

*Aspergillus terrestris* [36].

## Antiviral Agents

Many acyclic (carboxylic) nucleoside derivatives induce antiviral activities. For the treatment of HSV-1 and HSV-2 infections and for VZV infections (varicella and herpes zoster), Acyclovir and valaciclovir are effective. Ganciclovir and valganciclovir act against CMV infections found in immunosuppressed patients. Topical use of penciclovir is used for treating the HSV infections which are superficial mucocutaneous. Analogues of guanosine inhibit HSV-1, HSV-2, VZV, CMV, and herpesviruses like HHV-6 (human herpesvirus type 6) [37]. Similarly, regarding acyclic nucleoside phosphonates, their antiviral activity is also reported. In AIDS patients with CMV retinitis, Cidofovir is used for treatment. Cidofovir also has use in human papilloma virus (HPV) infections, poxvirus, adenovirus, herpesvirus, and polyomavirus. Adefovir dipivoxil, a prodrug of adefovir, is effective in the treatment of chronic HBV infections as it has been reported to reduce HBV DNA load. Prodrug form of tenofovir, disoproxil fumarate (TDF), acts against HIV infections (AIDS) [37]. A potent and explicit inhibitor of the CMV UL97 kinase, maribavir has been thoroughly studied [38]. β-Carboline derivatives such as 9-methyl-norharmane, 9-methyl-harmane, and 6-methox--harmane have been studied to show novel antiviral properties against HSV-1 and HSV-2 [39]. Potential inhibition of human immunodeficiency virus (HIV), herpes simplex virus (HSV), coxsackievirus B3 (CVB3), cytomegalovirus (CMV), influenza virus, and hepatitis virus has been shown by naturally occurring polysaccharides and those polysaccharides which are modified chemically [40]. Amantadine and rimantadine which are the derivatives of adamantan are available for treatment against infections of influenza A virus. Zanamivir and oseltamivir are two leading neuraminidase inhibitors that are used for the therapy and prophylaxis of influenza A and B virus infections. In response to various zanamivir and oseltamivir-resistant influenza A and B viruses, pyrrolidine derivatives peramivir and A-315675 are active. Ribavirin shows activity against both influenza viruses, human and avian (H5N1). Inhibiting the attachment of the influenza virus to the cells, sialylglycopolymers play an important role. A substituted pyrazine, T-705 exhibits *in vitro* as well as *in vivo* anti-influenza virus capabilities. PEGylated interferon when combined with ribavirin acts as a standard treatment for chronic HCV infections [41]. Various organotin derivatives show partial as well as potent antiviral activity [42]. Ganciclovir, an antiviral agent, is the first drug of choice for CMV infection. In clinical use, maribavir, also called GW1263W94, is treated as the most active anti-CMV drug [43]. An isolate from *Ampullariella regularis* is known as neplanocin A which is a carbocyclic nucleoside and acts as a potent antiviral agent [44]. Compounds isolated from artesunate have been investigated to possess antiviral properties and the ability to inhibit the NF-κB pathway. Artemisinin shows strong antiherpesviral activities [45]. The infection of some DNA and RNA viruses is inhibited by lithium chloride (LiCl). LiCl inhibits the viruses like porcine coronavirus, an avian coronavirus, infectious bronchitis virus, porcine reproductive and respiratory syndrome virus, transmissible gastroenteritis virus (TGEV), canine parvovirus, feline calicivirus, pseudorabies herpesvirus, and herpes simplex virus [46]. Daclatasvir selectively inhibits the *in vitro* HCV NS5A replication complex. Asunaprevir is an extensive protease inhibitor of HCV NS3. Both antiviral agents show a vigorous decrease in HCV RNA levels in persons with HCV genotype 1 infections [47]. Many L-nucleoside analogues have shown antiviral activities such as lamivudine, entecavir, and adefovir. Clevudine acts on viral polymerase and inhibits HBV replication. Telbivudine and valtorcitabine, which are also analogues of L-nucleosides, demonstrate strong anti-HBV properties specifically and selectively as well [48]. Metal nanoparticles have shown immense potential to be effective antiviral mediums against many viruses some of which include HIV-1, Tacaribe virus, respiratory syncytial virus, hepatitis B virus, monkeypox virus, herpes simplex virus, and influenza virus [49]. Baicalein, a flavone that is present in the roots of *Scutellaria baicalensis* produces a metabolite namely baicalin, which has shown inhibitory effects on replication of chikungunya virus (CHIKV) [50]. In a docked analysis, nicotinic acetylcholine receptor (nAChRα-1 subunit) peptides proved to minimize the infections caused by Rabies virus (RABV) in neuron cells [51]. An analogue of deoxycytidine known as gemcitabine acts against rhinovirus by inhibiting cytidine triphosphate (CTP) synthetase and also acts on enterovirus [52].

## Antiparasitic Agents

Extracts of many plants including *Sophora flavescens, Areca catechu, Dandrenthema indicum, Cyrtomium rhizome, Scutellaria baicalensis,* and *Celastrus angulatus* have been studied to possess antiparasitic properties against *Cryptocaryon irritans (C. irritans)*. Matrine, oxymatrine, epigallocatechin gallate, dihydroartemisinin, celangulin, L-DOPA, and caprylic acid which are phytochemicals are very effective against *C. irritans*. A product of *Magnolia officinalis,* which is magnolol acts against *Ichthyophthirius multifilis.* Oleanolic acid which is extracted from *Olea europaea* L. exhibits antiparasitic properties in response to *Leishmania braziliensis, Leishmania chagasi,* and *Trypanosoma cruzi.* A component is extracted from *Magnolia officinalis* called honokiol. Honokiol has been reported to show anti *C. irritans* effects, preventing fish from getting infected [53]. Coumarin, present in the extract of *Esenbeckiea febrifuga,* which is rutaceae family, *Calophyllum brasiliense,* and some others, demonstrates important activity against *Leishmania* species [54]. The lapachol-ruthenium complexes are capable of inducing potent activities against *Leishmania amazonensis* and *Plasmodium falciparum* [55]. Vanadyl containing compounds in conjugation with [VO(L1-2H)(phen)] and [VO(L3-2H)(phen)] forming a complex has been noted to exhibit high anti-trypanosomal and anti-leishmanial activity in an *in vitro* study [56]. Quinoxaline complexes inhibit kinetoplastid by acting against *Trypanosoma cruzi* and *Leishmania amazonensis* [57]. Vinyl sulfones are effective inhibitors of papain family that resemble cysteine proteases that have a proteolytic role in parasites like *Trypanosoma cruzi, Trypanosoma brucei,* and *Plasmodium falciparum* [58]. Nitroimidazole carboxamides acts against *Giardia lamblia* and *Entamoeba histolytica* [59]. Menadione (MEN) is a Vitamin K3 provitamin that metabolizes in the liver to Vitamin K. Menadione has been prospectively studied to act against *Schistosoma mansoni* [60]. *Ichthyophthirius multifiliis,* the causative agent of Ichthyophthiriasis, is acted upon by commercially available curcumin [61]. Phosphonium lipocations derived from naphthoquinones have been studied to show inhibitory effects on *Trypanosoma cruzi* and *Plasmodium falciparum* [62]. Leaf extracts of *Psidium guajava* and *Psidium brownianum* have *in vitro* antiparasitic activity in response to epimastigote forms of *Trypanosoma cruzi* and promastigote forms of *Leishmania braziliensis* and *Leishmania infantum* [63]. *Physalis angulate (*EEPA) causes cell death by necrosis in *Trypanosoma cruzi* [64]. Betulinic acid has anti *Trypanosoma cruzi* effects. Reports of antiparasitical activities of betulinic acid against *Plasmodium falciparum* and *Leishmania* species are also reported [65]. Gold complex [Au(PPh$_3$)(CQ)]PF$_6$ causes potent inhibition of *Plasmodium berghei* and also acts against *Plasmodium falciparum.* Another gold complex, [Au(dppz)$_2$]Cl$_3$, has been studied to show great anti-leishmanial effects. Gold drug auranofin is a very strong inhibitor of *Schintosome* TGR (multifunctional enzyme) [66].

## ANTIMICROBIALS FROM NATURAL SOURCES

### Essential Oils

Essential oils extracted from commercially aromatic plants like *Melaleuca alternifolia* (tea tree), *Thymus vulgaris* (thyme), *Mentha piperita* (peppermint), and *Rosmarinus officinalis* (rosemary) are used for the treatment of infections caused by bacteria and fungi. *P. graveolens* oil when combined with norfloxacin shows a synergistic effect against *Staphylococcus aureus* and *Bacillus cereus.* Amphotericin B combined with *M. alternifolia* oil displays dominant antagonistic activity against *C. albicans* [67]. Essential oils from cardamom, basil, rosemary, anise, coriander, dill, parsley, and angelica also possess antipathogenic and saprophytic effects. Oregano, basil, and coriander essential oils inhibit *P. aeruginosa, S. aureus,* and *Yersinia enterocolitica.* Oregano essential oil shows effects in response to *S. typhimurium*. *Achillea clavennae* essential oil shows inhibitory results against *Klebsiella pneumonia, Streptococcus pneumonia, Haemophilus influenza,* and *P. aeruginosa*. Oregano, savory, and thyme essential oils show strong inhibition of *Clostridium botulinum* and *Clostridium perfringens*. Pathogens like *S. aureus* and *Providencia stuartii* have been inhibited by the essential oil extracted from *Salvia officinalis*. Thyme and mint essential oil extract present antibacterial properties against *S. aureus, S. typhimurium, Vibrioparahaemolyticus, L. monocytogenes, E. coli, C. botulinum, C. perfringens, Shigella sonnei, Sarcina lutea,* and *Micrococcus flavus* [68]. Lemongrass essential oil (LGEO) possesses inhibitory activities against species like *Candida albicans, Candida tropicalis,* and *C. parapsilosis*. LGEO also shows effects on molds like *A. niger* and *Penicillium* species [69]. The essential oil from *Bidens pilosa* has been studied to show substantial antifungal and antibacterial effects [70]. Eugenol, a component of the essential oil from clove, shows broad bactericidal activity in microorganisms like *Escherichia coli, Staphylococcus aureus, Pseudomonas aeruginosa,* and *Listeria monocytogenes* [71]. Essential oils from lemon balm (*Melissa officinalis*) and marjoram (*Origanum majorana*) demonstrate a quantitative antimicrobial activity in response to Gram-positive and Gram-negative bacteria. The essential oils isolated from the plants usually have been reported to be active against Gram-positive bacteria in comparison to Gram-negative bacteria [72]. Basil essential oil shows strong activity against many microorganisms including the bacteria such as *Staphylococcus aureus* and *Escherichia coli* and fungi like *Aspergillus niger* and *Fusarium solani* [73]. The essential oil of *Artemisia biensis* has shown antidermatophytic activity, and also against *Cryptococcus neofromans, Fonsecaea pedrosoni,* and *Aspergillus niger* while as the isolated essential oil of *Artemisia absinthium* is very vigorous against *Staphylococcus* species [74]. *Eucalyptus globulus* Labill (Myrtaceae) is the main source of eucalyptus oil and it has been reported to show potential antibacterial activities [75]. Citrus related essential oils are exceptional antimicrobial means against the bacteria *Salmonella* [76]. The essential oils of oregano and garlic are capable to inhibit *S. aureus, S. enteritidis, L. monocytogenes, E. coli,* and *L. plantarum* [77]. *Cinnamomum osmopholeum* leaf essential oils contain a compound known as cinnamaldehyde, which inhibits the bacterial growth, yeast, filamentous molds and shows potential antifungal properties [78]. *Lavandula luisieri* essential oil has promising antifungal properties [79].

## Antimicrobial Pesticides

Phenyl isothiocyanate (PEITC) which is isolated from horseradish possesses pesticide and antimicrobial properties acting against a number of fungi and bacteria [80]. Lichens are rich in terphenylquinones and pulvinic acids which help lichens have immense antimicrobial pesticide activities [81]. *Nostoc* strain ATCC

53789 which is a cryptophycin producer has demonstrated a wide range of pesticidal activities including antifungal, antibacterial, and insecticidal [82]. Rotenone is isolated from family *Leguminosae* and exhibits biopesticidal activities against many microorganisms [83]. *Bacillus thuringiensis* has been used to control insects in many developed countries [84]. Derivatives of strobilurins are used in fungal management. An isolate of actinomycete *Streptomyces kasugaensis* is kasugamycin which has fungicidal properties. Copper octanoate has also been reported to show antifungal activities [85]. Eucalyptus, cumin, and oregano essential oils have been studied to show potent antimicrobial activity and are a major content of many pesticides [86]. For the use of new pesticides, antimicrobial peptides (AMPs) have displayed a wide range of actions in response to bacteria, viruses, parasites, and fungi [87]. Organotin containing compounds have long been used in agricultural purposes for their fungicidal and bactericidal activities [88].

## PHYSICAL AGENTS

### Heat

Heat treatment affects the growth rate of bacteria and fungi [89]. Heating has for long been used to reduce the microorganisms in the milk as a process of pasteurization [90]. Heat treatment causes deglycosylation of natural ginsenosides which are converted to low polarity ginsenosides improving its antimicrobial activity against *F. nucleatum, C. perfringens,* and *P. gingivalis* [91]. Heating the silver nanoparticles whilst oxidation has shown to increase the antimicrobial activity of silver hydroxyapatite coatings and thus makes sure the antimicrobial activity remains steady [92].

### Radiation

Radiation-induced graft polymerization of N-vinyl pyrrolidone leads to the synthesis of antimicrobial fabric which may be used in the face masks [93]. Radiolytically synthesized silver nanoparticles gain tremendous antimicrobial activities in response to bacteria and fungi and thus irradiation procedure is used in many antimicrobial textile industries [94]. UV and VUV irradiations have been studied to possess antimicrobial effects and reduce the number of microorganisms like *S. aureus, B. atrophaeus,* and *E. coli* [95]. The antimicrobial approach involves photodynamic therapy, which results in the reduction of highly reactive oxygen species. Photodynamic therapy is an efficient strategy in helping to eradicate oral pathogenic bacteria [96]. Both *in vitro* and *in vivo* studies reveal that UV radiation causes the induction of antimicrobial peptides [97]. A very useful method is gamma irradiation, which is used in preventing contamination and control pathogenic microorganisms that affect fruits and vegetables [98].

## ANTIMICROBIALS USE IN FOODS

Bacteriocins have been thoroughly studied as food preservatives due to bio-preservative activity. Nisin, a bacteriocin produced by *Lactococcus lactis* subsp. *Lactis* has been used to preserve food. Liposomes have been presented as pediocin AcH vectors in dairy and meat products like non-fat dry milk, beef muscle tissue or beef tallow, and butter fat. As antimicrobials, nisin loaded liposomes meet the need for controlling spoiling and bacterial pathogens of food, which are typically faced during food processing [99]. Chitosan, a polysaccharide derivative of chitin which is known to possess a range of antimicrobial and antifungal properties. Bio-films of chitosan act as packaging material and have shown excellent results in preserving a number of foods and extending the food shelf life. Chitosan films inhibit the growth of lactic acid bacteria, *Enterobacteriaceae, Lactobacillus sakei,* and *Serratia liquifaciens* [100]. Cinnamaldehyde possesses antimicrobial activity against bacteria, molds, and yeasts. The incorporation of cinnamaldehyde in Gliadin films is very active in various food systems in reducing fungal growth. Gliadin-cinnamaldehyde films are being produced in food packaging for cheese spread and sliced bread [101]. Essentials oils are used as potential antimicrobials with attributes of natural food additives. Apart from being used in fruits and vegetables, essential oils possess antimicrobial activities in meat products also [103]. The addition of marjoram essential oil derived from *Origanum majorana* L. to fresh sausage depicted bacteriostatic activity at minimal concentrations and bactericidal activity at high concentrations [102]. Bacteriocins are combined with foods such as cheese to preserve food against *Clostridium* and *Listeria* [104]. Encapsulated essential oils from *Melaleuca alternifolia* and D-limonene enhance the quality and safety by acting as preservatives in foods. Nanoencapsulation of terpenes showed a delay in the microbial growth or complete inactivation of microorganisms while producing changes in the organoleptic properties of the fruit juices [105]. Silver nanoparticles have been studied to show antimicrobial properties against a number of microorganisms, which makes it useful in commercial food packaging as it has the capacity of inhibiting a number of bacteria and yeast [106]. The antimicrobial compounds from lactic acid bacteria have been used to prevent spoilage and in food preservation using natural fermentation methods. They have shown applications in baking products, meat, vegetables. The bacteriocins from lactic acid bacteria can be used as food preservatives. They also possess organoleptic properties which help in aroma generation, enhanced sweetness, and exopolysaccharide production. They have technological benefit of preventing over acidification in yoghurt [107]. Essential oils are known for their antimicrobial properties in combination with inducing aromas and flavors in the foods. They are considered as essential preservatives. The citrus oils are used as antimicrobials in foods and they have shown organoleptic effects [108]. Bacteriolytic enzymes, lysozymes extracted from eggs of hen have shown to inhibit the growth of spores of *Clostridium tyrobutyricum* in cheese. Lysozymes act as quality preservatives in alcohol-containing beverages. Another lysozyme that is available commercially has shown effective properties against the growth of *Listeria monocytogenes* during the shelf life of salmon roe and minced tuna raw products [109]. Lactoferrin has been used in commercial products, which include sports beverages, dietary supplements, and human infant formulas and it is known to improve function of immune system. Ovotransferrin, a metalloproteinase isolated from egg white albumin possesses antimicrobial properties against a wide range of pathogenic and spoilage bacteria like *S. aureus, Salmonella enteritidis, Pseudomonas aeruginosa,* and *Bacillus cereus* [109]. Reutarin has been investigated to have biopreservative actions in meat and dairy products. Cultures produced using pediocin for sausage and cheddar cheese fermentation inhibits the growth of *L. monocytogenes.* Similarly, cystibiotic is added in food products to control the microorganisms growing during storage of foods [109]. The essential oils of clary, juniper, lemon, majoram, and sage have been applied to preserve apple juice. Naturally found antibacterial compounds like extracts of herbs, spices, organic acids, bacteriocins, salts, and essential oils have been reported to improve shelf life of meat. Chitosan and cinnamon derived essential oils improved shell life of trout fillet in addition to enhance odor, texture, and color [110]. Polyethylene film loaded with ZnO (Zinc Oxide) nanoparticles, which possess biocidal activities, bears preventive activities and can be used in food packaging [111]. The antimicrobial compounds like acetic acid, acetates, dehydroacetic acid, and diacetates are used to target yeasts and bacteria and are applied in baked goods, dairy products, condiments, fats, oils meat, and sauces. Parabenes are used against yeasts and molds and show applications in baked goods, dry sausage, and syrups. Recent studies have shown that the use of nanoemulsions carrying functional lipids like antioxidants, colors, flavors, and antimicrobials can improve the safety and quality of food products [112]. The classification of all antimicrobial agents has been mentioned in Fig. (**1**).

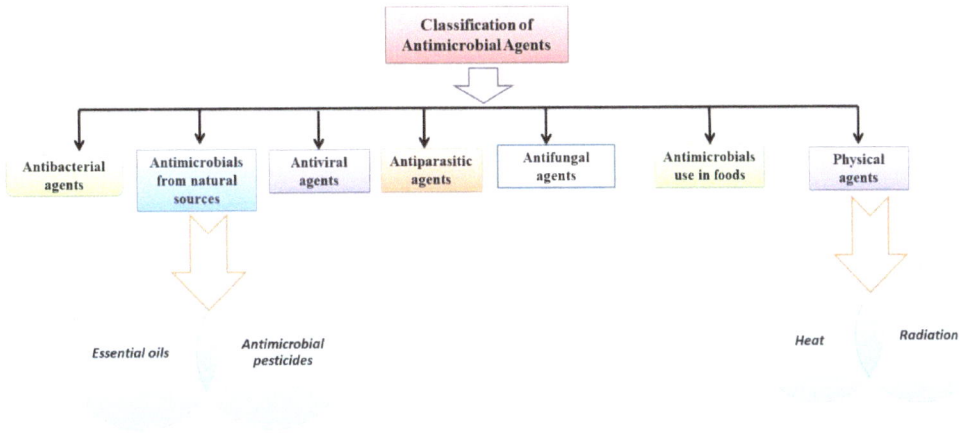

**Fig. (1).** Classification of antimicrobial agents.

## CONCLUSION

There are a huge number of antimicrobial agents around the globe for treating the infections caused by bacteria, fungi, viruses, and parasites. Antimicrobial peptides show effective antimicrobial activity against many bacterial strains including multidrug-resistant bacteria, Gram-positive, and Gram-negative bacteria. In recent years nanoparticles have revolutionized antimicrobial therapies. Many agents are active against *Staphylococcus, Streptococcus,* and *E. coli.* Among the fungi related antimicrobials, drugs against *Aspergillus, Cryptococcus,* and *Dermatophytes* have been developed and some have fungistatic activity. Antiviral drugs are effective against HIV, HSV, and CMV like viruses. *Trypanosoma, Leishmania,* and *Plasmodium* are being effectively treated in a number of ways. Metal complexes are a new way of reducing parasitical infections. Many of the food-derived antimicrobials such as bacteriocins, chitin, cinnamaldehyde, essential oils, terpenes, lactoferrin, ovotransferrin, and reutarin are used to preserve the foods products and eradicate/inhibit the growth of microbes to prevent them from spoilage. Essential oils from a number of plants act on bacteria and a number of fungi. Antimicrobial pesticides are being used as insecticides, bactericides, and fungicides. High temperature has a potential effect on microbial growth while irradiation has shown tremendous results in the last few decades of inhibiting bacterial colonial growth.

## CONSENT FOR PUBLICATION

Not applicable.

## CONFLICT OF INTEREST

There is no conflict of interest.

## ACKNOWLEDGEMENTS

All the authors of the manuscript thank and acknowledge their respective universities and institutes.

## REFERENCES

[1]     Burnett-Boothroyd S, McCarthy B. Antimicrobial treatments of textiles for hygiene and infection control applications: an industrial perspective.Textiles for Hygiene and Infection Control. Elsevier 2011; pp. 196-209.
        [http://dx.doi.org/10.1533/9780857093707.3.196]

[2]     Cowan MM. Plant products as antimicrobial agents. Clin Microbiol Rev 1999; 12(4): 564-82.
        [http://dx.doi.org/10.1128/CMR.12.4.564] [PMID: 10515903]

[3]     Roscia G, Falciani C, Bracci L, Pini A. The development of antimicrobial peptides as new antibacterial drugs. Curr Protein Pept Sci 2013; 14(8): 641-9.
        [http://dx.doi.org/10.2174/13892037140813122715 5308] [PMID: 24384032]

[4]     Apfel C, Banner DW, Bur D, *et al.* Hydroxamic acid derivatives as potent peptide deformylase inhibitors and antibacterial agents. J Med Chem 2000; 43(12): 2324-31.
        [http://dx.doi.org/10.1021/jm000018k] [PMID: 10882358]

[5]     Bax BD, Chan PF, Eggleston DS, *et al.* Type IIA topoisomerase inhibition by a new class of antibacterial agents. Nature 2010; 466(7309): 935-40.
        [http://dx.doi.org/10.1038/nature09197] [PMID: 20686482]

[6]     Fenton M, Ross P, McAuliffe O, O'Mahony J, Coffey A. Recombinant bacteriophage lysins as antibacterials. Bioeng Bugs 2010; 1(1): 9-16.
        [http://dx.doi.org/10.4161/bbug.1.1.9818] [PMID: 21327123]

[7]     Fischetti VA. Bacteriophage lysins as effective antibacterials. Curr Opin Microbiol 2008; 11(5): 393-400.
        [http://dx.doi.org/10.1016/j.mib.2008.09.012] [PMID: 18824123]

[8]     Gao WW, Gopala L, Bheemanaboina RRY, Zhang GB, Li S, Zhou CH. Discovery of 2-aminothiazolyl berberine derivatives as effectively antibacterial agents toward clinically drug-resistant Gram-negative Acinetobacter baumanii. Eur J Med Chem 2018; 146: 15-37.
        [http://dx.doi.org/10.1016/j.ejmech.2018.01.038] [PMID: 29396362]

[9]     Hajipour MJ, Fromm KM, Ashkarran AA, *et al.* Antibacterial properties of nanoparticles. Trends Biotechnol 2012; 30(10): 499-511.
        [http://dx.doi.org/10.1016/j.tibtech.2012.06.004] [PMID: 22884769]

[10]    Hatvani N. Antibacterial effect of the culture fluid of Lentinus edodes mycelium grown in submerged liquid culture. Int J Antimicrob Agents 2001; 17(1): 71-4.
        [http://dx.doi.org/10.1016/S0924-8579(00)00311-3] [PMID: 11137653]

[11]    Liu Q, Li J, Zhong X, *et al.* Enhanced antibacterial activity and mechanism studies of Ag/Bi2O3 nanocomposites. Adv Powder Technol 2018; 29(9): 2082-90.
        [http://dx.doi.org/10.1016/j.apt.2018.05.015]

[12]    Moghimi R, Aliahmadi A, Rafati H, Abtahi HR, Amini S, Feizabadi MM. Antibacterial and anti-biofilm activity of nanoemulsion of Thymus daenensis oil against multi-drug resistant Acinetobacter baumannii. J Mol Liq 2018; 265: 765-70.

[http://dx.doi.org/10.1016/j.molliq.2018.07.023]

[13]    Patra M, Gasser G, Metzler-Nolte N. Small organometallic compounds as antibacterial agents. Dalton Trans 2012; 41(21): 6350-8.
       [http://dx.doi.org/10.1039/c2dt12460b] [PMID: 22411216]

[14]    Chang EL, Simmers C, Knight DA. Cobalt complexes as antiviral and antibacterial agents. Pharmaceuticals (Basel) 2010; 3(6): 1711-28.
       [http://dx.doi.org/10.3390/ph3061711] [PMID: 27713325]

[15]    Radisavljevic A, Stojanovic DB, Perisic S, *et al.* Cefazolin-loaded polycaprolactone fibers produced *via* different electrospinning methods: Characterization, drug release and antibacterial effect. Eur J Pharm Sci 2018; 124: 26-36.
       [http://dx.doi.org/10.1016/j.ejps.2018.08.023] [PMID: 30130639]

[16]    Ren L, Hemar Y, Perera CO, Lewis G, Krissansen GW, Buchanan PK. Antibacterial and antioxidant activities of aqueous extracts of eight edible mushrooms. Bioact Carbohydr Dietary Fibre 2014; 3(2): 41-51.
       [http://dx.doi.org/10.1016/j.bcdf.2014.01.003]

[17]    Ruangsri J, Salger SA, Caipang CM, Kiron V, Fernandes JM. Differential expression and biological activity of two piscidin paralogues and a novel splice variant in Atlantic cod (Gadus morhua L.). Fish Shellfish Immunol 2012; 32(3): 396-406.
       [http://dx.doi.org/10.1016/j.fsi.2011.11.022] [PMID: 22178249]

[18]    Jansen M, Wahida A, Latz S, *et al.* Enhanced antibacterial effect of the novel T4-like bacteriophage KARL-1 in combination with antibiotics against multi-drug resistant Acinetobacter baumannii. Sci Rep 2018; 8(1): 14140.
       [http://dx.doi.org/10.1038/s41598-018-32344-y] [PMID: 30237558]

[19]    Elias LM, Fortkamp D, Sartori SB, *et al.* The potential of compounds isolated from Xylaria spp. as antifungal agents against anthracnose. Braz J Microbiol 2018; 49(4): 840-7.
       [http://dx.doi.org/10.1016/j.bjm.2018.03.003] [PMID: 29631892]

[20]    da Silva PM, de Moura MC, Gomes FS, *et al.* PgTeL, the lectin found in Punica granatum juice, is an antifungal agent against Candida albicans and Candida krusei. Int J Biol Macromol 2018; 108: 391-400.
       [http://dx.doi.org/10.1016/j.ijbiomac.2017.12.039] [PMID: 29225175]

[21]    Shaker DS, Ismail S, Hamed S, El-Shishtawy EM. Butoconazole nitrate vaginal sponge: Drug release and antifungal efficacy. J Drug Deliv Sci Technol 2018; 48: 274-87.
       [http://dx.doi.org/10.1016/j.jddst.2018.09.011]

[22]    Sheehan DJ, Hitchcock CA, Sibley CM. Current and emerging azole antifungal agents. Clin Microbiol Rev 1999; 12(1): 40-79.
       [http://dx.doi.org/10.1128/CMR.12.1.40] [PMID: 9880474]

[23]    Arif T, Bhosale JD, Kumar N, *et al.* Natural products--antifungal agents derived from plants. J Asian Nat Prod Res 2009; 11(7): 621-38.
       [http://dx.doi.org/10.1080/10286020902942350] [PMID: 20183299]

[24]    Bernier KM, Morrison LA. Antifungal drug ciclopirox olamine reduces HSV-1 replication and disease in mice. Antiviral Res 2018; 156: 102-6.
       [http://dx.doi.org/10.1016/j.antiviral.2018.06.010] [PMID: 29908958]

[25]    Campos LM, De Melo L, Lemos AS, *et al.* Mitracarpus frigidus: A promising antifungal in the treatment of vulvovaginal candidiasis. Ind Crops Prod 2018; 123: 731-9.
       [http://dx.doi.org/10.1016/j.indcrop.2018.07.038]

[26]    Chen SCA, Slavin MA, Sorrell TC. Echinocandin antifungal drugs in fungal infections: a comparison. Drugs 2011; 71(1): 11-41.
       [http://dx.doi.org/10.2165/11585270-000000000-00000] [PMID: 21175238]

[27]   Foggi CC, Fabbro MT, Santos LP, *et al.* Synthesis and evaluation of α-Ag2WO4 as novel antifungal agent. Chem Phys Lett 2017; 674: 125-9.
[http://dx.doi.org/10.1016/j.cplett.2017.02.067]

[28]   Nasrollahi A, Pourshamsian K, Mansourkiaee P. Antifungal activity of silver nanoparticles on some of fungi. Int J Nanodimens 2011; 1(3): 233-9.

[29]   Jia R, Duan Y, Fang Q, Wang X, Huang J. Pyridine-grafted chitosan derivative as an antifungal agent. Food Chem 2016; 196: 381-7.
[http://dx.doi.org/10.1016/j.foodchem.2015.09.053] [PMID: 26593505]

[30]   Kubiça TF, Denardi LB, Azevedo MI, *et al.* Antifungal activities of tacrolimus in combination with antifungal agents against fluconazole-susceptible and fluconazole-resistant Trichosporon asahii isolates. Braz J Infect Dis 2016; 20(6): 539-45.
[http://dx.doi.org/10.1016/j.bjid.2016.08.008] [PMID: 27697432]

[31]   Matsubara VH, Bandara HM, Mayer MP, Samaranayake LP. Probiotics as antifungals in mucosal candidiasis. Clin Infect Dis 2016; 62(9): 1143-53.
[http://dx.doi.org/10.1093/cid/ciw038] [PMID: 26826375]

[32]   Miceli MH, Kauffman CA. Isavuconazole: a new broad-spectrum triazole antifungal agent. Clin Infect Dis 2015; 61(10): 1558-65.
[http://dx.doi.org/10.1093/cid/civ571] [PMID: 26179012]

[33]   Samadi FM, Suhail S, Sonam M, *et al.* Antifungal efficacy of herbs. J Oral Biol Craniofac Res 2019; 9(1): 28-32.
[http://dx.doi.org/10.1016/j.jobcr.2018.06.002] [PMID: 30197861]

[34]   Wang S, Bao L, Wang W, Song D, Wang J, Cao X. Heterocyclic pyrrolizinone and indolizinones derived from natural lactam as potential antifungal agents. Fitoterapia 2018; 129: 257-66.
[http://dx.doi.org/10.1016/j.fitote.2018.07.013] [PMID: 30056185]

[35]   Wani MY, Ahmad A, Kumar S, Sobral AJ. Flucytosine analogues obtained through Biginelli reaction as efficient combinative antifungal agents. Microb Pathog 2017; 105: 57-62.
[http://dx.doi.org/10.1016/j.micpath.2017.02.006] [PMID: 28189732]

[36]   Zargaran M, Taghipour S, Kiasat N, *et al.* Luliconazole, an alternative antifungal agent against Aspergillus terreus. J Mycol Med 2017; 27(3): 351-6.
[http://dx.doi.org/10.1016/j.mycmed.2017.04.011] [PMID: 28483449]

[37]   De Clercq E, Neyts E. Antiviral agents acting as DNA or RNA chain terminators, in Antiviral Strategies. 2009; 53-84.

[38]   Chou S, Ercolani RJ, Derakhchan K. Antiviral activity of maribavir in combination with other drugs active against human cytomegalovirus. Antiviral Res 2018; 157: 128-33.
[http://dx.doi.org/10.1016/j.antiviral.2018.07.013] [PMID: 30040968]

[39]   Gonzalez MM, Cabrerizo FM, Baiker A, *et al.* β-Carboline derivatives as novel antivirals for herpes simplex virus. Int J Antimicrob Agents 2018; 52(4): 459-68.
[http://dx.doi.org/10.1016/j.ijantimicag.2018.06.019] [PMID: 30006037]

[40]   Chen L, Huang G. The antiviral activity of polysaccharides and their derivatives. Int J Biol Macromol 2018; 115: 77-82.
[http://dx.doi.org/10.1016/j.ijbiomac.2018.04.056] [PMID: 29654857]

[41]   De Clercq E. Antiviral agents active against influenza A viruses. Nat Rev Drug Discov 2006; 5(12): 1015-25.
[http://dx.doi.org/10.1038/nrd2175] [PMID: 17139286]

[42]   Carraher CE Jr, Roner MR. Organotin polymers as anticancer and antiviral agents. J Organomet Chem 2014; 751: 67-82.
[http://dx.doi.org/10.1016/j.jorganchem.2013.05.033]

[43]   Biron KK. Antiviral drugs for cytomegalovirus diseases. Antiviral Res 2006; 71(2-3): 154-63.
[http://dx.doi.org/10.1016/j.antiviral.2006.05.002] [PMID: 16765457]

[44]   Cho JH, Bernard DL, Sidwell RW, Kern ER, Chu CK. Synthesis of cyclopentenyl carbocyclic nucleosides as potential antiviral agents against orthopoxviruses and SARS. J Med Chem 2006; 49(3): 1140-8.
[http://dx.doi.org/10.1021/jm0509750] [PMID: 16451078]

[45]   Hahn F, Fröhlich T, Frank T, *et al.* Artesunate-derived monomeric, dimeric and trimeric experimental drugs - Their unique mechanistic basis and pronounced antiherpesviral activity. Antiviral Res 2018; 152: 104-10.
[http://dx.doi.org/10.1016/j.antiviral.2018.02.013] [PMID: 29458133]

[46]   Li HJ, Gao DS, Li YT, Wang YS, Liu HY, Zhao J. Antiviral effect of lithium chloride on porcine epidemic diarrhea virus *in vitro*. Res Vet Sci 2018; 118: 288-94.
[http://dx.doi.org/10.1016/j.rvsc.2018.03.002] [PMID: 29547727]

[47]   Lok AS, Gardiner DF, Lawitz E, *et al.* Preliminary study of two antiviral agents for hepatitis C genotype 1. N Engl J Med 2012; 366(3): 216-24.
[http://dx.doi.org/10.1056/NEJMoa1104430] [PMID: 22256805]

[48]   Mathé C, Gosselin G. L-nucleoside enantiomers as antivirals drugs: a mini-review. Antiviral Res 2006; 71(2-3): 276-81.
[http://dx.doi.org/10.1016/j.antiviral.2006.04.017] [PMID: 16797735]

[49]   Galdiero S, Falanga A, Vitiello M, Cantisani M, Marra V, Galdiero M. Silver nanoparticles as potential antiviral agents. Molecules 2011; 16(10): 8894-918.
[http://dx.doi.org/10.3390/molecules16108894] [PMID: 22024958]

[50]   Oo A, Rausalu K, Merits A, *et al.* Deciphering the potential of baicalin as an antiviral agent for Chikungunya virus infection. Antiviral Res 2018; 150: 101-11.
[http://dx.doi.org/10.1016/j.antiviral.2017.12.012] [PMID: 29269135]

[51]   Sajjanar B, Dhusia K, Saxena S, *et al.* Nicotinic acetylcholine receptor alpha 1(nAChRα1) subunit peptides as potential antiviral agents against rabies virus. Int J Biol Macromol 2017; 104(Pt A): 180-8.
[http://dx.doi.org/10.1016/j.ijbiomac.2017.05.179] [PMID: 28587964]

[52]   Song JH, Kim SR, Heo EY, *et al.* Antiviral activity of gemcitabine against human rhinovirus in vitro and in vivo. Antiviral Res 2017; 145: 6-13.
[http://dx.doi.org/10.1016/j.antiviral.2017.07.003] [PMID: 28705625]

[53]   Zhong ZH, Guo WL, Lei Y, *et al.* Antiparasitic efficacy of honokiol against Cryptocaryon irritans in pompano, Trachinotus ovatus. Aquaculture 2018.

[54]   De Alcantara FC, Lozano VF, Velosa AS, dos Santos MR, Pereira RM. New coumarin complexes of Zn, Cu, Ni and Fe with antiparasitic activity. Polyhedron 2015; 101: 165-70.
[http://dx.doi.org/10.1016/j.poly.2015.09.010]

[55]   Barbosa MI, Corrêa RS, de Oliveira KM, *et al.* Antiparasitic activities of novel ruthenium/lapachol complexes. J Inorg Biochem 2014; 136: 33-9.
[http://dx.doi.org/10.1016/j.jinorgbio.2014.03.009] [PMID: 24727183]

[56]   Benítez J, Becco L, Correia I, *et al.* Vanadium polypyridyl compounds as potential antiparasitic and antitumoral agents: new achievements. J Inorg Biochem 2011; 105(2): 303-12.
[http://dx.doi.org/10.1016/j.jinorgbio.2010.11.001] [PMID: 21194632]

[57]   Cogo J, Cantizani J, Cotillo I, *et al.* Quinoxaline derivatives as potential antitrypanosomal and antileishmanial agents. Bioorg Med Chem 2018; 26(14): 4065-72.
[http://dx.doi.org/10.1016/j.bmc.2018.06.033] [PMID: 30100019]

[58]   Kerr ID, Lee JH, Farady CJ, *et al.* Vinyl sulfones as antiparasitic agents: a structural basis for drug design. J Biol Chem 2009. p. jbc. M109. 014340

[59]  Jarrad AM, Debnath A, Miyamoto Y, *et al.* Nitroimidazole carboxamides as antiparasitic agents targeting Giardia lamblia, Entamoeba histolytica and Trichomonas vaginalis. Eur J Med Chem 2016; 120: 353-62.
[http://dx.doi.org/10.1016/j.ejmech.2016.04.064] [PMID: 27236016]

[60]  Kapadia GJ, Soares IAO, Rao GS, *et al.* Antiparasitic activity of menadione (vitamin K$_3$) against Schistosoma mansoni in BABL/c mice. Acta Trop 2017; 167: 163-73.
[http://dx.doi.org/10.1016/j.actatropica.2016.12.001] [PMID: 28017859]

[61]  Liu YM, Zhang QZ, Xu DH, Fu YW, Lin DJ, Zhou SY. Antiparasitic efficacy of commercial curcumin against Ichthyophthirius multifiliis in grass carp (Ctenopharyngodon idellus). Aquaculture 2017; 480: 65-70.
[http://dx.doi.org/10.1016/j.aquaculture.2017.07.041]

[62]  Long TE, Lu X, Galizzi M, Docampo R, Gut J, Rosenthal PJ. Phosphonium lipocations as antiparasitic agents. Bioorg Med Chem Lett 2012; 22(8): 2976-9.
[http://dx.doi.org/10.1016/j.bmcl.2012.02.045] [PMID: 22414614]

[63]  Machado AJT, Santos ATL, Martins GMAB, *et al.* Antiparasitic effect of the Psidium guajava L. (guava) and Psidium brownianum MART. EX DC. (araçá-de-veado) extracts. Food Chem Toxicol 2018; 119: 275-80.
[http://dx.doi.org/10.1016/j.fct.2018.03.018] [PMID: 29548852]

[64]  Meira CS, Guimarães ET, Dos Santos JA, *et al. in vitro* and *in vivo* antiparasitic activity of Physalis angulata L. concentrated ethanolic extract against Trypanosoma cruzi. Phytomedicine 2015; 22(11): 969-74.
[http://dx.doi.org/10.1016/j.phymed.2015.07.004] [PMID: 26407938]

[65]  Meira CS, Barbosa-Filho JM, Lanfredi-Rangel A, Guimarães ET, Moreira DR, Soares MB. Antiparasitic evaluation of betulinic acid derivatives reveals effective and selective anti-Trypanosoma cruzi inhibitors. Exp Parasitol 2016; 166: 108-15.
[http://dx.doi.org/10.1016/j.exppara.2016.04.007] [PMID: 27080160]

[66]  Navarro M. Gold complexes as potential anti-parasitic agents. Coord Chem Rev 2009; 253(11-12): 1619-26.
[http://dx.doi.org/10.1016/j.ccr.2008.12.003]

[67]  van Vuuren SF, Suliman S, Viljoen AM. The antimicrobial activity of four commercial essential oils in combination with conventional antimicrobials. Lett Appl Microbiol 2009; 48(4): 440-6.
[http://dx.doi.org/10.1111/j.1472-765X.2008.02548.x] [PMID: 19187494]

[68]  Swamy MK, Akhtar MS, Sinniah UR. Antimicrobial properties of plant essential oils against human pathogens and their mode of action: an updated review. Evid Based Complement Alternat Med 2016; 20163012462
[http://dx.doi.org/10.1155/2016/3012462] [PMID: 28090211]

[69]  Boukhatem MN, Ferhat MA, Kameli A, Saidi F, Kebir HT. Lemon grass (Cymbopogon citratus) essential oil as a potent anti-inflammatory and antifungal drugs. Libyan J Med 2014; 9(1): 25431.
[http://dx.doi.org/10.3402/ljm.v9.25431] [PMID: 28156278]

[70]  Deba F, Xuan TD, Yasuda M, Tawata S. Chemical composition and antioxidant, antibacterial and antifungal activities of the essential oils from Bidens pilosa Linn. var. Radiata Food Control 2008; 19(4): 346-52.
[http://dx.doi.org/10.1016/j.foodcont.2007.04.011]

[71]  Devi KP, Nisha SA, Sakthivel R, Pandian SK. Eugenol (an essential oil of clove) acts as an antibacterial agent against Salmonella typhi by disrupting the cellular membrane. J Ethnopharmacol 2010; 130(1): 107-15.
[http://dx.doi.org/10.1016/j.jep.2010.04.025] [PMID: 20435121]

[72]  Gutierrez J, Barry-Ryan C, Bourke P. Antimicrobial activity of plant essential oils using food model

media: efficacy, synergistic potential and interactions with food components. Food Microbiol 2009; 26(2): 142-50.
[http://dx.doi.org/10.1016/j.fm.2008.10.008] [PMID: 19171255]

[73] Hussain AI, Anwar F, Hussain Sherazi ST, Przybylski R. Chemical composition, antioxidant and antimicrobial activities of basil (Ocimum basilicum) essential oils depends on seasonal variations. Food Chem 2008; 108(3): 986-95.
[http://dx.doi.org/10.1016/j.foodchem.2007.12.010] [PMID: 26065762]

[74] Lopes-Lutz D, Alviano DS, Alviano CS, Kolodziejczyk PP. Screening of chemical composition, antimicrobial and antioxidant activities of Artemisia essential oils. Phytochemistry 2008; 69(8): 1732-8.
[http://dx.doi.org/10.1016/j.phytochem.2008.02.014] [PMID: 18417176]

[75] Mulyaningsih S, Sporer F, Reichling J, Wink M. Antibacterial activity of essential oils from Eucalyptus and of selected components against multidrug-resistant bacterial pathogens. Pharm Biol 2011; 49(9): 893-9.
[http://dx.doi.org/10.3109/13880209.2011.553625] [PMID: 21591991]

[76] O'Bryan CA, Crandall PG, Chalova VI, Ricke SC. Orange essential oils antimicrobial activities against Salmonella spp. J Food Sci 2008; 73(6): M264-7.
[http://dx.doi.org/10.1111/j.1750-3841.2008.00790.x] [PMID: 19241555]

[77] Seydim A, Sarikus G. Antimicrobial activity of whey protein based edible films incorporated with oregano, rosemary and garlic essential oils. Food Res Int 2006; 39(5): 639-44.
[http://dx.doi.org/10.1016/j.foodres.2006.01.013]

[78] Shreaz S, Wani WA, Behbehani JM, *et al.* Cinnamaldehyde and its derivatives, a novel class of antifungal agents. Fitoterapia 2016; 112: 116-31.
[http://dx.doi.org/10.1016/j.fitote.2016.05.016] [PMID: 27259370]

[79] Zuzarte M, Gonçalves MJ, Cruz MT, *et al.* Lavandula luisieri essential oil as a source of antifungal drugs. Food Chem 2012; 135(3): 1505-10.
[http://dx.doi.org/10.1016/j.foodchem.2012.05.090] [PMID: 22953886]

[80] Chen H, Wang C, Ye J, Zhou H, Chen X. Antimicrobial activities of phenethyl isothiocyanate isolated from horseradish. Nat Prod Res 2012; 26(11): 1016-21.
[http://dx.doi.org/10.1080/14786419.2010.535148] [PMID: 21815843]

[81] Dayan FE, Romagni JG. Lichens as a potential source of pesticides. Pestic Outlook 2001; 12(6): 229-32.
[http://dx.doi.org/10.1039/b110543b]

[82] Biondi N, Piccardi R, Margheri MC, Rodolfi L, Smith GD, Tredici MR. Evaluation of Nostoc strain ATCC 53789 as a potential source of natural pesticides. Appl Environ Microbiol 2004; 70(6): 3313-20.
[http://dx.doi.org/10.1128/AEM.70.6.3313-3320.2004] [PMID: 15184126]

[83] Cavoski I, Caboni P, Miano T. Natural pesticides and future perspectives.Pesticides in the Modern World-Pesticides Use and Management. InTech 2011.
[http://dx.doi.org/10.5772/17550]

[84] Butt TM, Harris JG, Powell KA. Microbial biopesticides, in Biopesticides: use and delivery 1999; 23-44.

[85] Cantrell CL, Dayan FE, Duke SO. Natural products as sources for new pesticides. J Nat Prod 2012; 75(6): 1231-42.
[http://dx.doi.org/10.1021/np300024u] [PMID: 22616957]

[86] Isman MB. Plant essential oils for pest and disease management. Crop Prot 2000; 19(8-10): 603-8.
[http://dx.doi.org/10.1016/S0261-2194(00)00079-X]

[87] Montesinos E, Bardají E. Synthetic antimicrobial peptides as agricultural pesticides for plant-disease

control. Chem Biodivers 2008; 5(7): 1225-37.
[http://dx.doi.org/10.1002/cbdv.200890111] [PMID: 18649311]

[88]   Crowe AJ. Organotin compounds in agriculture since 1980. Part I. Fungicidal, bactericidal and herbicidal properties. Appl Organomet Chem 1987; 1(2): 143-55.
[http://dx.doi.org/10.1002/aoc.590010206]

[89]   Pietikäinen J, Pettersson M, Bååth E. Comparison of temperature effects on soil respiration and bacterial and fungal growth rates. FEMS Microbiol Ecol 2005; 52(1): 49-58.
[http://dx.doi.org/10.1016/j.femsec.2004.10.002] [PMID: 16329892]

[90]   Cosentino C, Labella C, Elshafie HS, *et al.* Effects of different heat treatments on lysozyme quantity and antimicrobial activity of jenny milk. J Dairy Sci 2016; 99(7): 5173-9.
[http://dx.doi.org/10.3168/jds.2015-10702] [PMID: 27157571]

[91]   Xue P, Yao Y, Yang XS, Feng J, Ren GX. Improved antimicrobial effect of ginseng extract by heat transformation. J Ginseng Res 2017; 41(2): 180-7.
[http://dx.doi.org/10.1016/j.jgr.2016.03.002] [PMID: 28413322]

[92]   Zhang X, Chaimayo W, Yang C, Yao J, Miller BL, Yates MZ. Silver-hydroxyapatite composite coatings with enhanced antimicrobial activities through heat treatment. Surf Coat Tech 2017; 325: 39-45.
[http://dx.doi.org/10.1016/j.surfcoat.2017.06.013]

[93]   Aoki S, Fujiwara K, Sugo T, Suzuki K. Antimicrobial fabric adsorbed iodine produced by radiation-induced graft polymerization. Radiat Phys Chem 2013; 84: 242-5.
[http://dx.doi.org/10.1016/j.radphyschem.2012.05.003]

[94]   Bera A, Garai P, Singh R, *et al.* Gamma radiation synthesis of colloidal AgNPs for its potential application in antimicrobial fabrics. Radiat Phys Chem 2015; 115: 62-7.
[http://dx.doi.org/10.1016/j.radphyschem.2015.05.041]

[95]   Brandenburg R, Lange H, von Woedtke T, *et al.* Antimicrobial effects of UV and VUV radiation of nonthermal plasma jets. IEEE Trans Plasma Sci 2009; 37(6): 877-83.
[http://dx.doi.org/10.1109/TPS.2009.2019657]

[96]   Garcez AS, Nuñez SC, Hamblin MR, Ribeiro MS. Antimicrobial effects of photodynamic therapy on patients with necrotic pulps and periapical lesion. J Endod 2008; 34(2): 138-42.
[http://dx.doi.org/10.1016/j.joen.2007.10.020] [PMID: 18215668]

[97]   Gläser R, Navid F, Schuller W, *et al.* UV-B radiation induces the expression of antimicrobial peptides in human keratinocytes *in vitro* and *in vivo*. J Allergy Clin Immunol 2009; 123(5): 1117-23.
[http://dx.doi.org/10.1016/j.jaci.2009.01.043] [PMID: 19342087]

[98]   Tawema P, Han J, Vu KD, Salmieri S, Lacroix M. Antimicrobial effects of combined UV-C or gamma radiation with natural antimicrobial formulations against Listeria monocytogenes, Escherichia coli O157: H7, and total yeasts/molds in fresh cut cauliflower. Lebensm Wiss Technol 2016; 65: 451-6.
[http://dx.doi.org/10.1016/j.lwt.2015.08.016]

[99]   Da Silva Malheiros P, Daroit DJ, Brandelli A. Food applications of liposome-encapsulated antimicrobial peptides. Trends Food Sci Technol 2010; 21(6): 284-92.
[http://dx.doi.org/10.1016/j.tifs.2010.03.003]

[100]  Aider M. Chitosan application for active bio-based films production and potential in the food industry. Lebensm Wiss Technol 2010; 43(6): 837-42.
[http://dx.doi.org/10.1016/j.lwt.2010.01.021]

[101]  Balaguer MP, Lopez-Carballo G, Catala R, Gavara R, Hernandez-Munoz P. Antifungal properties of gliadin films incorporating cinnamaldehyde and application in active food packaging of bread and cheese spread foodstuffs. Int J Food Microbiol 2013; 166(3): 369-77.
[http://dx.doi.org/10.1016/j.ijfoodmicro.2013.08.012] [PMID: 24029024]

[102]  Busatta C, Vidal RS, Popiolski AS, *et al.* Application of Origanum majorana L. essential oil as an

antimicrobial agent in sausage. Food Microbiol 2008; 25(1): 207-11.
[http://dx.doi.org/10.1016/j.fm.2007.07.003] [PMID: 17993397]

[103] Calo JR, Crandall PG, O'Bryan CA, Ricke SC. Essential oils as antimicrobials in food systems–A review. Food Control 2015; 54: 111-9.
[http://dx.doi.org/10.1016/j.foodcont.2014.12.040]

[104] Cleveland J, Montville TJ, Nes IF, Chikindas ML. Bacteriocins: safe, natural antimicrobials for food preservation. Int J Food Microbiol 2001; 71(1): 1-20.
[http://dx.doi.org/10.1016/S0168-1605(01)00560-8] [PMID: 11764886]

[105] Donsì F, Annunziata M, Sessa M, Ferrari G. Nanoencapsulation of essential oils to enhance their antimicrobial activity in foods. Lebensm Wiss Technol 2011; 44(9): 1908-14.
[http://dx.doi.org/10.1016/j.lwt.2011.03.003]

[106] Duncan TV. Applications of nanotechnology in food packaging and food safety: barrier materials, antimicrobials and sensors. J Colloid Interface Sci 2011; 363(1): 1-24.
[http://dx.doi.org/10.1016/j.jcis.2011.07.017] [PMID: 21824625]

[107] Rattanachaikunsopon P, Phumkhachorn P. Lactic acid bacteria: their antimicrobial compounds and their uses in food production. Ann Biol Res 2010; 1(4): 218-28.

[108] Fisher K, Phillips C. Potential antimicrobial uses of essential oils in food: is citrus the answer? Trends Food Sci Technol 2008; 19(3): 156-64.
[http://dx.doi.org/10.1016/j.tifs.2007.11.006]

[109] Juneja VK, Dwivedi HP, Yan X. Novel natural food antimicrobials. Annu Rev Food Sci Technol 2012; 3: 381-403.
[http://dx.doi.org/10.1146/annurev-food-022811-101241] [PMID: 22385168]

[110] Lucera A, Costa C, Conte A, Del Nobile MA. Food applications of natural antimicrobial compounds. Front Microbiol 2012; 3: 287.
[http://dx.doi.org/10.3389/fmicb.2012.00287] [PMID: 23060862]

[111] Tankhiwale R, Bajpai SK. Preparation, characterization and antibacterial applications of ZnO-nanoparticles coated polyethylene films for food packaging. Colloids Surf B Biointerfaces 2012; 90: 16-20.
[http://dx.doi.org/10.1016/j.colsurfb.2011.09.031] [PMID: 22015180]

[112] Weiss J, Gaysinsky S, Davidson M, McClements J. Nanostructured encapsulation systems: food antimicrobials, in Global Issues Food Sci Technol. 2009; 425-79.

# CHAPTER 6

# Essential Oils

**Regiane Ribeiro-Santos[1,*], Mariana Andrade[2] and Ana Sanches-Silva[3,4]**

[1] *Federal Institute of Education, Science and Technology of Pernambuco, IFPE Campus Vitória de Santo Antão, PE, Brazil*

[2] *Department of Food and Nutrition, National Institute of Health Dr. Ricardo Jorge, I.P., Lisbon, Portugal*

[3] *National Institute for Agricultural and Veterinary Research (INIAV), Vairão, Vila do Conde, Portugal*

[4] *Center for Study in Animal Science (CECA), ICETA, University of Oporto, Oporto, Portugal*

**Abstract:** Essential oils are natural compounds obtained from plants with powerful biological activities. Several studies have reported their use as food additives due to their actions as antimicrobial and antioxidant agents. Despite some limitations, such as aroma and toxicity related to high doses, the use of essential oils in foods is promising and makes it possible to reduce the use of synthetic additives in food applications. In this chapter, the most common extraction methods, as well as the antioxidant and antimicrobial activities of some essential oils are addressed. The legal aspects and the general health effects of essential oils are also covered.

**Keywords:** Antioxidant capacity, Antimicrobial activity, Essential oils, Food additives.

## INTRODUCTION

Essential oils (EOs) are extracted and used by human civilization since ancient times. They were used for medicinal purposes against infections, religious rituals, as fragrances, and for cooking as flavoring agents [1]. EOs are lipophilic and highly volatile secondary metabolites produced naturally by plants, generally belonging to Angiosperm families (plants with flower). The most commonly found chemical compounds present in these oils are mono and sesquiterpenes but, allyl and isoallyl phenols, aldehydes, esters, and alcohols can also be commonly found, depending on the plant species [1 - 3]. The natural role of EOs is the natural plant's defence against predators, UV radiation, fungus, or other pathoge-

* **Corresponding author Regiane Ribeiro-Santos:** Federal Institute of Education, Science and Technology of Pernambuco, IFPE Campus Vitória de Santo Antão, PE, Brazil

**Seyed Mohammad Nabavi et al. (Eds.)**

nic organisms and used for the plant's pollination. They can be obtained through several extraction methods and from all plant parts such as flowers, buds, leaves, stems, barks, and seeds [4 - 8]. The extraction method and the part of the plant used for the EOs extraction have a direct impact on the chemical constitution of the EOs. Since the biological properties are directly correlated with the presence and quantity of these compounds, consequently, these properties are affected by these factors [2, 9, 10].

Regarding the extraction techniques, the phenolic compounds present in EOs can be sensitive to light and temperature so, the choice of the extraction method is very important since it will determine how powerful the oil activity will be. The most conventional and used methods for obtaining EOs are cold expression (cold pressing), solvent extraction, the "Enfleurage" method, distillation (water, steam or a combination of the two), and extraction with supercritical gases [11]. With the passage of time and the development of new technologies, more efficient and "eco-friendly" extraction methods have emerged. Microwave-assisted extraction (MAE) resorts to heat,caused by the friction between molecules at specific atmospheric conditions, having a reasonable cost, leading to higher extraction yields when compared to the conventional extraction methods [11, 12]. Another method for extraction EOs is the Controlled Pressure Drop Process, which consists of submitting determined biomass, for a short time period, to high-pressured saturated steam followed by a sudden pressure drop, towards vacuum. This extraction method allows for a higher yield and a higher quality [11, 13]. Ultrasound-Assisted Extraction is another "eco-friendly" extraction method that allows a reduction in the use of organic solvents, a time-reduction and as a minimal effect on the extractable compounds, enabling an EO with possible higher biological activities [11, 14].

## ANTIMICROBIAL AND ANTIOXIDANT EOS

The food industry is always trying to find new ways to preserve and improve the nutritional and organoleptic properties of food. Generally, this industry resorts to synthetic additives, which are more chemically stable , economic and more easily applied than the natural ones. Recently, the use of certain synthetic additives, such as butylated hydroxyanisole (BHA) and hydroxytoluene (BHT), has been called into question since its long-term effects on human health are still unknown. Also, the prolonged exposure to these additives has been associated with the onset of neurodegenerative diseases and carcinogenesis [15 - 17]. This, in association with the consumer demand for natural products, has led to the search for natural additives. EOs, since they are known for their powerful antimicrobial and antioxidant properties, are great candidates for being studied as natural food additives that can be applied directly or indirectly to food. In fact, the use of EOs as food additives has been the object of several researches studies [8, 10 - 13].

*In vitro* and *in vivo* studies have shown the positive action of EOs as antimicrobial and antioxidant agents. In several studies, EOs have shown their action against several bacteria and fungus such as *Escherichia coli, Staphylococcus aureus, Listeria monocytogenes,* and *Penicillium* species (spp). This antimicrobial power can prevent foodborne diseases and food spoilage. Also, the antioxidant power of EOs has shown the potential to prevent lipid oxidation in fatty foods [2, 18 - 20]. In Table **1**, some antimicrobial and antioxidant activities in the food of some EOs are exhibited. It is thought that EOs act against bacteria by the disruption and penetration of the lipid structure's cell membrane of bacteria, which leads to protein denaturation and cell membrane destruction. These actions are due to their major compounds, terpenes [21].

**Table 1. Essential oils against different microrganisms\*.**

| Common name and scientific name (Plant species) | Microorganisms | Ref. |
|---|---|---|
| Basil (*Ocimum basilicum*) | *Enterococcus faecalis; Micrococcus luteus; Sarcina* sp; *Staphylococcus Aureus; Staphylococcus epidermidis; Streptococcus mutan, Acinetobacter* sp.; *Aeromonas* sp.; *Citrobacter freundii; Escherichia coli; Klebsiella pneumoniae; Proteus mirabilis; Proteus vulgaris; Salmonella choleraesuis; Serratiamarcescens; Shigella flexneri; Yersinia enterocolitica; Candida albicans; Trichophyton mentagrophytes; Trichophyton tonsurans; Trichophyton rubrum; Epidermophyton floccosum; Microsporum canis; Aspergillus niger; Bacillus subtilis Pasteurella multocida; Mucor Mucedo; Fusarium. solani; Botryodiplodia theobromae; Rhizoctonia solani* | [22 - 24] |
| Bergamot (*Citrus bergamia*) | *Staphylococcus aureus; Bacillus subtilis; Escherichia coli; Saccharomyces cerevisiae* | [25] |
| Black Cumin (*Nigella sativa*) | *Streptococcus* spp. *Enterococcus faecalis; Gemella haemolysins; Gemella morbillorum* | [26] |
| "Casca de anta" (*Drimys Angustifolia*) | *Bacillus cereus; Staphylococcus aureus; Acinetobacter baumanii; Escherichia coli; Pseudomonas aeruginosa* | [27] |
| Cinnamon (*Cinnamomum cassia*) with Cinnamaldehyde 85.6% | *Escherichia coli; Enterobacter arugenus; Vibrio cholera; Vibrio; Salmonella; Proteus vulgaris; Pseudomonas; Staphylococcus aureus;Candida* sp.; *Fusarium solani; Aspergillus sp., Microsporumgypseum; Tricophyton rubrum; Tricophyton mentagrophytes.* | [28] |
| Clove (*Eugenia aryophyllus*) | *Staphylococcus aureus; Bacillus subtilis; Klebsiella pneumoniae; Proteus vulgaris; Pseudomonas* aeruginosa; *Escherichia coli* | [29] |
| *Etlingera fimbriobracteata* | *Escherichia coli; Bacillus subtilis; Bacillus spizienii; Staphylococcus aureus; Candida albicans; Saccharomyces cerevisiae* | [30] |

| Common name and scientific name (Plant species) | Microorganisms | Ref. |
|---|---|---|
| Garlic *(Allium sativum)* | *Escherichia coli; Salmonella entérica; Listeria monocytogenes; Bacillus cereus; Shigella* sp.; *Vibrio* sp. *Yersinia enterocolitica; Campylobacter* sp.; *Bacteroides fragilis; Bacillus subtilus; Enterobacter aerogenes; Enterococcus faecalis; Klebsiella aerogenes; Proteus vulgaris; Lactobacillus acidophilus; Streptococcus faecalis* | [31] |
| Geranium *(Pelargonium graveolens)* | *Staphylococcus aureus; Bacillus subtilis; Klebsiella pneumonia; Proteus vulgaris; Pseudomonas aeruginosa; Escherichia coli* | [29] |
| Lemon *(Citrus limon)* | *Bacillus subtilis; Staphylococcus aureus* | [29] |
| Lemongrass *(Cymbopogon citratus)* | *Escherichia coli; Staphylococcus aureus; Bacillus cereus; Bacillus subtilis; Klebsiella pneumoniae* | [32] |
| Lime *(Citrus aurantium)* | *Staphylococcus. aureus; Bacillus subtilis; Klebsiella pneumoniae; Proteus vulgaris; Pseudomonas aeruginosa; Escherichia coli* | [29] |
| Onion *(Allium cepa)* | *Staphylococcus. aureus; Bacillus subtilis; Escherichia coli; Rhodotorula glutinis; Saccharomyces cerevisiae; Candida tropicalis; Aspergillus niger; Monascus purpureus; Aspergillus terreus* | [33] |
| Orange *(Citrus sinensis)* | *Staphylococcus. aureus; Bacillus subtilis; Klebsiella pneumoniae; Proteus vulgaris; Pseudomonas aeruginosa; Escherichia coli* | [29] |
| Oregano *(Origanum vulgare)* | *Staphylococcus aureus; Bacillus subtilis; Escherichia coli; Saccharomyces cerevisiae* | [25] |
| Pennyroyal *(M. pulegium L.)* | *Salmonella typhimurium; Staphylococcus aureus; Staphylococcus epidermidis; Escherichia coli; Bacillus cereus Vibrio cholera; Aspergillus niger; Listeria monocytogenes; Candida albicans* | [34] |
| Perilla *(Perilla arguta)* | *Staphylococcus aureus; Bacillus subtilis; Escherichia coli; Saccharomyces cerevisiae* | [25] |
| Rosemary *(Rosmarinus officinalis L)* | *Staphylococcus aureus; Bacillus subtilis; Klebsiella pneumoniae; Proteus vulgaris; Pseudomonas aeruginosa; Escherichia coli; Salmonella Typhimurium; Listeria monocytogenes; Enterococcus. faecalis* | [35, 36] |
| Salvia *(Salvia officinalis L)* | *Ashbiya gossypii; Aspergillus niger; Bacillus liqueniformis Candida albicans; Enterococcus hirae; Phanerochaete chrysosporium; Pichia subpeliucolosa; Trichoderma reesei; Escherichia coli; Proteus mirabili; Salmonella typhimurium; Aeromonas hydrophila; Aeromonas sóbria; Klebsiella oxytoca; Citrobacter* sp.; *Serratia marcescens; Bacillus megatherium; Bacillus cereus; Bacillus subtilis; Pseudomonas aeruginosa; Pseudomonas fluorescens; Staphylococcus aureus; Staphylococcus epidermidis* | [37, 38] |

*(Table 1) cont.....*

| Common name and scientific name (Plant species) | Microorganisms | Ref. |
|---|---|---|
| Thyme (*Thymus vulgaris* L) | *Staphylococcus aureus; Staphylococcus epidermidis; Streptococcus* sp. *Pantoa* sp.; *Escherichia coli; Aspergillus* sp.; *Penicillium* sp; *Alternaria* sp.; *Ulocladium* spp.; *Absidia* spp.; *Mucor* spp.; *Cladosporium* sp.; *Trichoderma* spp.; *Rhizopus* spp.; *Chaetomium globosum; Stachybotrys chartarum* | [19] |
| *Antimicrobial activity depends on the part of the plant used (Adapted from [39]).* | | |

Regarding the antioxidant capacity, it is thought that it is related to the synergistic effect that can occur between the major and minor compounds of EOs. The antioxidant capacity of EOs is attributed to the terpenolic and phenolic compounds present in the EOs constitution [21].

## LEGAL ASPECTS AND LIMITATIONS

Numerous research studies have documented and stated the effectiveness of the biological properties of several EOs. Although, there is still no specific legislation for the use of EOs and/or its constituents as food, even though several EOs are considered GRAS (Generally Recognized as Safe) food additives by the Food and Drug Administration (FDA) and are also approved by the European Commission [40, 41].

As previously said, EOs can be applied directly or indirectly to foods Table **2**. The direct form can present some disadvantages since EOs have a very strong taste and aroma, which may induce changes in the organoleptic properties of foods. Therefore, the indirect form can be the wisest way to apply EOs, since it can provide all the desirable effects without the undesirable effects. The encapsulation of EOs can be an alternative to the direct form, as is the incorporation of EOs in the active packages matrix. Thus, the compounds responsible for the biological properties may migrate to food, preventing the degradation of food. Also, the choice of the EO has to be in accordance with the food to prevent a negative sensory property [18, 21, 42].

In addition to the powerful smell and aroma, their low solubility in water and susceptibility for oxidation are also obstacles that can also limit their use. Encapsulation can also be an alternative that can minimize this problem [42].

The toxicity of the EOs can also represent a limitation in the application of these oils.

**Table 2. Essential oils used in food\*.**

| Food group/Food items | Essential oils | Biological properties | References |
|---|---|---|---|
| Fruits | | | |
| "Formosa" plum | Oregano (*Origanum vulgare*), Bergamot (*Citrus bergamia*) | Antimicrobial | [43] |
| Papaya | Oregano (*O. vulgare*), Cinnamon (*Cinnamomum zeylanicum*), Lemongrass (*Cymbopogon flexuosus*) | Antimicrobial | [44] |
| Strawberries | Clove (*Syzygium aromaticum*), Mustard (*Brassica nigra*), Lemon (*Citrus limon* L.) | Antifungal | [45, 46] |
| Vegetable | | | |
| Broccoli | Asian spice; Italian spice | Antimicrobial | [47] |
| Fresh cabbage | Thyme (*Thymus vulgaris*), Oregano (*O. vulgare)*, Lemongrass (*Cymbopogon flexuosus*) | Antibacterial | [48] |
| Minimally processed | *Oregano (O. vulgare)*, Rosemary (*Rosmarinus officinalis*) | Antimicrobial | [49] |
| Swiss chard leaves | Eucalyptus *(Eucalyptus globulus)*, Tea tree *(Melaleuca alternifolia)*, Clove *(Syzygium aromaticum)* | Antimicrobial | [50] |
| Seafood | | | |
| Mediterranean octopus | Oregano (*O. vulgare*) | Antimicrobial | [51] |
| Fish | Clove (*Syzygium aromaticum*) | Antimicrobial; Antioxidant | [52, 53] |
| Rainbow trout fillets | *Zataria multiflora* Boiss. | Antimicrobial; Antioxidant | [54] |
| Sardine | *Mentha suaveolens* | Antimicrobial | [55] |
| Swordfish fillets | Thyme (*T. vulgaris*) | Antimicrobial; Antioxidant | [56] |
| Meat and Chicken | | | |
| Beef patties | Thyme (*T. vulgaris*), Oregano (*O. vulgare*). | Antimicrobial | [57] |
| Beef muscle | Oregano (*O. vulgare)*; Pimento. | Antimicrobial | [58] |
| Bologna and ham | Cinnamon (*Cinnamomum cassia*); Winter savory (*Saturej amontana*). | Antimicrobial | [59] |
| Chicken | Oregano (*O. vulgare*). | Antimicrobial | [60] |
| Chicken breast cuts | Rosemary (*R. officinalis*) | Antimicrobial | [61] |
| Meat | Oregano (*O. vulgare*). | Antimicrobial | [62] |

(Table 2) cont.....

| Food group/Food items | Essential oils | Biological properties | References |
|---|---|---|---|
| Sausage | Basil *(Ocimum basilicum)*. | Antibacterial | [24] |
| Others foods | | | |
| Cheese | Oregano *(O. vulgare)* | Antimicrobial | [63] |
| Rice | *Laurus nobilis*; *Syzygium aromaticum* | Antifungal | [64] |
| Bakery | Cinnamon; clove | Antimicrobial | [65] |
| Pizza | Oregano *(O. vulgare)*. | Antimicrobial | [66] |
| *Essential oils added directly to food or in food packaging (Adapted from Ribeiro-Santos *et al.* 2017d). | | | |

## POSITIVE AND ADVERSE HEALTH EFFECTS

EOs have been used since the beginning of civilizations in traditional medicines, such as Indian (Ayurveda) and Chinese (Zhong Yo) medicines, being a natural alternative to conventional therapy and medication parentheses (Table **3**) [8]. Nevertheless, some of the chemical compounds present in EOs have proved to be harmful to human health or present a hazard when used in certain concentrations [67]. Most of the times, this toxicity is undervalued since essential oils are naturally produced from plants. Also, since they have been used since ancient times for several utilities including medicinal uses, toxicity may be taken lightly [68].

Table 3. Positive effects of different essential oils.

| Scientific name | Common name | Biological activity of the corresponding essential oil | Reference |
|---|---|---|---|
| *Allium cepa* L. | Onion | Antimicrobial | |
| *Aquilaria crassna* Pierre exLecomte | Agarwood | Anti-pancreatic cancer | [69] |
| *Artemisia campestris* | Field wormwood | Insecticidal | [70] |
| *Cinnamomum cassia* (Nees & T. Nees) J.Presl. | Chinese cinnamon | Antimicrobial | [71] |
| *Cinnamomum zeylanicum* Blume | Cinnamon | Antimicrobial | [23] |
| *Cinnamomum* sp. | Cinnamon | Insecticidal, acaricide | [72] |
| *Cuminum cyminum* L. | Cumin | Hepatoprotective | [73] |
| *Elaeoselinum asclepium* (L.) Bertol. | - | Antioxidant and antimicrobial | [74] |
| *Eucalyptus globulus* Labill. | Tasmanian blue gum | Antioxidant | [75] |
| *Eucalyptus globulus* | Tasmanian blue gum | Antimicrobial | [76] |
| *Eucalyptus lehmani* | - | Insecticidal | [77] |

*(Table 3) cont.....*

| Scientific name | Common name | Biological activity of the corresponding essential oil | Reference |
|---|---|---|---|
| *Eucalyptus sideroxylon* | Red iron bark | Antioxidant | [78] |
| *Foeniculum vulgare* Mill | Fennel | Insecticidal | [79] |
| *Illicium verum* Hook.f. | Star anise | Colon cancer | [80] |
| *Juniperus phoenicea* | Phoenicean juniper | Antioxidant | [81] |
| *Lavandula angustifolia* Mill. | Lavender | Analgesic | [82] |
| *Melissa officinalis* L. | Lemon balm | Anti-diabetic | [83] |
| *Mentha pulegium*L. | Pennyroyal | Insecticidal | [84] |
| *Mentha rotundifolia*L. | Apple mint | Insecticidal | |
| *Nigella sativa* L. | Black Cumin | Breast cancer | [85] |
| *Ocimum basilicum* L. | Basil | Antifungal and antibacterial | [24] |
| *Ocimum gratissimum* L. | Basil | Antitrypanosomal and antiplasmodial | [86] |
| *Origanum vulgare* L. | Oregano | Antioxidant | [87] |
| *Origanum vulgare* L. | Oregano | Anti-inflammatory | [88] |
| *Rosmarinus officinalis* L. | Rosemary | Antioxidant, antimicrobial, ant-cancer, anti-inflammatory, anti-diabetic | [37, 86] |
| *Salvia lavandulifolia* Vahl | Spanish sage | Treatment of neurodegenerative diseases | [89] |
| *Salvia officinalis* L. | Sage | Antimicrobial and antioxidant | [39] |
| *Satureja hortensis* L. | Savory | Antifungal | [90] |
| *Skimmia laureola* Franch. | Nazar Panra | Antinociceptive and antipyretic | [91] |
| *Thymus serpyllum* | Wild Thyme | Antioxidant | [87] |
| *Thymus vulgaris* L. | Thyme | Antioxidant and antimicrobial | [22] |

The biological responses of essential oils are due to their chemical composition in which their volatile substances react with biomolecules, producing a biological response. In consequence, the higher the dose, the higher the biological response should be which this may lead to toxicological effects in human organs, for instance, liver necrosis. Given this, it is necessary to maintain a balance between the effective EO dose and the risk of toxicity [21, 68]. For instance, some EOs are considered safe for human consumption at low concentrations [92].

Also, the toxicity of EOs not only relies on the dose intake but also on the used frequency of an essential oil or a specific chemical essential oil compound. The individual susceptibility to a potentially toxic substance is also a factor to consider [92, 93]. EOs interactions can occur between one and more of their constituents, as well as among a component and a drug or a food item [93].

## CONCLUSION

Essential oils represent an incredible potential to be applied directly or indirectly as a food additive due to their powerful biological activities, like antioxidant and antimicrobial capacities. Although, the food industry together with the scientific community has some challenges to overcome regarding these substances. Synergetic and antagonist effects between minor and major compounds have to be studied in further detail, as well as, the optimal concentration that must be added in order to ensure consumer safety.

## CONSENT FOR PUBLICATION

Not applicable.

## CONFLICT OF INTEREST

All authors declare there is no conflict of interest.

## ACKNOWLEDGEMENTS

This work was supported by the research project "i.FILM – Multifunctional Films for Intelligent and Active Applications" (no. 17921) cofounded by European Regional Development Fund (FEDER) through the Competitiveness and Internationalization Operational Program under the "Portugal 2020" Program, Call no. 33/SI/2015, Co-Promotion Projects. Mariana Andrade is grateful for their research grant (2016/iFILM/BM) in the frame of the iFILM project.

## REFERENCES

[1]   Ríos J-L. Essential Oils: What They Are and How the Terms Are Used and Defined.Essent Oils Food Preserv Flavor Saf. 1st ed. Elsevier 2016; pp. 3-10.
      [http://dx.doi.org/10.1016/B978-0-12-416641-7.00001-8]

[2]   Ribeiro-Santos R, Andrade M, de Melo NR, dos Santos FR, Neves I de A, de Carvalho MG, *et al.* Biological activities and major components determination in essential oils intended for a biodegradable food packaging. Ind Crops Prod 2017; 97: 201-10.
      [http://dx.doi.org/10.1016/j.indcrop.2016.12.006]

[3]   Hossain MA, Shah MD, Sang SV, Sakari M. Chemical composition and antibacterial properties of the essential oils and crude extracts of Merremia borneensis J King Saud Univ - Sci 2012; 24: 243-9.
      [http://dx.doi.org/10.1016/j.jksus.2011.03.006]

[4]   Dvaranauskaite A, Venskutonis P, Raynaud C, Talou T, Viškelis P, Sasnauskas A. Variations in the essential oil composition in buds of six blackcurrant (Ribes nigrum L.) cultivars at various development phases. Food Chem 2009; 114: 671-9.
      [http://dx.doi.org/10.1016/j.foodchem.2008.10.005]

[5]   Aidi Wannes W, Mhamdi B, Sriti J, *et al.* Antioxidant activities of the essential oils and methanol extracts from myrtle (Myrtus communis var. italica L.) leaf, stem and flower. Food Chem Toxicol

2010; 48(5): 1362-70.
[http://dx.doi.org/10.1016/j.fct.2010.03.002] [PMID: 20211674]

[6]     Lv J, Huang H, Yu L, *et al.* Phenolic composition and nutraceutical properties of organic and conventional cinnamon and peppermint. Food Chem 2012; 132(3): 1442-50.
[http://dx.doi.org/10.1016/j.foodchem.2011.11.135] [PMID: 29243634]

[7]     Hill LE, Gomes C, Taylor TM. Characterization of beta-cyclodextrin inclusion complexes containing essential oils (trans-cinnamaldehyde, eugenol, cinnamon bark, and clove bud extracts) for antimicrobial delivery applications. Lebensm Wiss Technol 2013; 51: 86-93.
[http://dx.doi.org/10.1016/j.lwt.2012.11.011]

[8]     Nakatsu T, Lupo AT, Chinn JW, Kang RKL. Biological Activity of Essential Oils and Their Constituents (Part B). In: Rahman Atta-ur, Ed. Stud Nat Prod Chem. Elsevier B.V 2000; 21: pp. 571-631.

[9]     Elzaawely AA, Xuan TD, Koyama H, Tawata S. Antioxidant activity and contents of essential oil and phenolic compounds in flowers and seeds of Alpinia zerumbet (Pers.). BL Burtt & RM Sm Food Chem 2007; 104: 1648-53.
[http://dx.doi.org/10.1016/j.foodchem.2007.03.016]

[10]    Bendahou M, Muselli A, Grignon-Dubois M, Benyoucef M, Desjobert J-M, Bernardini A-F, *et al.* Antimicrobial activity and chemical composition of Origanum glandulosum Desf. essential oil and extract obtained by microwave extraction: Comparison with hydrodistillation. Food Chem 2008; 106: 132-9.
[http://dx.doi.org/10.1016/j.foodchem.2007.05.050]

[11]    Stratakos AC, Koidis A. Methods for Extracting Essential Oils.Essent Oils Food Preserv Flavor Saf. Elsevier 2016; pp. 31-8.
[http://dx.doi.org/10.1016/B978-0-12-416641-7.00004-3]

[12]    Cooke M, Poole CF, Wilson ID, Adlard ER, Eds. Encyclopedia of Separation Science. Academic Press 2000.

[13]    Rashidi S, Eikani MH, Ardjmand M. Extraction of Hyssopus officinalis L. essential oil using instant controlled pressure drop process. J Chromatogr A 2018; 1579: 9-19.
[http://dx.doi.org/10.1016/j.chroma.2018.10.020] [PMID: 30430990]

[14]    Vilkhu K, Mawson R, Simons L, Bates D. Applications and opportunities for ultrasound assisted extraction in the food industry — A review. Innov Food Sci Emerg Technol 2008; 9: 161-9.
[http://dx.doi.org/10.1016/j.ifset.2007.04.014]

[15]    Carocho M, Morales P, Ferreira ICFR. Natural food additives: Quo vadis? Trends Food Sci Technol 2015; 45: 284-95.
[http://dx.doi.org/10.1016/j.tifs.2015.06.007]

[16]    Pereira de Abreu DA, Losada PP, Maroto J, Cruz JM. Evaluation of the effectiveness of a new active packaging film containing natural antioxidants (from barley husks) that retard lipid damage in frozen Atlantic salmon (Salmo salar L.). Food Res Int 2010; 43: 1277-82.
[http://dx.doi.org/10.1016/j.foodres.2010.03.019]

[17]    Sanches-Silva A, Costa D, Albuquerque TG, *et al.* Trends in the use of natural antioxidants in active food packaging: a review. Food Addit Contam Part A Chem Anal Control Expo Risk Assess 2014; 31(3): 374-95.
[http://dx.doi.org/10.1080/19440049.2013.879215] [PMID: 24405324]

[18]    Ribeiro-Santos R, Sanches-Silva A, Motta JFG, Andrade M, Neves I de A, Teófilo RF, *et al.* Combined use of essential oils applied to protein base active food packaging: Study *in vitro* and in a food simulant. Eur Polym J 2017; 93: 75-86.
[http://dx.doi.org/10.1016/j.eurpolymj.2017.03.055]

[19]    Segvić Klarić M, Kosalec I, Mastelić J, Piecková E, Pepeljnak S. Antifungal activity of thyme

(Thymus vulgaris L.) essential oil and thymol against moulds from damp dwellings. Lett Appl Microbiol 2007; 44(1): 36-42.
[http://dx.doi.org/10.1111/j.1472-765X.2006.02032.x] [PMID: 17209812]

[20] Teixeira B, Marques A, Ramos C, Batista I, Serrano C, Matos O, *et al.* European pennyroyal (Mentha pulegium) from Portugal: Chemical composition of essential oil and antioxidant and antimicrobial properties of extracts and essential oil. Ind Crops Prod 2012; 36: 81-7.
[http://dx.doi.org/10.1016/j.indcrop.2011.08.011]

[21] Sánchez-González L, Vargas M, González-Martínez C, Chiralt A, Cháfer M. Use of Essential Oils in Bioactive Edible Coatings: A Review. Food Eng Rev 2011; 3: 1-16.
[http://dx.doi.org/10.1007/s12393-010-9031-3]

[22] Bozin B, Mimica-Dukic N, Simin N, Anackov G. Characterization of the volatile composition of essential oils of some lamiaceae spices and the antimicrobial and antioxidant activities of the entire oils. J Agric Food Chem 2006; 54(5): 1822-8.
[http://dx.doi.org/10.1021/jf051922u] [PMID: 16506839]

[23] Hussain AI, Anwar F, Hussain Sherazi ST, Przybylski R. Chemical composition, antioxidant and antimicrobial activities of basil (Ocimum basilicum) essential oils depends on seasonal variations. Food Chem 2008; 108(3): 986-95.
[http://dx.doi.org/10.1016/j.foodchem.2007.12.010] [PMID: 26065762]

[24] Gaio I, Saggiorato AG, Treichel H, Cichoski AJ, Astolfi V, Cardoso RI, *et al.* Antibacterial activity of basil essential oil (Ocimum basilicum L.) in Italian-type sausage. J Für Verbraucherschutz Und Leb 2015; 10: 323-9.
[http://dx.doi.org/10.1007/s00003-015-0936-x]

[25] Lv F, Liang H, Yuan Q, Li C. *In vitro* antimicrobial effects and mechanism of action of selected plant essential oil combinations against four food-related microorganisms. Food Res Int 2011; 44: 3057-64.
[http://dx.doi.org/10.1016/j.foodres.2011.07.030]

[26] Jrah Harzallah H, Kouidhi B, Flamini G, Bakhrouf A, Mahjoub T. Chemical composition, antimicrobial potential against cariogenic bacteria and cytotoxic activity of Tunisian Nigella sativa essential oil and thymoquinone. Food Chem 2011; 129: 1469-74.
[http://dx.doi.org/10.1016/j.foodchem.2011.05.117]

[27] Santos TG, Dognini J, Begnini IM, Rebelo RA, Verdi M, de Gasper AL, *et al.* Chemical characterization of essential oils from Drimys angustifolia miers (Winteraceae) and antibacterial activity of their major compounds. J Braz Chem Soc 2013; 24: 164-70.
[http://dx.doi.org/10.1590/S0103-50532013000100020]

[28] Ooi LSM, Li Y, Kam S-L, Wang H, Wong EYL, Ooi VEC. Antimicrobial activities of cinnamon oil and cinnamaldehyde from the Chinese medicinal herb Cinnamomum cassia Blume. Am J Chin Med 2006; 34(3): 511-22.
[http://dx.doi.org/10.1142/S0192415X06004041] [PMID: 16710900]

[29] Prabuseenivasan S, Jayakumar M, Ignacimuthu S. *In vitro* antibacterial activity of some plant essential oils. BMC Complement Altern Med 2006; 6: 39.
[http://dx.doi.org/10.1186/1472-6882-6-39] [PMID: 17134518]

[30] Ud-Daula AFMS, Demirci F, Abu Salim K, Demirci B, Lim LBL, Baser KHC, *et al.* Chemical composition, antioxidant and antimicrobial activities of essential oils from leaves, aerial stems, basal stems, and rhizomes of Etlingera fimbriobracteata (K.Schum.) R.M.Sm. Ind Crops Prod 2016; 84: 189-98.
[http://dx.doi.org/10.1016/j.indcrop.2015.12.034]

[31] Ross ZM, O'Gara EA, Hill DJ, Sleightholme HV, Maslin DJ. Antimicrobial properties of garlic oil against human enteric bacteria: evaluation of methodologies and comparisons with garlic oil sulfides and garlic powder. Appl Environ Microbiol 2001; 67(1): 475-80.
[http://dx.doi.org/10.1128/AEM.67.1.475-480.2001] [PMID: 11133485]

[32]   Naik MI, Fomda BA, Jaykumar E, Bhat JA. Antibacterial activity of lemongrass (Cymbopogon citratus) oil against some selected pathogenic bacterias. Asian Pac J Trop Med 2010; 3: 535-8.
       [http://dx.doi.org/10.1016/S1995-7645(10)60129-0]

[33]   Ye C-L, Dai D-H, Hu W-L. Antimicrobial and antioxidant activities of the essential oil from onion (Allium cepa L.). Food Control 2013; 30: 48-53.
       [http://dx.doi.org/10.1016/j.foodcont.2012.07.033]

[34]   Mahboubi M, Haghi G. Antimicrobial activity and chemical composition of Mentha pulegium L. essential oil. J Ethnopharmacol 2008; 119(2): 325-7.
       [http://dx.doi.org/10.1016/j.jep.2008.07.023] [PMID: 18703127]

[35]   Ojeda-Sana AM, van Baren CM, Elechosa MA, Juárez MA, Moreno S. New insights into antibacterial and antioxidant activities of rosemary essential oils and their main components. Food Control 2013; 31: 189-95.
       [http://dx.doi.org/10.1016/j.foodcont.2012.09.022]

[36]   Jordán MJ, Lax V, Rota MC, Lorán S, Sotomayor JA. Effect of bioclimatic area on the essential oil composition and antibacterial activity of Rosmarinus officinalis L. Food Control 2013; 30: 463-8.
       [http://dx.doi.org/10.1016/j.foodcont.2012.07.029]

[37]   Bouaziz M, Yangui T, Sayadi S, Dhouib A. Disinfectant properties of essential oils from Salvia officinalis L. cultivated in Tunisia. Food Chem Toxicol 2009; 47(11): 2755-60.
       [http://dx.doi.org/10.1016/j.fct.2009.08.005] [PMID: 19682532]

[38]   Longaray Delamare AP, Moschen-Pistorello IT, Artico L, Atti-Serafini L, Echeverrigaray S. Antibacterial activity of the essential oils of Salvia officinalis L. and Salvia triloba L. cultivated in South Brazil. Food Chem 2007; 100: 603-8.
       [http://dx.doi.org/10.1016/j.foodchem.2005.09.078]

[39]   Ribeiro-Santos R, Andrade M, Sanches-Silva A. Application of encapsulated essential oils as antimicrobial agents in food packaging. Curr Opin Food Sci 2017; 14: 78-84.
       [http://dx.doi.org/10.1016/j.cofs.2017.01.012]

[40]   Food And Drug Administration (FDA). 182.20 Essential oils, oleoresins (solvent-free), and natural extractives (including distillates). Title 21 Food Drugs 2017.

[41]   European Parliament and the Council of the European Union. Regulation (EU) No 1334/2008. Off J. Eur Union 2008; 34-50.

[42]   Ribeiro-Santos R, Andrade M, de Melo NR, Sanches-Silva A. Use of essential oils in active food packaging: Recent advances and future trends. Trends Food Sci Technol 2017; 61: 132-40.
       [http://dx.doi.org/10.1016/j.tifs.2016.11.021]

[43]   Choi WS, Singh S, Lee YS. Characterization of edible film containing essential oils in hydroxypropyl methylcellulose and its effect on quality attributes of 'Formosa' plum (Prunus salicina L.). Lebensm Wiss Technol 2016; 70: 213-22.
       [http://dx.doi.org/10.1016/j.lwt.2016.02.036]

[44]   Espitia PJP, Soares N de FF, Botti LCM, de Melo NR, Pereira OL, da Silva WA. Assessment of the efficiency of essential oils in the preservation of postharvest papaya in an antimicrobial packaging system. Braz J Food Technol 2012; 15: 333-42.
       [http://dx.doi.org/10.1590/S1981-67232012005000027]

[45]   Aguilar-González AE, Palou E, López-Malo A. Antifungal activity of essential oils of clove (Syzygium aromaticum) and/or mustard (Brassica nigra) in vapor phase against gray mold (Botrytis cinerea) in strawberries. Innov Food Sci Emerg Technol 2015; 32: 181-5.
       [http://dx.doi.org/10.1016/j.ifset.2015.09.003]

[46]   Perdones Á, Escriche I, Chiralt A, Vargas M. Effect of chitosan-lemon essential oil coatings on volatile profile of strawberries during storage. Food Chem 2016; 197(Pt A): 979-86.
       [http://dx.doi.org/10.1016/j.foodchem.2015.11.054] [PMID: 26617043]

[47]  Takala PN, Vu KD, Salmieri S, Khan RA, Lacroix M. Antibacterial effect of biodegradable active packaging on the growth of Escherichia coli, Salmonella typhimurium and Listeria monocytogenes in fresh broccoli stored at 4 °C. Lebensm Wiss Technol 2013; 53: 499-506.
[http://dx.doi.org/10.1016/j.lwt.2013.02.024]

[48]  Hyun J-E, Bae Y-M, Yoon J-H, Lee S-Y. Preservative effectiveness of essential oils in vapor phase combined with modified atmosphere packaging against spoilage bacteria on fresh cabbage. Food Control 2015; 51: 307-13.
[http://dx.doi.org/10.1016/j.foodcont.2014.11.030]

[49]  de Azeredo GA, Stamford TLM, Nunes PC, Gomes Neto NJ, de Oliveira MEG, de Souza EL. Combined application of essential oils from Origanum vulgare L. and Rosmarinus officinalis L. to inhibit bacteria and autochthonous microflora associated with minimally processed vegetables. Food Res Int 2011; 44: 1541-8.
[http://dx.doi.org/10.1016/j.foodres.2011.04.012]

[50]  Ponce AG, del Valle CE, Roura SI. Natural essential oils as reducing agents of peroxidase activity in leafy vegetables. Lebensm Wiss Technol 2004; 37: 199-204.
[http://dx.doi.org/10.1016/j.lwt.2003.07.005]

[51]  Atrea I, Papavergou A, Amvrosiadis I, Savvaidis IN. Combined effect of vacuum-packaging and oregano essential oil on the shelf-life of Mediterranean octopus (Octopus vulgaris) from the Aegean Sea stored at 4 ° C. Food Microbiol 2009; 26(2): 166-72.
[http://dx.doi.org/10.1016/j.fm.2008.10.005] [PMID: 19171258]

[52]  Gómez-Estaca J, López de Lacey A, López-Caballero ME, Gómez-Guillén MC, Montero P. Biodegradable gelatin-chitosan films incorporated with essential oils as antimicrobial agents for fish preservation. Food Microbiol 2010; 27(7): 889-96.
[http://dx.doi.org/10.1016/j.fm.2010.05.012] [PMID: 20688230]

[53]  Salgado PR, López-Caballero ME, Gómez-Guillén MC, Mauri AN, Montero MP. Sunflower protein films incorporated with clove essential oil have potential application for the preservation of fish patties. Food Hydrocoll 2013; 33: 74-84.
[http://dx.doi.org/10.1016/j.foodhyd.2013.02.008]

[54]  Raeisi M, Tajik H, Aliakbarlu J, Mirhosseini SH, Hosseini SMH. Effect of carboxymethyl cellulose-based coatings incorporated with Zataria multiflora Boiss. essential oil and grape seed extract on the shelf life of rainbow trout fillets. Lebensm Wiss Technol 2015; 64: 898-904.
[http://dx.doi.org/10.1016/j.lwt.2015.06.010]

[55]  Petretto GL, Fancello F, Zara S, et al. Antimicrobial activity against beneficial microorganisms and chemical composition of essential oil of Mentha suaveolens ssp. insularis grown in Sardinia. J Food Sci 2014; 79(3): M369-77.
[http://dx.doi.org/10.1111/1750-3841.12343] [PMID: 24506214]

[56]  Kykkidou S, Giatrakou V, Papavergou A, Kontominas MG, Savvaidis IN. Effect of thyme essential oil and packaging treatments on fresh Mediterranean swordfish fillets during storage at 4°C. Food Chem 2009; 115: 169-75.
[http://dx.doi.org/10.1016/j.foodchem.2008.11.083]

[57]  Emiroğlu ZK, Yemiş GP, Coşkun BK, Candoğan K. Antimicrobial activity of soy edible films incorporated with thyme and oregano essential oils on fresh ground beef patties. Meat Sci 2010; 86(2): 283-8.
[http://dx.doi.org/10.1016/j.meatsci.2010.04.016] [PMID: 20580990]

[58]  Oussalah M, Caillet S, Salmiéri S, Saucier L, Lacroix M. Antimicrobial and antioxidant effects of milk protein-based film containing essential oils for the preservation of whole beef muscle. J Agric Food Chem 2004; 52(18): 5598-605.
[http://dx.doi.org/10.1021/jf049389q] [PMID: 15373399]

[59]  Oussalah M, Caillet S, Salmiéri S, Saucier L, Lacroix M. Antimicrobial effects of alginate-based films

containing essential oils on Listeria monocytogenes and Salmonella typhimurium present in bologna and ham. J Food Prot 2007; 70(4): 901-8.
[http://dx.doi.org/10.4315/0362-028X-70.4.901] [PMID: 17477259]

[60]   Fernández-Pan I, Carrión-Granda X, Maté JI. Antimicrobial efficiency of edible coatings on the preservation of chicken breast fillets. Food Control 2014; 36: 69-75.
[http://dx.doi.org/10.1016/j.foodcont.2013.07.032]

[61]   de Melo AA, Geraldine RM, Silveira MF, *et al.* Microbiological quality and other characteristics of refrigerated chicken meat in contact with cellulose acetate-based film incorporated with rosemary essential oil. Braz J Microbiol 2012; 43(4): 1419-27.
[http://dx.doi.org/10.1590/S1517-83822012000400025] [PMID: 24031972]

[62]   Skandamis PN, Nychas G-JE. Preservation of fresh meat with active and modified atmosphere packaging conditions. Int J Food Microbiol 2002; 79(1-2): 35-45.
[http://dx.doi.org/10.1016/S0168-1605(02)00177-0] [PMID: 12382683]

[63]   Otero V, Becerril R, Santos JA, Rodríguez-Calleja JM, Nerín C, García-López M-L. Evaluation of two antimicrobial packaging films against Escherichia coli O157:H7 strains *in vitro* and during storage of a Spanish ripened sheep cheese (Zamorano). Food Control 2014; 42: 296-302.
[http://dx.doi.org/10.1016/j.foodcont.2014.02.022]

[64]   Pilar Santamarina M, Roselló J, Giménez S, Amparo Blázquez M. Commercial Laurus nobilis L. and Syzygium aromaticum L. Merr. & Perry essential oils against post-harvest phytopathogenic fungi on rice. Lebensm Wiss Technol 2016; 65: 325-32.
[http://dx.doi.org/10.1016/j.lwt.2015.08.040]

[65]   Souza AC, Goto GEO, Mainardi JA, Coelho ACV, Tadini CC. Cassava starch composite films incorporated with cinnamon essential oil: Antimicrobial activity, microstructure, mechanical and barrier properties. Lebensm Wiss Technol 2013; 54: 346-52.
[http://dx.doi.org/10.1016/j.lwt.2013.06.017]

[66]   Botre DA, Soares N de FF, Espitia PJP, de Sousa S, Renhe IRT. Avaliação de filme incorporado com óleo essencial de orégano para conservação de pizza pronta. Rev Ceres 2010; 57: 283-91.
[http://dx.doi.org/10.1590/S0034-737X2010000300001]

[67]   European Commission. Commission Implementing Regulation (EU) Nº 872/2012. Off J. Eur Union 2012; 1-161.

[68]   Baser KHC, Buchbauer G, Eds. Handbook of Essential Oils: Science, Technology and Applications. CRC Press 2010.

[69]   Dahham SS, Tabana YM, Ahmed Hassan LE, Khadeer Ahamed MB, Abdul Majid AS, Abdul Majid AMS. *In vitro* antimetastatic activity of Agarwood (Aquilaria crassna) essential oils against pancreatic cancer cells. Alexandria J Med 2016; 52: 141-50.
[http://dx.doi.org/10.1016/j.ajme.2015.07.001]

[70]   Titouhi F, Amri M, Messaoud C, Haouel S, Youssfi S, Cherif A, *et al.* Protective effects of three Artemisia essential oils against Callosobruchus maculatus and Bruchus rufimanus (Coleoptera: Chrysomelidae) and the extended side-effects on their natural enemies. J Stored Prod Res 2017; 72: 11-20.
[http://dx.doi.org/10.1016/j.jspr.2017.02.007]

[71]   Ghabraie M, Vu KD, Tata L, Salmieri S, Lacroix M. Antimicrobial effect of essential oils in combinations against five bacteria and their effect on sensorial quality of ground meat. Lebensm Wiss Technol 2016; 66: 332-9.
[http://dx.doi.org/10.1016/j.lwt.2015.10.055]

[72]   Ribeiro-Santos R, Andrade M, Madella D, Martinazzo AP, de Aquino Garcia Moura L, de Melo NR, *et al.* Revisiting an ancient spice with medicinal purposes: Cinnamon. Trends Food Sci Technol 2017; 62: 154-69.
[http://dx.doi.org/10.1016/j.tifs.2017.02.011]

[73] Mostafa DM, Kassem AA, Asfour MH, Al Okbi SY, Mohamed DA, Hamed TE-S. Transdermal cumin essential oil nanoemulsions with potent antioxidant and hepatoprotective activities: In-vitro and in-vivo evaluation. J Mol Liq 2015; 212: 6-15.
[http://dx.doi.org/10.1016/j.molliq.2015.08.047]

[74] Bouchekrit M, Laouer H, Hajji M, Nasri M, Haroutounian SA, Akkal S. Essential oils from Elaeoselinum asclepium: Chemical composition, antimicrobial and antioxidant properties. Asian Pac J Trop Biomed 2016; 6: 851-7.
[http://dx.doi.org/10.1016/j.apjtb.2016.07.014]

[75] Luís Â, Duarte A, Gominho J, Domingues F, Duarte AP. Chemical composition, antioxidant, antibacterial and anti-quorum sensing activities of Eucalyptus globulus and Eucalyptus radiata essential oils. Ind Crops Prod 2016; 79: 274-82.
[http://dx.doi.org/10.1016/j.indcrop.2015.10.055]

[76] Harkat-Madouri L, Asma B, Madani K, Bey-Ould Si Said Z, Rigou P, Grenier D, et al. Chemical composition, antibacterial and antioxidant activities of essential oil of Eucalyptus globulus from Algeria. Ind Crops Prod 2015; 78: 148-53.
[http://dx.doi.org/10.1016/j.indcrop.2015.10.015]

[77] Hamdi SH, Hedjal-Chebheb M, Kellouche A, Khouja ML, Boudabous A, Ben Jemâa JM. Management of three pests' population strains from Tunisia and Algeria using Eucalyptus essential oils. Ind Crops Prod 2015; 74: 551-6.
[http://dx.doi.org/10.1016/j.indcrop.2015.05.072]

[78] Shahwar D, Raza MA, Bukhari S, Bukhari G. Ferric reducing antioxidant power of essential oils extracted from Eucalyptus and Curcuma species. Asian Pac J Trop Biomed 2012; 2: S1633-6.
[http://dx.doi.org/10.1016/S2221-1691(12)60467-5]

[79] Pavela R, Žabka M, Bednář J, Tříska J, Vrchotová N. New knowledge for yield, composition and insecticidal activity of essential oils obtained from the aerial parts or seeds of fennel (Foeniculum vulgare Mill.). Ind Crops Prod 2016; 83: 275-82.
[http://dx.doi.org/10.1016/j.indcrop.2015.11.090]

[80] Asif M, Yehya AHS, Al-Mansoub MA, Revadigar V, Ezzat MO, Khadeer Ahamed MB, et al. Anticancer attributes of Illicium verum essential oils against colon cancer. S Afr J Bot 2016; 103: 156-61.
[http://dx.doi.org/10.1016/j.sajb.2015.08.017]

[81] Keskes H, Mnafgui K, Hamden K, Damak M, El Feki A, Allouche N. In vitro anti-diabetic, anti-obesity and antioxidant proprieties of Juniperus phoenicea L. leaves from Tunisia. Asian Pac J Trop Biomed 2014; 4: S649-55.
[http://dx.doi.org/10.12980/APJTB.4.201414B114]

[82] Ghods AA, Abforosh NH, Ghorbani R, Asgari MR. The effect of topical application of lavender essential oil on the intensity of pain caused by the insertion of dialysis needles in hemodialysis patients: A randomized clinical trial. Complement Ther Med 2015; 23(3): 325-30.
[http://dx.doi.org/10.1016/j.ctim.2015.03.001] [PMID: 26051566]

[83] Yen H-F, Hsieh C-T, Hsieh T-J, Chang F-R, Wang C-K. In vitro anti-diabetic effect and chemical component analysis of 29 essential oils products. Yao Wu Shi Pin Fen Xi 2015; 23(1): 124-9.
[http://dx.doi.org/10.1016/j.jfda.2014.02.004] [PMID: 28911435]

[84] Brahmi F, Abdenour A, Bruno M, Silvia P, Alessandra P, Danilo F, et al. Chemical composition and in vitro antimicrobial, insecticidal and antioxidant activities of the essential oils of Mentha pulegium L. and Mentha rotundifolia (L.) Huds growing in Algeria. Ind Crops Prod 2016; 88: 96-105.
[http://dx.doi.org/10.1016/j.indcrop.2016.03.002]

[85] Periasamy VS, Athinarayanan J, Alshatwi AA. Anticancer activity of an ultrasonic nanoemulsion formulation of Nigella sativa L. essential oil on human breast cancer cells. Ultrason Sonochem 2016; 31: 449-55.

[http://dx.doi.org/10.1016/j.ultsonch.2016.01.035] [PMID: 26964971]

[86]   Kpadonou Kpoviessi BGH, Kpoviessi SDS, Yayi Ladekan E, *et al*. *In vitro* antitrypanosomal and antiplasmodial activities of crude extracts and essential oils of Ocimum gratissimum Linn from Benin and influence of vegetative stage. J Ethnopharmacol 2014; 155(3): 1417-23.
[http://dx.doi.org/10.1016/j.jep.2014.07.014] [PMID: 25058875]

[87]   Lin C-W, Yu C-W, Wu S-C, Yih K-H. DPPH Free-Radical Scavenging Activity, Total Phenolic Contents and Chemical Composition Analysis of Forty-Two Kinds of Essential Oils. Yao Wu Shi Pin Fen Xi 2009; 17: 386-95.

[88]   Ocaña-Fuentes A, Arranz-Gutiérrez E, Señorans FJ, Reglero G. Supercritical fluid extraction of oregano (Origanum vulgare) essentials oils: anti-inflammatory properties based on cytokine response on THP-1 macrophages. Food Chem Toxicol 2010; 48(6): 1568-75.
[http://dx.doi.org/10.1016/j.fct.2010.03.026] [PMID: 20332013]

[89]   Porres-Martínez M, González-Burgos E, Accame MEC, Gómez-Serranillos MP. Phytochemical composition, antioxidant and cytoprotective activities of essential oil of Salvia lavandulifolia Vahl. Food Res Int 2013; 54: 523-31.
[http://dx.doi.org/10.1016/j.foodres.2013.07.029]

[90]   Razzaghi-Abyaneh M, Shams-Ghahfarokhi M, Yoshinari T, *et al*. Inhibitory effects of Satureja hortensis L. essential oil on growth and aflatoxin production by Aspergillus parasiticus. Int J Food Microbiol 2008; 123(3): 228-33.
[http://dx.doi.org/10.1016/j.ijfoodmicro.2008.02.003] [PMID: 18353477]

[91]   Muhammad N, Barkatullah , Ibrar M, *et al*. *In vivo* screening of essential oils of Skimmia laureola leaves for antinociceptive and antipyretic activity. Asian Pac J Trop Biomed 2013; 3(3): 202-6.
[http://dx.doi.org/10.1016/S2221-1691(13)60050-7] [PMID: 23620838]

[92]   Raut JS, Karuppayil SM. A status review on the medicinal properties of essential oils. Ind Crops Prod 2014; 62: 250-64.
[http://dx.doi.org/10.1016/j.indcrop.2014.05.055]

[93]   Unlu M, Ergene E, Unlu GV, Zeytinoglu HS, Vural N. Composition, antimicrobial activity and *in vitro* cytotoxicity of essential oil from Cinnamomum zeylanicum Blume (Lauraceae). Food Chem Toxicol 2010; 48(11): 3274-80.
[http://dx.doi.org/10.1016/j.fct.2010.09.001] [PMID: 20828600]

CHAPTER 7

# Colouring Agents

**Natália Martins** and **Isabel C.F.R. Ferreira**[*]

*Centro de Investigação de Montanha (CIMO), Instituto Politécnico de Bragança, 5300-253 Bragança, Portugal*

**Abstract:** The world of food colorants has experienced a very exciting development in the last few years. The demand for increasingly organoleptic appealing, a safer, secure and healthy foodstuff is evident for consumers. Among them, the health-promoting ability of food products containing colouring agents is considered the most important. Linked with this, natural food colorants have been proposed as the most promising and safe alternatives. Numerous side effects and related toxicity have been increasingly associated with the consumption of synthetic colorants, some being already forbidden, while for others, the adequate daily intake (ADI) was re-adjusted. Thus, the aim of the present chapter is to provide an overview on the field of food colouring agents, namely highlighting the currently available natural and synthetic sources of colouring agents, the main representative groups and corresponding physicochemical properties, legislation and regulatory practices, and finally the latest pharmacokinetic data.

Phenolic compounds, including anthocyanins, carotenoids, and betalains, comprise the most commonly used food colouring agents from natural origin. At the same time, increasingly strict regulatory practices have been applied for the quality assurance of those from natural and synthetic origins. Naturally-derived food colorants seem to have higher quality and efficiency than those from synthetic sources, apart from playing a significant role as health promoters. Concerning synthetic food colorants, due to the increase in the reported side effects and toxicity, they have been progressively substituted by those obtained from natural origin. Allergic reactions, behavioral and neurocognitive effects are among the most frequent side effects, both at medium and long-terms.

Overall, a marked change in attitude and priorities has been observed in consumers, not only related to food and nutrition science, but also pharmaceutical, nutraceutical and cosmetic industries. It drives manufacturers to find new, natural and healthy sources of colors and flavors and other organoleptic attributes for the currently marketed food products.

**Keywords:** Colorant additives, Health-related impact, Natural pigments, Organoleptic features, Synthetic pigments.

---

[*] **Corresponding author Isabel C.F.R. Ferreira:** Centro de Investigação de Montanha (CIMO), Instituto Politécnico de Bragança, 5300-253 Bragança, Portugal; E-mail: iferreira@ipb.pt

**Seyed Mohammad Nabavi *et al.* (Eds.)**

# INTRODUCTORY SECTION

Color food additives are amongst the most interesting case-studies at the biotechnological and scientific levels [1, 2]. There are no doubts that color has an impressive and direct contribution in the delightful attributes of foodstuff, and therefore exerts a large influence on consumers' perceptions, opinions, and consequent modulation of their food preferences, selection and eating desires [3 - 5].

In a broad sense, food colorants are commonly defined as *"any dye, pigment or substance which when added or applied to a food, drug or cosmetic, or to the human body, is capable (alone or through reactions with other substances) of imparting color"* [6]. But, apart from their colouring attributes, food dyes can also be effectively used to contribute to flavoring assurance, safety, quality and maintenance of organoleptic characteristics of numerous food products, as well as to ensure consumer satisfaction. The high delivery of products with multiple formats, colors, tastes, smells and textures available in markets and supermarkets is surprising [1, 2, 7]. Biotechnological industries have largely contributed to current advances observed in the area of food science and technology, but it is also important to emphasize that most of them derive from consumer desires and specific needs [1, 4, 5]. These improvements, apart from increasing appealing and sensorial attractiveness (such as visual perception, color and smell) of numerous foodstuff, confer important benefits on its shelf life, microbiological quality and security and also added-value to food products [1, 8].

Despite that natural foodstuff having their organoleptic characteristics, color intensity and physicochemical attributes, storage and processing conditions/ practices exert a pronounced influence on their final coloration, leading to some unpleasant features that modern consumers do not appreciate. Thus, colouring agents appeared as an effective strategy to overcome these problems/constraints. Being increasingly appreciated and selected for multiple purposes, food colorants have also been targeted by highly strict regulatory legislation, and at the same time, a progressive replacement of synthetic dyes from natural sources has been observed. All these improvements firstly aimed to ensure consumer safety and security are moved by the increasing scientific knowledge about all these food ingredients, and by the good manufacturing practices followed by food industries [2, 9, 10]. The European Food and Safety Authority (EFSA) and Food and Drug Administration (FDA) are the most important regulatory organizations endowed with the responsibility to ensure the quality and security of food products and to promote human health and wellbeing [1, 11].

Currently, due to the increasing knowledge on the field of food science and technology, several food colorants that were used for decades are no longer available, because of the doubtless evidences of their side effects and toxicity at middle-, medium- and even long-terms. Several organic disturbances were described, up to the point that beyond it, different food ingredients were forbidden, maximum levels and toxicological data were also established. It is important to emphasize is that not only synthetic food colorants but also commercial plant-animal sources have been progressively suspended by those regulatory authorities [11 - 13]. However, the formulation of food products containing natural ingredients has received pivotal attention for three different reasons. The first one is because a particular interest of natural pigments on daily food has been shown by modern consumers' that are increasingly informed about the latest advances on food science and health promotion [12, 14, 15]. Secondly, manufacturing industries, moved by the increasing consumer requests for healthy food products containing natural pigments in detriment of the synthetic ones, and by the strict regulatory guidelines, have adapted/replaced a broad variety of formulation techniques and food ingredients [16, 17]. Finally, recent investigations have demonstrated that natural food colorants are safer and provide health benefits besides conferring organoleptic features, related to different biological functions and disease-preventing properties [1, 8, 12].

Based on these aspects, the present chapter aims to provide an overview on the field of food colorants, as shown in Fig. (1). It emphasises on the currently available natural and synthetic sources of colouring agents, the main representative groups and corresponding physicochemical properties, legislation and regulatory guidelines, including safe and maximum levels, toxicological data and their positive and/or side effects.

## FOOD ADDITIVES: THE PARTICULAR CASE OF COLOURING AGENTS

Food additives have received great attention in the last few decades, and presently achieved a renowned status at industrial and scientific levels. Consumers' demands have exerted a pivotal impact on these advances, even triggered the emergence of very interesting opportunities in the food industry [14, 15]. In spite of their ancient use, particularly food colorants have received marked attention, and most specifically, natural food colorants reached the top of demands. It is unquestionable their prominent ability to color foods, but in the last years, its ability to provide health-related benefits has also been largely highlighted [5, 8, 18]. Modern consumers are not so much focused on delightful, attractive and pleasant foodstuffs, but instead, a great interest has been given to its ability for health promotion, disease prevention and to be used as add-value ingredients [15,

19, 20].

In spite, the assurance of consumers' requirements satisfaction at a level of organoleptic characteristics triggers the growing interest for synthetic food colorants, presently and considering the latest demands related to health maintenance, the addition of natural pigments to food products, in detriment of synthetic ones, has been increasingly requested. These marked changes are mainly related to the fact that clearly evident side effects, signals of toxicity at short-, middle- and even long-terms, and also health impairment abilities, including possible carcinogenic effects, have been attributed to synthetic colorants consumption [1, 11].

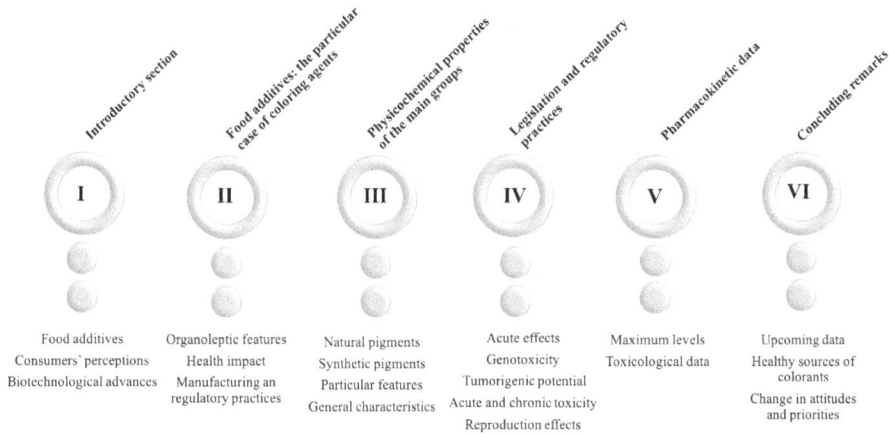

**Fig. (1).**  Brief overview of the structure and contents of this chapter.

Synthetic colorants are no longer available, but even the other ones in which no associated negative effects were reported, have been increasingly avoided by worldwide consumers. Thus, natural ones apart from being markedly requested, doubtless evidences have revealed that they are more effective as those derived from chemical synthesis. Furthermore, they are also able to provide considerable health benefits besides their prominent organoleptic features, being more safe and feasible to confer functional properties to foodstuffs, at the same time, that present a marked ability to exert more than two single benefits as food ingredients (*i.e.*, colouring attributes plus antioxidant and even preservative effects) [1, 8, 12]. Not least interesting to highlight is that data have revealed that health concerns of modern consumers are more likely related to the choice of functional foods for its disease-preventing properties and not so much for its risk-reducing or appearance-enhancing abilities [21]. This is in accordance with the latest reported data related to consumers' demands for industries, accompanied by the highly specific regulatory guidelines that have been implemented in order to ensure consumers' safety and quality of life [22 - 24]. But, beyond these aspects, another main goal of legislation practices is to ensure adequate labeling information of marketed foodstuffs [25], considering that inappropriate labels have been occasionally found in different food products.

Thus, proper manufacturing and legislation of current foodstuffs are of the utmost importance not only to ensure the final quality of final products, consumers' safety and satisfaction, and simultaneously the general recognition of agro-industrial and biotechnological procedures.

## PHYSICOCHEMICAL PROPERTIES OF THE MAIN GROUPS

Due to consumers' requirements and factors for advancements, there are no doubts that increasing market pressure has been put on food and biotechnological industries [1, 19]. Among other goals, it is clearly evident that agro-industrial and biotechnological industries mainly aim to ensure consumers' expectations and increasingly specific needs [1, 7]. However, to achieve significant advances, a strict collaboration with food science and technology research units is of the utmost importance, and in order to obtain scientific research data that allow food industries to elaborate more specific, healthier, safer, highly-valuable and nutritionally-enriched food products/ingredients. Not least interesting to point out is that scientific research centers perform increasingly deepen investigations not only to discover more effective and safer ingredients but to assess the real bioactive effects of numerous promisor molecules with a feasible impact on health and wellbeing. The achievement of their physical and chemical characteristics is also assessed in order to establish optimum processing and storage conditions; the assessment of their pharmacokinetics and pharmacodynamics effects are also determined, both at short-middle and long-terms, to ensure consumers' safety and security [1, 15, 26]. Through this data, increasingly strict regulatory legislation on food additives has been created, distinguishing permitted ones from the forbidden ones and safer ones from the harmful food ingredients; food colorants represent an optimum example, being the list of permitted and prohibited food pigments progressively updated [27, 28], in spite to the existence of enormous discrepancies between several countries of European Union (EU) and other non-EU countries [29 - 31]. On top of these contradictions are synthetic food colorants; several reports highlight its health impairment effects while other does not observe the same findings. The highest alarming fact is why they are completely forbidden in some countries, while, in other ones, no associated risk with their use/consumption has been questioned [11, 32]. Thus, it still remains crucial to the standardization of these methodological procedures. In the following section, the currently available natural and synthetic food colorants, including some particular characteristics of the main groups, is briefly explained.

## Colouring Agents from Natural Origin

Due to the increasing evidences that naturally-occurring food colorants are safer and health promoters, at the same time, with no toxic effects, numerous studies have been carried out to provide more detailed, effective and specific/selective information about these promising molecules. Anthocyanins, betalains and carotenoids have been intensively investigated, while the information available for annatto, carminic acid, chlorophyll and curcumin is slightly more limited (Table 1). However, all these natural pigment classes are already allowed and its associated E codes established. On the other hand, many other naturally-derived molecules are still under investigation and despite their promising potential, E codes were not yet authorized (Table 2), being essential to achieve more detailed and strength information.

Anthocyanins represent the most widely investigated natural ingredients for colorant purposes, being the richest sources of pigments, flowers, fruits, leaves and even whole plants. The real potential of anthocyanins from commercial sources has also been assessed, namely those from cyanidin 3-glucoside, pelargonidin 3-glucoside and peonidin 3-glucoside. However, it is crucial to point out that in spite of the upcoming potential of anthocyanins, they are largely susceptible to external influences, such as those derived from variations on pH, temperature, humidity, salinity, stress and even storage conditions. To sediment and even to clearly explain this aspect, Cabrita *et al.* (2000) evaluating the effect of pH and temperature during storage conditions on anthocyanins color and stability, reached pronounced variations on assessed characteristics depending on the parameters established. Thus, the authors observed that while the strong acidic medium reddish color was the most predominant, at relative neural conditions, it dominates the bluish color. More interestingly, other authors found that the stability of anthocyanin 3-glucosides is maximum at pH values 8-9, while other anthocyanin pigments reached at pH values ranging from 5-7 [33]. Therefore, it is clearly evident that anthocyanin color may vary from red to purple and even blue color depending on the manufacturing parameters used.

Betalain pigments with a red-purple color possess very interesting abilities to be used as effective food ingredients. Being already approved with E162 code, they can be effectively used in a wide variety of products, such as burgers, desserts, ice creams, jams, jellies, soups, sauces, sweets, drinks, dairy products and yogurts.

**Table 1. Approved natural food colorants belonging to different classes.**

| Class | E code | Colorant constituents | Source | Part used | Reference |
|---|---|---|---|---|---|
| Annato | E160b | Annato (bixin and/or norbixin) | *Bixa orellana* L. | Seeds | [75 - 78] |
| | | | Commercial | | [79 - 81] |
| Anthocyanins | E163 | 3-Deoxyanthocyanidins | *Sorghum bicolor* (L.) Moench | Seeds | [82] |
| | | Anthocyanin-derived extracts | *Acacia decurrens* Willd. | Bark | [83] |
| | | | *Ajuga reptans* L. | Flowers | [84] |
| | | | *Brassica oleracea* L. spp. | Leaves | [85, 86] |
| | | | *Canna indica* L. | Flowers | [87] |
| | | | *Celosia cristata* L. | Flowers | [83] |
| | | | *Coffea arabica* L. | Husks | [88] |
| | | | *Daucus carota* L. | Roots | [89] |
| | | | *Euterpe oleracea* Mart. | Fruits | [90] |
| | | | *Hibiscus rosa-sinensis* L. | Flowers | [91] |
| | | | *Hippeastrum reticulatum* var. *striatifolium* | Bulb | [92] |
| | | | *Ipomoea batatas* (L.) Lam. | Tubers | [93] |
| | | | *Mirabilis jalapa* L. | Flowers | [83] |
| | | | *Musa paradisiaca* Linnaeus | Bracts | [94] |
| | | | *Oryza sativa* L. | Grains | [95] |
| | | | *Oxalis triangularis* ssp. *papilionaceae* | Leaves | [96] |
| | | | *Punica granatum* L. | Rind | [83] |
| | | | *Rhoeo spathacea* (Swartz) Stearn | Leaves | [97] |
| | | | *Rubus glaucus* Benth | Fruits | [98] |
| | | | *Sambucus nigra* L. | | [86] |
| | | | *Tulipa gesneriana* L. varieties | Flowers | [20] |
| | | | *Tagetes erecta* L. | Flowers | [83] |
| | | | *Vaccinium ashei* var. Rabbiteye | Fruits | [52] |
| | | | *Vaccinium pahalae* Skottsb. | Shots | [99] |

*(Table 1) cont.....*

| Class | E code | Colorant constituents | Source | Part used | Reference |
|-------|--------|----------------------|--------|-----------|-----------|
| | | | *Vitis vinifera* L. | Marc | [100] |
| | | | *Zea mays* L. cv Zihei | Cob, grains | [101, 102] |
| | | Cyanidin 3-glucoside | *Pistacia lentiscus* L. | Fruits | [103] |
| | | | *Santalum album* L. | Fruits | [104] |
| | | | Commercial | | [17] |
| | | Cyanidin 3-rutinoside | *Phillyrea latifolia* L. | Fruits | [103] |
| | | | *Rubia peregrina* L. | Fruits | [103] |
| | | Delphinidin 3-rutinoside | *Abies koreana* E. H. Wilson | | [33] |
| | | | *Solanum melongeana* L. | Fruits | [105] |
| | | Malvidin 3-glucoside | *Vaccinium* spp. | | [33] |
| | | Methyl pyrano-anthocyanidins | *Vitis vinifera* L. | Skin | [106] |
| | | Pelargonidin 3-glucoside | *Fragaria ananassa* L. *maximus* | | [33] |
| | | | Commercial | | [107] |
| | | Peonidin 3-glucoside | Commercial | | [17] |
| | | | *Oriza sativa* L. | | [33] |
| | | Petunidin 3-glucoside | *Abies koreana* E. H. Wilson | | [33] |
| Betalains | E162 | Betacyanins | *Hylocereus polyrhizus* (Weber) Britton & Rose | Fruits | [34] |
| | | Betalains | *Beta vulgaris* L. | Roots | [108] |
| | | | *Opuntia ficus-indica* [L.] Miller | Fruits | [35, 109] |
| | | | *Opuntia stricta* (Haw.) Haw. | Fruits | [37] |
| | | | *Rivina humilis* L. | Fruits | [38] |
| Carminic acid | E120 | Carminic acid | Commercial | | [17, 46 - 48] |
| Carotenoids | E160a | α-Carotene | *Daucus carota* L. | Roots | [110] |
| | E160a | β-Carotene | *Blakeslea trispora* | Fungus | [45] |
| | | | Commercial | | [79, 111] |
| | | | *Daucus carota* L. | Roots | [110] |
| | E160a | *trans*-β-Carotene | Commercial | | [107] |
| | E161b | Lutein (or xanthophylls) | Commercial | | [81, 111] |
| | | | *Daucus carota* L. | Roots | [110] |

*(Table 1) cont.....*

| Class | E code | Colorant constituents | Source | Part used | Reference |
|---|---|---|---|---|---|
| | | | *Tagetes erecta* L. | Flowers | [112] |
| | | | *Tagetes* spp. | Flowers | [113] |
| | E161j | Astaxanthin | *Scenedesmus* sp. | Microalgae | [42] |
| | | | *Xanthophyllomyces dendrorhous* | Yeast | [42] |
| | | | *Haematococcus pluvialis* | Aquatic animal | [43] |
| Chlorophyll | E140 | Chlorophyll | *Spinacea oleracea* L. | Leaves | [114] |
| | | | *Spirulina pratensis* | Algae | [44] |
| Curcumin | E100 | Curcumin | *Curcuma longa* L. | Rhizomes | [115, 116] |
| | | | Commercial | | [17, 107, 117 - 120] |

**Table 2. Other natural food colorants, under investigation, belonging to different classes.**

| Class | Colorant constituents | Source | Part used | Reference |
|---|---|---|---|---|
| Carotenoids | Crocetin | Commercial | | [59, 60] |
| | | *Crocus sativus* L. | | [121] |
| | Crocin | Commercial | | [59] |
| | | | | [60] |
| Phenolic compounds | 4',5,7-trihydroxyflavone | Commercial | | [107] |
| | Apigenin | Commercial | | [107] |
| | Fisetin | Commercial | | [107] |
| | Myricetin | *Myrica cerifera* L. | Roots | [107] |
| | Myricitrin | *Myrica cerifera* L. | Roots | [107] |
| | Naringin | Commercial | | [107] |
| | Quercetin | Commercial | | [107] |
| | Rutin | Commercial | | [107] |
| Other phenolics | Carthamin | *Carthamus tinctorius* L. | Flowers | [122] |
| | | Commercial | | [107] |
| | Flavonoids and total phenolics | *Senna bicapsularis* L. | Flowers | [91] |
| | Phenolics | *Euterpe oleracea* Mart. | Fruits | [90] |
| | Phloridzin | *Malus domestica* Borkh. | Fruits | [123] |
| | Pigment* | *Cinnamomum burmannii* (Nees & T. Nees) Blume | Fruits | [124] |

*(Table 2) cont.....*

| Class | Colorant constituents | Source | Part used | Reference |
|-------|----------------------|--------|-----------|-----------|
| | Polyphenols | *Mastisia cordata* Bonpl. | Fruits | [125] |
| | Safflomin A | Commercial | | [107] |
| | Safflomin B | Commercial | | [107] |
| Other pigments | C-Phycocyanin | *Arthrospira platensis* | Cyanobacterium | [53] |
| | C-Phycoerythrin | Blue-green algae | Cyanobacteria | [54] |
| | Fennel | *Crithmum maritimum* L. | Aerial parts | [55] |
| | Genipin | Commercial | | [59, 60, 126] |
| | | *Gardenia jasminoides* Ellis | Fruits | [56, 57] |
| | | *Genipa americana* L. | Fruits | [58] |
| | Geniposide | Commercial | | [59] |
| | Madder color | *Rubia tinctorum* L. | Roots | [127, 128] |
| | Melanin | *Auricularia auricular* | Mushroom | [129] |
| | Monascorubrin | Commercial | | [60] |
| | Purple corn color | Commercial | | [61] |
| | Violacein | *Chromobacterium violaceum* UTM 5 | *Bacteria* | [62] |

* may be a melanin or phenolic pigment; studied phenolic compounds presented a color spectrum varying from yellow-orange to red or even dark purple.

In spite of the fact that beetroot (*Beta vulgaris* L.) still continues being the most common source, *Hylocereus polyrhizus* (Weber) Britton & Rose [34], *Opuntia ficus-indica* [L.] Miller [35, 36], *Opuntia stricta* (Haw.) Haw [37]. and *Rivina humilis* L [38]. fruits are also rich in these pigments. However, and in the same line of anthocyanins, betalains stability may be also markedly affected by temperature, pH, water activity, oxygen, light, chelating agents, co-presence of compounds, pigment concentration, storage and processing conditions [39, 40].

Carotenoids comprise another very interesting group of phytochemicals with important colouring abilities. In spite of being widely recognized for its renowned antioxidant potential acting on large scale as natural preservatives, the use for cosmetic, pharmaceutical and nutraceutical purposes is still increasing [12, 41]. Commonly applied in food products with high contents of fatty acids, such as butter and margarines, cakes, milk products and soft drinks, carotenoids are also applied in products with moderate to low fatty acids concentration. Overall, most of the food products are susceptible to oxidation, which explains its increasingly widespread use by food industries. Plant flowers, roots, leaves and even whole plants are interesting sources of carotenoids, but algae/microalgae, fungus/yeasts and even aquatic animals have been increasingly used as raw materials to isolate carotenoid pigments [42 - 45]. More interestingly to emphasize is that while some carotenoid pigments maybe both found in plant and/or animals, other ones are only present in animal sources, such as astaxanthin (E161j) mainly isolated from *Scenedesmus* sp. (microalgae), *Xanthophyllomyces dendrorhous* (yeast) and *Haematococcus pluvialis* (aquatic animal) (Table **1**).

Annato (E160b) is also a very interesting yellow-red pigment extracted from *Bixa orellana* L. seeds with a long history of use. Bixin and norbixin comprises the main components widely applied in cakes, biscuits, rice, flour, soft drinks, smoked fish, sausages, meat products, dairy products, snack foods and ice creams. Carminic acid (E120) is another yellow to red-orange pigment with colouring abilities, which already exists from commercial origin being stablished an adequate daily intake (ADI) of 5 mg/kg b.w., in order to ensure its safely inclusion in cakes, cookies, beverages, jam, jelly, ice creams, sausages, pies, dried fish, yogurt, gelatins, cider, tomato, dairy products, cherries, non-carbonated drinks, chewing gums, pills and cough drops [17, 46 - 48]. The green pigment chlorophyll (E140) has been also applied in beverages, fruit juices, pasta, dairy products, soups, sweeter preparations, being mainly isolated from *Spinacea oleracea* L. leaves. Lastly, curcumin (E100), the yellow-orange pigment isolated from *Curcuma longa* L. rhizomes is also the most widely known pigment belonging to the curcuminoids group. Both from natural and commercial sources, this pigment is used by food industries for multiple purposes, such as fish and baked products, dairy products, ice cream, yoghurts, yellow cakes, biscuits, sweets, cereals, sauces and gelatins [3].

On the other hand, phenolic compounds represent another promising class of natural pigments Table **2**. Their colorant abilities have been intensively studied, and despite very interesting findings have been reached concerning to its safety, stability and spectrum of activity, many other phenolic molecules still continue scarcely exploited [49 - 51]. Despite its renowned health-promoting and functional abilities, this group of bioactive molecules may also exert many other biotechnological benefits apart from its colouring abilities [15, 52]. Up to now, naringin (flavanone), 4',5,7-trihydroxyflavones and apigenin (flavones) and fisetin, myricetin, myricitin, quercetin and rutin (flavonols) are among those from which color abilities have been investigated. However, only myricetin and myricitrin were from plant origin (*Myrica cerifera* L. roots), being commercial sources of phenolic compounds the most commonly used.

Other naturally-derived food pigments remain under investigation, such as the blue pigment c-phycocyanin, isolated from *Arthrospira platensis* (cyanobacteria) [53]; the red-orange pigment c-phycoerythrin, from blue-green algae [54]; the grey and green colors provided by hot-air and freeze-dried aerial parts of

*Crithmum maritimum* L., respectively [55]; the blue pigment genipin, derived both from *Gardenia jasminoides* Ellis and *Genipa americana* L. fruits; the red pigment madder color, isolated from *Rubia tinctorum* L. roots also revealed promissory and very attractive potentialities when added, respectively to beverages, juices, nectars, desserts and gels [56 - 58], and hams, sausages, boiled fish, paste, beverages and some confectionaries products. Moreover, geniposide, monascorubrin and purple corn color [59 - 61] have also been studied, but only from the commercial origin. A violet pigment, violacein, isolated from *Chromobacterium violaceum* UTM 5 bacteria has also been used in yogurt and jelly products [62].

Based on the latest findings, it is clearly evident that naturally-derived food colorants are markedly safer, specific and non-toxic in comparison with synthetic ones, at the same time have the ability to act as health-promoters and exert functional properties [1, 2]. Recently, a secondary metabolite produced by the *Monascus* genus (pigment named by monascin) has revealed very interesting food colouring abilities, as also considerable health benefits as anti-inflammatory, antidiabetic, anti-cholesterolemic and antitumor [63, 64]. However, there is not a general consensus about its safe use, therefore, no E code was attributed in the EU. More interestingly to highlight is that while in Germany, its use is considered illegal, in Asian countries, this naturally-derived molecule has been effectively applied in food products [65]. Thus, such studies shall be developed in order to clearly improve this expansive and renowned area of knowledge.

## Colouring Agents from Synthetic Origin

While naturally-derived food pigments have been increasingly exploited for its multiple benefits and biotechnological potentialities, synthetic food colorants have been also investigated due to its short-middle and even long-terms side effects and even toxicity.

Since the boom of colorant agents, synthetic food colorants became widely used for multiple purposes, related to a marked increase of foodstuffs acceptability. However, over the years, multiple changes have been progressively observed, and a considerable amount of them was removed and even forbidden. Table **3** shows the most commonly used and markedly studied synthetic food colorants in terms of side effects, security, short-, middle- and long-terms toxicity and even health impact. The ADI values of these food colorants have been progressively re-evaluated and current doses were established by FDA and EFSA.

Based on the established ADI values, caramel (E150), followed by blue, yellow, green and lastly white food colorants seems to be less dangerous. Interestingly, vegetable carbon (E153) and titanium dioxide (E171) have not established ADI, being applied in jam and jelly crystals [66] and in confectionery, baked goods, cheeses, icings and toppings, respectively. Otherwise, the lowest ADI values were stablished for red to orange colorants, such as erythrosine – E127 (0.1 mg/kg b.w.), red 2G – E128 (0.1 mg/kg b.w.) and amaranth – E123 (0.8 mg/kg b.w.), and for brown FK – E154 (0.15 mg/kg b.w.), which mean that a strong possibility of side effects and related toxicity occurrence exists.

Apart from these particularly highlighted harmful synthetic colorants, it is also important to point out that the occurrence of cumulative effects is also possible, due to its daily intake in different types of foods. Most of the foodstuffs in which those synthetic food colorants are used are also daily consumed in beverages, cocktails, alcoholic drinks, fish and meat products, and candied cherries (mainly by children and teenagers). Therefore, it is feasible to infer that the risk of organic saturation, side effects occurrence and related toxicity is eminent. Finally, it is also crucial to emphasize that sugar products and beverages (both alcoholic and non-alcoholic) have large amounts of these food colorants, which besides triggering the occurrence of adverse effects, also incites their additive consumption.

**Table 3. Synthetic food colorants approved and currently allowed by the European Union.**

| Color class | E code | Colorant | ADI | References |
|---|---|---|---|---|
| Black | E151 | Brilliant black | 1 mg/kg b.w. | [130] |
| | E153 | Vegetable carbon | Not specified | [66] |
| Blue | E133 | Brilliant blue FCF | 10 mg/kg b.w. | [32, 47, 48, 72, 131 - 142] |
| | E132 | Indigo carmine (syn.: indigotine) | 5 mg/kg b.w. | [32, 47, 48, 71, 131, 136, 138, 139, 141 - 144] |
| | E131 | Patent blue V | 15 mg/kg b.w. | [136, 141, 143, 145] |
| Brown | E154 | Brown FK | 0.15 mg/kg b.w. | [146] |
| | E155 | Brown HT | 1.5 mg/kg b.w. | [147] |
| Caramel | E150 | Caramel | 160-200 mg/kg b.w. | [148] |
| Green | E141ii | Copper chlorophyllin-complexes | 7.5 mg/kg b.w. | [149 - 151] |
| | E142 | Green S | 5 mg/kg b.w. | [136, 152] |
| Red-orange | E129 | Allura Red AC | 7 mg/kg b.w. | [17, 26, 32, 47, 48, 131, 132, 136, 138, 139, 141, 142, 153 - 157] |
| | E123 | Amaranth | 0.8 mg/kg b.w. | [131, 132, 136 - 139, 141, 142, 144, 154 - 156, 158 - 164] |
| | E160a | β-carotene | 5 mg/kg b.w. | [165 - 168] |

*(Table 3) cont.....*

| Color class | E code | Colorant | ADI | References |
|---|---|---|---|---|
| | E120 | Carminic acid | 5 mg/kg b.w. | [32, 70, 133] |
| | E122 | Carmoisine (syn.: azorubine) | 4 mg/kg b.w. | [17, 136, 141, 154, 155, 158, 169 - 172] |
| | E127 | Erythrosine | 0.1 mg/kg b.w. | [26, 32, 131, 132, 136, 138, 139, 154 - 156, 158, 162, 173 - 175] |
| | E180 | Litholrubine BK | 1.5 mg/kg b.w. | [32, 176] |
| | E124 | Ponceau 4R | 4 mg/kg b.w. | [26, 47, 48, 131, 132, 136 - 139, 141, 142, 154 - 156, 158 - 161, 177, 178] |
| | E128 | Red 2G (syn.: azophloxine) | 0.1 mg/kg b.w. | [26, 73, 136, 141, 154, 155, 158] |
| Yellow | E104 | Quinoline yellow | 10 mg/kg b.w. | [17, 32, 136, 141, 159, 179, 180] |
| | E110 | Sunset yellow FCF | 2.5 mg/kg b.w. | [17, 26, 32, 47, 48, 131 - 142, 144, 153, 154, 156, 159 - 161, 177, 181, 182] |
| | E102 | Tartrazine | 7.5 mg/kg b.w. | [17, 47, 48, 69, 132 - 143, 153, 159 - 162, 177, 183] |
| White | E171 | Titanium dioxide | Not specified | [184, 185] |

# LEGISLATION AND REGULATORY PRACTICES

Beyond the large impact of consumers' demands in the food industry, increasingly strict and specific regulatory practices have been progressively implemented and updated. In contrary to the broad consensus, current legislation does not exist to difficult and/or to restrict the activity of food and biotechnological industries, but instead to ameliorate and to improve the safety assessment of numerous marketed foodstuffs [3]. Moreover, it also opens very interesting opportunities for the future food market, once promotes the development of a wide variety of formulation, presentation and types of foodstuffs, which consequently contributes to ensure the consumers' expectations and satisfaction.

In general, the available legislation improves the general knowledge about the safety, stability, security, bioavailability, bioefficacy, maximum doses and even adequate daily intake towards their healthy consumption. Moreover, these regulatory practices for food industries also provide the latest insights concerning the toxicological data, positive and/or adverse effects which also refers to the safe use of food colorants, emphasizing those that are available and non-toxic, available but relatively non-toxic, available but slight toxic and, lastly, those that are no longer available.

Therefore, through these advances, it is possible to properly develop and to ensure good manufacturing practices at industrial levels, and simultaneously achieve consumers' safety and health maintenance at short-, middle- and even long-terms [3, 5]. As shown in Table **3**, several food synthetic colorants are still allowed, but current ADIs are different than the initial ones. In fact, both positive and negative effects of food colorants have been increasingly assessed not only for their upcoming applications in food, pharmaceutical and cosmetic industries but in many other areas [11]. For example, Carocho *et al.* [1] highlighted the lack of uniformity of worldwide legislation concerning additives, namely preservatives, nutritional additives, colouring, flavoring, texturizing, and miscellaneous agents. They were analyzed in terms of safety and toxicity apart from conflicting results in several studies. In a similar manner, Martins *et al.* [3] also reported these aspects but mainly focused on the main classes of natural food colorants, namely those that can be used at large scale; those that only received approval, as well as many others, that are still under investigation. In fact, current laws concerning food colorants not only focus on the type of colorant that can be used and its approval source, but also its level of purity, type of food in which it can be used and adequate levels towards a safe consumption [67].

Thus, and apart from the latest advances on this field of regulatory guidelines, more deepen studies should be carried out in order to determine the acute and short-, middle- and long-term effects, genotoxic and tumorigenic potential, likelihood of acute and chronic toxicity occurrence, and not least important its effects during pregnancy and early developmental stages, and reproduction [68]. Finally, it is also important to emphasize that ADI levels during these particular stages should also be determined/assessed.

## PHARMACOKINETIC DATA

### Maximum Levels

Based on the last findings provided by pharmacokinetic and pharmacodynamics data related to colorants application, in terms of safety, quality and health impact at short-, middle-, and even long-terms, several restrictions of their use have been applied and consequently, their respective ADI quantities (mg/kg b.w.) have been properly adjusted.

As shown in Table **3**, the more stringent regulations have been applied to synthetic food colorants. The term acceptable daily intake (ADI) was introduced by FAO/WHO Expert Committee on Food Additives in 1961, to establish the daily amount of an additive in food that could be ingested over time without causing an appreciable health risk [28]. Therefore, the determination of ADI may be considered the starting point to establish the maximum levels of certain additives included in food products. However, European Food Safety Authority (EFSA) determines that no maximum levels should be established to those substances, but instead highlighted that they should be applied/used according to good manufacturing practices, always ensuring that their intended use do not overlap consumers' safety and security, without causing any associated risk due to their consumption [28].

Thus, considering the ADI data provided in Table **3**, it is possible to stablish three different levels of food colorants security. In this sense, caramel (E150, ADI = 160-200 mg/kg b.w.), vegetable carbon (E153, ADI not specified) and titanium dioxide (E171, ADI not specified) may be considered safe, while brilliant blue (E133, ADI = 10 mg/kg b.w.), patent blue (E131, ADI = 15 mg/kg b.w.), copper chlorophyllin-complexes (E141ii, ADI = 7.5 mg/kg b.w.), allura red AC (E129, ADI = 7 mg/kg b.w.), quinolone yellow (E104, ADI = 10 mg/kg b.w.) and tartrazine (E102, ADI = 7.5 mg/kg b.w.) may be considered as moderately safe. Lastly, brilliant blue (E151, ADI = 1 mg/kg b.w.), indigo carmine (E132, ADI = 5 mg/kg b.w.), brown FK (E154, ADI = 0.15 mg/kg b.w.), litholrubine BK (E180, ADI = 1.5 mg/kg b.w.), carmoisine (E122, ADI = 4 mg/kg b.w.), erythrosine (E127, ADI = 0.1 mg/kg b.w.), brown HT (E155, ADI = 1.5 mg/kg b.w.), green S (E142, ADI = 5 mg/kg b.w.), amaranth (E123, ADI = 0.8 mg/kg b.w.), β-carotene (E160a, ADI = 5 mg/kg b.w.), carminic acid (E120, ADI = 5 mg/kg b.w.), ponceau 4R (E124, ADI =4 mg/kg b.w.), red 2G (E128, ADI =0.1 mg/kg b.w.) and sunset yellow FCT (E110, ADI = 2.5 mg/kg b.w.), that present the lowest ADI, should be considered as potentially toxic. In fact, there is an increasing number of studies based on low-to-severe side effects and even toxicity related to synthetic colorants consumption. However, despite that for natural food colorants no ADI was already established, it is important to emphasize that a proper and conscientious rationalization of their use should be also performed.

## Toxicological Data

Several toxicological data have been obtained in order to assess the likelihood of side effects occurrence, acute oral, short-term and sub-chronic toxicity, genotoxicity, chronic toxicity and even carcinogenic effects, reproductive and developmental toxicity, hypersensitive and intolerance reactions as well as other specific studies.

In the following sub-sections, a brief description of toxicological aspects is presented for the synthetic food colorants that present the most relevant data.

## Brilliant Blue FCF

Brilliant Blue FCF (E 133) is a triarylmethane dye authorized as a food additive in the EU, with a currently established ADI of 10 mg/kg b.w [72]. Initially, joint FAO/WHO Expert Committee on Food Additives and EU Scientific Committee for Food established an ADI of 12.5 mg/kg b.w. as safe, but based on the latest long-term studies, namely assessing its genotoxic, sub-chronic, reproductive, developmental and long-term toxicity potential, including the likelihood of carcinogenic effects, important reasons were given to revise ADI for 10 mg/kg b.w. in 1984 [72]. More recently, and through the application of an uncertainty factor of 100, a new ADI for Brilliant Blue FCT was established as 6 mg/kg b.w. to ensure its safer and healthy consumption [72].

## Carmines, Carminic Acid and Cochineal

Cochineal, carminic acid and carmines (E 120) are red anthraquinone dyes authorized as food additives in EU, with an established ADI of 5 mg/kg b.w. Based on the numerous studies already developed, no carcinogenic, genotoxic and relevant toxicological data have been reported [70]. However, concerning its allergenic, hypersensitive and intolerance abilities, the available scenario is completely different. Several patients that had consumed alcoholic beverages containing carmine presented acute urticaria and angioedema. Other patients that consumed a carmine-containing drink, ice-cream and even carmine-containing yogurt experienced an anaphylactic reaction being required emergency treatment, developing an immediate onset of nausea, pruritus, urticaria, hypotension and tachycardia within 3 hours of hospital admission. In fact, immunoglobulin E (IgE) sensitization was observed in patients by positive skin prick tests to carmine and by radioallergosorbent test (RAST) [70]. High serum levels of IgE antibodies were also found in non-atopic patients to carminic acid-albumin conjugates.

Generalized urticaria, angioedema and asthma were also observed in patients after consumption of yoghurt containing an estimated amount of 1.3 mg carmine, in spite, similar symptoms were also observed after consumption of other red-colored foods [70]. Irritation of larynx and edema of eyelids are also common, followed by urticaria, stomachache and diarrhea. In fact, numerous studies have reported a marked allergenic potential of cochineal extracts (mostly carmine and carminic acid) mostly related to incest proteins; therefore, protein contents in carmine dyes should be reduced as much as possible [70]. It may be ensured by using appropriate purification steps during manufacturing processes and, subsequently, avoiding cochineal proteinaceous compounds. On the other hand, it is also essential to consider that maximum limits for toxic elements (*i.e.* arsenic, cadmium, lead, and mercury) were also established by EU specifications, once a lower exposure to those toxics should be ensured in foods containing E120 dyes [70].

Finally, and not least important to point out is that the already established ADI of 5 mg/kg b.w. does not cover the minimum sensitizing doses for susceptible individuals, up to the point that allergic reactions may occur due to the exposure to cochineal extract and carmines. Therefore, strict control should be taken to avert the occurrence of hypersensitivity and even severe anaphylactic reactions.

## Indigo Carmine

Indigo Carmine (E132) is an indigoid colouring substance with a form of dark-blue powder or granules currently available in the EU as a food additive with a established ADI of 5 mg/kg b.w [71].

Despite in 1969, a temporary ADI of 0-2.5 mg/kg b.w./day was stablished, in 1975, it was increased to a full ADI of 0-5 mg/kg b.w./day based on the long-term studies developed. Similarly to other food additives, several side effects might occur, despite indigo carmine, no carcinogenic and toxicological effects were markedly reported. For example, in ageing mice, after microscopy analysis, slight neoplastic, degenerative, hyperplastic and inflammatory changes were observed in different tissues [71]. However, it is convenient to highlight that those changes occurred without having any relationship with the dose applied, and consequently, are unrelated to the dietary administration of Indigo Carmine. A moderate blue-green discoloration of the gastrointestinal tract, including liver, gall-bladder and urine was also found and closely related to the Indigo Carmine ingestion. No signals of genotoxicity and developmental of adverse effects were reported by the current studies [71]. The effects of Indigo Carmine on reproduction, the occurrence of modifications on hematological and biological parameters in chronic toxicity studies and subacute studies were not described, as well as allergic reactions [71]. However, despite those safer concerns, it was already proposed that the current specifications should be revised to ensure the proper and safer consumption by children and susceptible people, always ensuring that ADI established is not exceeded. Moreover, it is not clear if the occurred adverse effects were due to the indigo carmine itself or to the presence of impurities and/or contaminants in the material tested.

## Red 2G

Red 2G (E128), also known as azophloxine, is a mono-azo dye, currently authorized by the EU with an established ADI of 0.1 mg/kg b.w [73]. Several studies have been performed to access toxicological data related to their use. Despite many studies show significant results, with the currently available data, it is not possible to make feasible conclusions. In fact, Red 2G is extensively metabolized to aniline, which is a carcinogen and, therefore, a genotoxic mechanism cannot be excluded. Thus, special attention should be given to food products containing this food additive.

## Tartrazine

Tartrazine (E 102) is an azo dye allowed as a food additive in the EU, with an established ADI of 7.5 mg/kg b.w. It has been reported by several studies that adverse reactions may occur in humans, such as vasculitis and urticaria, in spite that no convincing conclusions have been reached concerning to its ability to induce immune-mediated (hypersensitivity) reactions [69]. Thus, those symptoms seem to be more closely related to intolerance reactions than those immune-mediated. Not least important to emphasize is that tartrazine is commonly used in combination with other mixtures of synthetic colorants, and therefore the side effects occurrence may be due to the exposure of the mixture or even caused by a single other synthetic dye. For example, a mixture of sodium benzoate with tartrazine was recognized to be able to produce adverse behavior reactions (*i.e.* increased hyperactivity) in children with 3-years old [69].

Apart from urticaria, periorbital edema, facial flushing, itching, angioedema and even asthma may also occur, despite being uncommon. But, it was reported that the use of 10% of ADI value does not cause adverse dermatologic reactions or aggravated atopic dermatitis symptoms, even in patients with allergic disorders [69]. Therefore, studies assessing the occurrence of other allergic reactions such as hay fever, allergic rhinitis and eczema should clearly identify and separate subjects with asthmatic conditions.

Intolerance reactions appear to be the most common side effects; however, according to the current information available only in a specific fraction of people, it can be reached. Those reactions may be present in specific people through the consumption of this food additive under normal conditions (*i.e.* less than milligram quantities) [69]. Thus, in these situations, once tartrazine may induce intolerance reactions at dose levels within ADI value, their presence in marketed products should be clearly labelled; in fact, essential information for intolerant people should be provided, both destined to human food consumption or pharmaceutical applications, to avoid the occurrence of undesirable situations.

Moreover, studies focused on the evaluation of the genotoxic, carcinogenic, semi-chronic, reproductive, developmental and long-term toxicity provided by tartrazine consumption concluded that significantly higher doses than ADI of 7.5 mg/kg b.w. were necessary to observe adverse reactions [69]. Thus, overall, the evaluation panel concluded that it is not necessary to revise the already established ADI, the possible occurrence of intolerance reaction in a small fraction of the population will be highlighted.

**Vegetable Carbon**

Vegetable carbon (E153) is an authorized food additive in the EU, but apart from its use as a food colorant, it is also widely known as a medicinal substance, namely as an antidote or intestinal adsorptive drug [66]. It is a carbonized raw material from vegetable origin, and the current legislation on this field refers to possible uses of vegetable carbon and its safety evaluation.

Considering its long history of safe use in medicine, vegetable carbon is absent of significant toxicological effects considering the concentrations used in pharmaceutical preparations, nearly 18 to 300 times higher than those daily exposed through dietary consumption [66]. No data are available concerning the genotoxic, chronic potential, carcinogenic, reproductive and developmental toxicity of vegetable carbon [66]. Only data related to its carcinogenic and genotoxic potential have been reported, but that can be closely attributed to the carcinogenic potential of polycyclic aromatic hydrocarbons (PAHs) adsorbed to carbon black [66]. These toxic compounds/impurities are derived from the source material used to produce vegetable carbon, being present in relatively low concentrations. Thus, aiming to control and to ensure the proper use and safety of vegetable carbon, residual quantities (*e.g.* with a limit of detection of 0.1 µg/kg) were fixed/specified and subsequently validated by analytical methods [66]. In fact, and despite these requirements, it is a fact that PAHs resulting from the use of vegetable carbon as a food colorant are much greater than those PAHs from diet. Moreover, it is also crucial to note that the carcinogenic potential and content of PAHs derived from carbon blacks are largely higher and more dangerous than those present in vegetable carbon.

In a broad sense, and despite several food dyes have presented significant side effects, the occurrence of allergic reactions and intolerances is still the most common, together with urticaria and vasculitis and, more extremely, anaphylactic reactions. Chronic urticaria and angioedema are uncommon, but it is also convenient to highlight that sensitive individual may also react to food additives at markedly lower dose levels than the ADI. Moreover, apart from allergic reactions, several effects on children's behavior were also reported, being attention deficit hyperactivity disorder (ADHD), the most commonly described, followed by negative effects on concentration activity [17, 52, 74]. ADHD is the most common, with six synthetic food colorants being currently indicated as having negative effects on the concentration activity [28], namely Tartrazine (E102), Quinolone Yellow (E104), Sunset Yellow FCF (E110), Carmoisine/

Azorubine (E122), Ponceau 4R (E124) and Allura Red AC (E129).

Thus, more than to proceed with these studies, it is also of the utmost importance to assess individual idiosyncrasies as well as pharmacokinetic and pharmacodynamics between individuals belonging to different populations. In all cases, the use of natural dyes seems to provide additional benefits to the use of synthetic ones, because apart from possessing biosimilar molecules and being easily recognized by the human body, they are easily metabolized and, therefore, secondary metabolites may also be produced, conferring multiple and multidimensional benefits to the human body (longevity and quality of life).

## CONCLUDING REMARKS

The interest for naturally-derived food additives is unquestionable, being even increasingly clear evident their real benefits at a level of health and longevity promotion, disease prevention and even maintenance of a good quality of life. Concerning synthetic food dyes, and despite the increasing interest of consumers by natural ones, increasingly deepen studies have revealed that they have marked abilities to cause adverse effects and even toxicity both at short-middle and even long-terms. Moreover, the currently available ADI values are completely different from the first ones, and despite that, ADI values were improved for some of them, for the majority, those values were markedly reduced and even prohibited. Moreover, different and contradictory legislation is available: while some food additives are authorized in EU, they are no longer available in the United States, and vice-versa. Therefore, it still remains the question about their real safety and security, and if economic interests are overlapping health issues. Furthermore, and not least important to point out is that completely different results have been reported concerning the biological and toxicological data of numerous food dyes. In fact, considering that markedly contradictory data have been analyzed by EFSA, it becomes difficult to conclude about the real safety and security of those food additives, possible health implications and adequate ADI. The quality, purity, methodological procedures, type of study and subjects selected, among many other aspects, largely influence the final data obtained, but it is also crucial to be in mind that exigency and quality of studies should be ensured. While this counter-information remains unsolved, the market of natural food additives has gained an increasing demand and visibility by worldwide consumers and food, pharmaceutical and cosmetic industries. In fact, it is not new that consumers have progressively avoided synthetic food colorants due to its negative health effects, and consequently demanded healthy foods, which do not contain those additives.

Thus, a change in attitude and priorities has been markedly observed by worldwide consumers, not only at a level of food and nutrition science, but also pharmaceutical, nutraceutical and cosmetic industries, driving manufacturers to find new, natural and healthy sources of colors and flavors and other organoleptic attributes for the currently marketed food products.

## CONSENT FOR PUBLICATION

Not applicable.

## CONFLICTS OF INTEREST

No conflicts of interest to declare.

## ACKNOWLEDGEMENTS

The authors are grateful to the Foundation for Science and Technology (FCT, Portugal) for financial support to CIMO (UIDB/00690/2020) research centre.

## REFERENCES

[1]     Carocho M, Barreiro MF, Morales P, Ferreira ICFR. Adding molecules to food, pros and cons: A review on synthetic and natural food additives. Compr Rev Food Sci Food Saf 2014; 13: 377-99.
[http://dx.doi.org/10.1111/1541-4337.12065]

[2]     Dias MI, Ferreira ICFR, Barreiro MF. Microencapsulation of bioactives for food applications. Food Funct 2015; 6: 1035-52.
[http://dx.doi.org/10.1039/C4FO01175A]

[3]     Martins N, Roriz CL, Morales P, Barros L, Ferreira ICFR. Food colorants: challenges, opportunities and current desires of agro-industries to ensure consumer expectations and regulatory practices. Trends Food Sci Technol 2016; 52: 1-15.
[http://dx.doi.org/10.1016/j.tifs.2016.03.009]

[4]     Ray S, Raychaudhuri U, Chakraborty R. An overview of encapsulation of active compounds used in food products by drying technology. Food Biosci 2015; 13: 76-83.
[http://dx.doi.org/10.1016/j.fbio.2015.12.009]

[5]     Shim S-M, Seo SH, Lee Y, Moon G-I, Kim M-S, Park J-H. Consumers' knowledge and safety perceptions of food additives: Evaluation on the effectiveness of transmitting information on preservatives. Food Control 2011; 22: 1054-60.
[http://dx.doi.org/10.1016/j.foodcont.2011.01.001]

[6]     FDA. Overview of Food Ingredients, Additives & Colors 2016. Available at: http://www.fda.gov/Food/IngredientsPackagingLabeling/FoodAdditivesIngredients/ucm094211.htm

[7]     Ayala-Zavala JF, Vega-Vega V, Rosas-Domínguez C, Palafox-Carlos H, Villa-Rodriguez JA, Siddiqui MW, *et al.* Agro-industrial potential of exotic fruit byproducts as a source of food additives. Food Res Int 2011; 44: 1866-74.
[http://dx.doi.org/10.1016/j.foodres.2011.02.021]

[8]     Delgado-Vargas F, Paredes-Lopez O. Natural Colorants for Food and Nutraceutical Uses. Trends Food Sci Technol 2003; 14: 438.
[http://dx.doi.org/10.1016/S0924-2244(03)00076-1]

[9]     Laokuldilok N, Thakeow P, Kopermsub P, Utama-ang N. Optimisation of microencapsulation of turmeric extract for masking flavour. Food Chem 2016; 194: 695-704.
[http://dx.doi.org/10.1016/j.foodchem.2015.07.150]

[10]    Bridle P, Timberlake CF. Anthocyanins as natural food colours—selected aspects. Food Chem 1997; 58: 103-9.
[http://dx.doi.org/10.1016/S0308-8146(96)00222-1]

[11]    Amchova P, Kotolova H, Ruda-Kucerova J. Health safety issues of synthetic food colorants. Regul Toxicol Pharmacol 2015; 73: 914-22.
[http://dx.doi.org/10.1016/j.yrtph.2015.09.026]

[12]    Rodriguez-Amaya DB. Natural food pigments and colorants. Curr Opin Food Sci 2016; 7: 20-6.
[http://dx.doi.org/10.1016/j.cofs.2015.08.004]

[13]    Tumolo T, Lanfer-Marquez UM. Copper chlorophyllin: A food colorant with bioactive properties? Food Res Int 2012; 46: 451-9.
[http://dx.doi.org/10.1016/j.foodres.2011.10.031]

[14]    Carocho M, Morales P, Ferreira ICFR. Natural food additives: Quo vadis? Trends Food Sci Technol 2015; 45: 284-95.
[http://dx.doi.org/10.1016/j.tifs.2015.06.007]

[15]    Shahid M. Shahid-ul-Islam;Mohammad F. Recent advancements in natural dye applications: a review. J Clean Prod 2013; 53: 310-31.
[http://dx.doi.org/10.1016/j.jclepro.2013.03.031]

[16]    Wissgott U, Bortlik K. Prospects for new natural food colorants. Trends Food Sci Technol 1996; 7: 298-302.
[http://dx.doi.org/10.1016/0924-2244(96)20007-X]

[17]    Masone D, Chanforan C. Study on the interaction of artificial and natural food colorants with human serum albumin: A computational point of view. Comput Biol Chem 2015; 56: 152-8.
[http://dx.doi.org/10.1016/j.compbiolchem.2015.04.006]

[18]    Gengatharan A, Dykes GA, Choo WS. Betalains: Natural plant pigments with potential application in functional foods. Lebensm Wiss Technol 2015; 64: 645-9.
[http://dx.doi.org/10.1016/j.lwt.2015.06.052]

[19]    Agócs A, Deli J. Pigments in your food. J Food Compos Anal 2011; 24: 757-9.
[http://dx.doi.org/10.1016/j.jfca.2011.07.001]

[20]    Sagdic O, Ekici L, Ozturk I, Tekinay T, Polat B, Tastemur B, *et al.* Cytotoxic and bioactive properties of different color tulip flowers and degradation kinetic of tulip flower anthocyanins. Food Chem Toxicol 2013; 58: 432-9.
[http://dx.doi.org/10.1016/j.fct.2013.05.021]

[21]    Siró I, Kápolna E, Kápolna B, Lugasi A. Functional food. Product development, marketing and consumer acceptance—A review. Appetite 2008; 51: 456-67.
[http://dx.doi.org/10.1016/j.appet.2008.05.060]

[22]    Bagchi D. Nutraceuticals and functional foods regulations in the United States and around the world Houston, TX, USA: Academic Press publications 2006; vol. 221.

[23]    Viuda-Martos M, Ruiz-Navajas Y, Fernández-López J, Pérez-Álvarez JA. Spices as Functional Foods. Crit Rev Food Sci Nutr 2010; 51: 13-28.
[http://dx.doi.org/10.1080/10408390903044271]

[24]    Jauho M, Niva M. Lay understandings of functional foods as hybrids of food and medicine. Food. Cult Soc An Int J Multidiscip 2013; 16: 43-63.
[http://dx.doi.org/10.2752/175174413X13500468045362]

[25]    Kammerer DR, Kammerer J, Valet R, Carle R. Recovery of polyphenols from the by-products of plant food processing and application as valuable food ingredients. Food Res Int 2014; 65: 2-12.
[http://dx.doi.org/10.1016/j.foodres.2014.06.012]

[26]    Zou T, He P, Yasen A, Li Z. Determination of seven synthetic dyes in animal feeds and meat by high

performance liquid chromatography with diode array and tandem mass detectors. Food Chem 2013; 138: 1742-8.
[http://dx.doi.org/10.1016/j.foodchem.2012.11.084]

[27]  Council Regulation (EC) 1129/2011. Council Regulation (EC) 1129/2011 of 11 November 2011 on amending Annex II to Regulation (EC) No 1333/2008 of the European Parliament and of the Council by establishing a Union list of food additives. n.d.

[28]  Council Regulation (EC) 1333/2008. Council Regulation (EC) 1333/2008 of 16 December 2008 on food additives. 2008. OJ L354/16. n.d.

[29]  Official Journal of the European Communities Legislation. Scope of EU's permitted food colorants list now covers medicinal products. 2009; Vol. 2009.

[30]  Chemical Engineering US spending on food colorants & adjuvants approaching $400 M 2002.

[31]  Europe EnvironmentEU rejects German appeal for more extensive restrictions on azo colorants 2005.

[32]  Kapadia GJ, Tokuda H, Sridhar R, Balasubramanian V, Takayasu J, Bu P, *et al.* Cancer chemopreventive activity of synthetic colorants used in foods, pharmaceuticals and cosmetic preparations. Cancer Lett 1998; 129: 87-95.
[http://dx.doi.org/10.1016/S0304-3835(98)00087-1]

[33]  Cabrita L, Fossen T, Andersen ØM. Colouring and stability of the six common anthocyanidin 3-glucosides in aqueous solutions. Food Chem 2000; 68: 101-7.
[http://dx.doi.org/10.1016/S0308-8146(99)00170-3]

[34]  Stintzing FC, Schieber A, Carle R. Betacyanins in fruits from red-purple pitaya, Hylocereus polyrhizus (Weber). Britton & Rose Food Chem 2002; 77: 101-6.
[http://dx.doi.org/10.1016/S0308-8146(01)00374-0]

[35]  Cassano A, Conidi C, Drioli E. Physico-chemical parameters of cactus pear (Opuntia ficus-indica) juice clarified by microfiltration and ultrafiltration processes. Desalination 2010; 250: 1101-4.
[http://dx.doi.org/10.1016/j.desal.2009.09.117]

[36]  Otálora MC, Carriazo JG, Iturriaga L, Nazareno MA, Osorio C. Microencapsulation of betalains obtained from cactus fruit (Opuntia ficus-indica) by spray drying using cactus cladode mucilage and maltodextrin as encapsulating agents. Food Chem 2015; 187: 174-81.
[http://dx.doi.org/10.1016/j.foodchem.2015.04.090]

[37]  Obón JM, Castellar MR, Alacid M, Fernández-López JA. Production of a red-purple food colorant from Opuntia stricta fruits by spray drying and its application in food model systems. J Food Eng 2009; 90: 471-9.
[http://dx.doi.org/10.1016/j.jfoodeng.2008.07.013]

[38]  Khan MI, Giridhar P. Enhanced chemical stability, chromatic properties and regeneration of betalains in Rivina humilis L. berry juice. Lebensm Wiss Technol 2014; 58: 649-57.
[http://dx.doi.org/10.1016/j.lwt.2014.03.027]

[39]  Khan MI. Stabilization of betalains: A review. Food Chem 2016; 197: 1280-5.
[http://dx.doi.org/10.1016/j.foodchem.2015.11.043]

[40]  Popa A, Moldovan B, David L. Betanin from red beet (Beta vulgaris L.) extraction conditions and evaluation of the thermal stability. J Chem 2015; 66: 413-6.

[41]  Dias MG, Camões MFGFC, Oliveira L. Carotenoids in traditional Portuguese fruits and vegetables. Food Chem 2009; 113: 808-15.
[http://dx.doi.org/10.1016/j.foodchem.2008.08.002]

[42]  Grewe C, Menge S, Griehl C. Enantioselective separation of all-E-astaxanthin and its determination in microbial sources. J Chromatogr A 2007; 1166: 97-100.
[http://dx.doi.org/10.1016/j.chroma.2007.08.002]

[43]  Hong HL, Suo QL, Han LM, Li CP. Study on precipitation of astaxanthin in supercritical fluid.

Powder Technol 2009; 191: 294-8.
[http://dx.doi.org/10.1016/j.powtec.2008.10.022]

[44] Danesi EDG, Rangel-Yagui CDO, Carvalho JCM, Sato S. An investigation of effect of replacing nitrate by urea in the growth and production of chlorophyll by Spirulina platensis. Biomass Bioenergy 2002; 23: 261-9.
[http://dx.doi.org/10.1016/S0961-9534(02)00054-5]

[45] Nabae K, Ichihara T, Hagiwara A, Hirota T, Toda Y, Tamano S, *et al.* A 90-day oral toxicity study of beta-carotene derived from Blakeslea trispora, a natural food colorant, in F344 rats. Food Chem Toxicol 2005; 43: 1127-33.
[http://dx.doi.org/10.1016/j.fct.2005.03.003]

[46] Bibi NS, Galvis L, Grasselli M, Fernández-Lahore M. Synthesis and sorption performance of highly specific imprinted particles for the direct recovery of carminic acid. Process Biochem 2012; 47: 1327-34.
[http://dx.doi.org/10.1016/j.procbio.2012.04.030]

[47] Huang H-Y, Chiu C-W, Sue S-L, Cheng C-F. Analysis of food colorants by capillary electrophoresis with large-volume sample stacking. J Chromatogr A 2003; 995: 29-36.
[http://dx.doi.org/10.1016/S0021-9673(03)00530-2]

[48] Huang H-Y, Shih Y-C, Chen Y-C. Determining eight colorants in milk beverages by capillary electrophoresis. J Chromatogr A 2002; 959: 317-25.
[http://dx.doi.org/10.1016/S0021-9673(02)00441-7]

[49] Grotewold E. The Science of Flavonoids. United States of America: The Ohio State University 2006.
[http://dx.doi.org/10.1007/978-0-387-28822-2]

[50] Robbins RJ. Phenolic acids in foods: an overview of analytical methodology. J Agric Food Chem 2003; 51: 2866-87.
[http://dx.doi.org/10.1021/jf026182t]

[51] Carocho M, Ferreira ICFR. A review on antioxidants, prooxidants and related controversy: natural and synthetic compounds, screening and analysis methodologies and future perspectives. Food Chem Toxicol 2013; 51: 15-25.
[http://dx.doi.org/10.1016/j.fct.2012.09.021]

[52] Jiménez-Aguilar DM, Ortega-Regules AE, Lozada-Ramírez JD, Pérez-Pérez MCI, Vernon-Carter EJ, Welti-Chanes J. Color and chemical stability of spray-dried blueberry extract using mesquite gum as wall material. J Food Compos Anal 2011; 24: 889-94.
[http://dx.doi.org/10.1016/j.jfca.2011.04.012]

[53] Martelli G, Folli C, Visai L, Daglia M, Ferrari D. Thermal stability improvement of blue colorant C-Phycocyanin from Spirulina platensis for food industry applications. Process Biochem 2014; 49: 154-9.
[http://dx.doi.org/10.1016/j.procbio.2013.10.008]

[54] Mishra SK, Shrivastav A, Pancha I, Jain D, Mishra S. Effect of preservatives for food grade C-Phycoerythrin, isolated from marine cyanobacteria Pseudanabaena sp. Int J Biol Macromol 2010; 47: 597-602.
[http://dx.doi.org/10.1016/j.ijbiomac.2010.08.005]

[55] Renna M, Gonnella M. The use of the sea fennel as a new spice-colorant in culinary preparations. Int J Gastron Food Sci 2012; 1: 111-5.
[http://dx.doi.org/10.1016/j.ijgfs.2013.06.004]

[56] Gao L-N, Zhang Y, Cui Y-L, Yan K. Evaluation of genipin on human cytochrome P450 isoenzymes and P-glycoprotein in vitro. Fitoterapia 2014; 98: 130-6.
[http://dx.doi.org/10.1016/j.fitote.2014.07.018]

[57] Hou YC, Tsai SY, Lai PY, Chen YS, Chao PDL. Metabolism and pharmacokinetics of genipin and

geniposide in rats. Food Chem Toxicol 2008; 46: 2764-9.
[http://dx.doi.org/10.1016/j.fct.2008.04.033]

[58]   Ramos-De-La-Peña AM, Renard CMGC, Wicker L, Montañez JC, García-Cerda LA, Contreras-Esquivel JC. Environmental friendly cold-mechanical/sonic enzymatic assisted extraction of genipin from genipap (Genipa americana). Ultrason Sonochem 2014; 21: 43-9.
[http://dx.doi.org/10.1016/j.ultsonch.2013.06.008]

[59]   Ozaki A, Kitano M, Furusawa N, Yamaguchi H, Kuroda K, Endo G. Genotoxicity of gardenia yellow and its components. Food Chem Toxicol 2002; 40: 1603-10.
[http://dx.doi.org/10.1016/S0278-6915(02)00118-7]

[60]   Wada M, Kido H, Ohyama K, Ichibangase T, Kishikawa N, Ohba Y, *et al.* Chemiluminescent screening of quenching effects of natural colorants against reactive oxygen species: Evaluation of grape seed, monascus, gardenia and red radish extracts as multi-functional food additives. Food Chem 2007; 101: 980-6.
[http://dx.doi.org/10.1016/j.foodchem.2006.02.050]

[61]   Nabae K, Hayashi S-M, Kawabe M, Ichihara T, Hagiwara A, Tamano S, *et al.* A 90-day oral toxicity study of purple corn color, a natural food colorant, in F344 rats. Food Chem Toxicol 2008; 46: 774-80.
[http://dx.doi.org/10.1016/j.fct.2007.10.004]

[62]   Venil CK, Aruldass CA, Halim MHA, Khasim AR, Zakaria ZA, Ahmad WA. Spray drying of violet pigment from Chromobacterium violaceum UTM 5 and its application in food model systems. Int Biodeterior Biodegradation 2015; 102: 1-6.
[http://dx.doi.org/10.1016/j.ibiod.2015.02.006]

[63]   Patakova P. Monascus secondary metabolites: Production and biological activity. J Ind Microbiol Biotechnol 2013; 40: 169-81.
[http://dx.doi.org/10.1007/s10295-012-1216-8]

[64]   Wang C, Chen D, Chen M, Wang Y, Li Z, Li F. Stimulatory effects of blue light on the growth, monascin and ankaflavin production in Monascus. Biotechnol Lett 2015; 37: 1043-8.
[http://dx.doi.org/10.1007/s10529-014-1763-3]

[65]   Wild D. Red mould rice (angkak). Analysis and detection in meat products. Fleischwirtschaft (Frankf) 2000; 80: 91-3.

[66]   EFSA. Scientific Opinion on the re-evaluation of vegetable carbon (E 153) as a food additive - EFSA Panel on Food Additives and Nutrient Sources added to Food (ANS). EFSA J 2012; 10: 1-34.

[67]   Moreno DA, García-Viguera C, Gil JI, Gil-Izquierdo A. Betalains in the era of global agri-food science, technology and nutritional health. Phytochem Rev 2008; 7: 261-80.
[http://dx.doi.org/10.1007/s11101-007-9084-y]

[68]   EFSA. Scientific Opinion on the re-evaluation of beetroot red (E 162) as a food additive - EFSA Panel on Food Additives and Nutrient Sources added to Food (ANS). EFSA J 2015; 13: 1-56.

[69]   EFSA. Scientific Opinion on the re-evaluation Tartrazine (E 102) - EFSA Panel on Food Additives and Nutrient Sources added to Food (ANS). EFSA J 2009; 7: 1-52.

[70]   EFSA. Scientific Opinion on the re-evaluation of cochineal, carminic acid, carmines (E 120) as a food additive - EFSA Panel on Food Additives and Nutrient Sources added to Food (ANS). EFSA J 2015; 13: 1-65.

[71]   EFSA. Scientific Opinion on the re-evaluation of Indigo Carmine (E 132) as a food additive - EFSA Panel on Food additives and Nutrient Sources added to Food (ANS). EFSA J 2014; 12: 1-51.

[72]   EFSA. Scientific Opinion on the re-evaluation of Brilliant Blue FCF (E 133) as a food additive - EFSA Panel on Food Additives and Nutrient Sources added to Food (ANS). EFSA J 2010; 8: 1-36.

[73]   EFSA. Opinion of the Scientific Panel on Food Additives, Flavourings, Processing Aids and Materials in Contact with Food on the food colouring Red 2G (E128) based on a request from the Commission

related to the re-evaluation of all permitted food additives. EFSA J 2007; 515: 1-28.

[74]  Gostner JM, Becker K, Ueberall F, Fuchs D. The good and bad of antioxidant foods: An immunological perspective. Food Chem Toxicol 2015; 80: 72-9.
[http://dx.doi.org/10.1016/j.fct.2015.02.012]

[75]  Agner AR, Barbisan LF, Scolastici C, Salvadori DMF. Absence of carcinogenic and anticarcinogenic effects of annatto in the rat liver medium-term assay. Food Chem Toxicol 2004; 42: 1687-93.
[http://dx.doi.org/10.1016/j.fct.2004.06.005]

[76]  Agner AR, Bazo AP, Ribeiro LR, Salvadori DMF. DNA damage and aberrant crypt foci as putative biomarkers to evaluate the chemopreventive effect of annatto (Bixa orellana L.) in rat colon carcinogenesis. Mutat Res Genet Toxicol Environ Mutagen 2005; 582: 146-54.
[http://dx.doi.org/10.1016/j.mrgentox.2005.01.009]

[77]  Anantharaman A, Priya RR, Hemachandran H, Sivaramakrishna A, Babu S, Siva R. Studies on interaction of norbixin with DNA: multispectroscopic and in silico analysis. Spectrochim Acta A Mol Biomol Spectrosc 2015; 144: 163-9.
[http://dx.doi.org/10.1016/j.saa.2015.02.049]

[78]  Bautista ARPL, Moreira ELT, Batista MS, Miranda MS, Gomes ICS. Subacute toxicity assessment of annatto in rat. Food Chem Toxicol 2004; 42: 625-9.
[http://dx.doi.org/10.1016/j.fct.2003.11.007]

[79]  Kohno Y, Asai S, Shibata M, Fukuhara C, Maeda Y, Tomita Y, *et al.* Improved photostability of hydrophobic natural dye incorporated in organo-modified hydrotalcite. J Phys Chem Solids 2014; 75: 945-50.
[http://dx.doi.org/10.1016/j.jpcs.2014.04.010]

[80]  Lima ROA, Azevedo L, Ribeiro LR, Salvadori DMF. Study on the mutagenicity and antimutagenicity of a natural food colouring (annatto) in mouse bone marrow cells. Food Chem Toxicol 2003; 41: 189-92.
[http://dx.doi.org/10.1016/S0278-6915(02)00208-9]

[81]  Sobral D, Costa RGB, Machado GM, Paula JCJ, Teodoro VAM, Nunes NM, *et al.* Can lutein replace annatto in the manufacture of Prato cheese? Lebensm Wiss Technol 2016; 68: 349-55.
[http://dx.doi.org/10.1016/j.lwt.2015.12.051]

[82]  Dykes L, Rooney WL, Rooney LW. Evaluation of phenolics and antioxidant activity of black sorghum hybrids. J Cereal Sci 2013; 58: 278-83.
[http://dx.doi.org/10.1016/j.jcs.2013.06.006]

[83]  Sivakumar V, Vijaeeswarri J, Anna JL. Effective natural dye extraction from different plant materials using ultrasound. Ind Crops Prod 2011; 33: 116-22.
[http://dx.doi.org/10.1016/j.indcrop.2010.09.007]

[84]  Terahara N, Callebaut A, Ohba R, Nagata T, Ohnishi-Kameyama M, Suzuki M. Acylated anthocyanidin 3-sophoroside-5-glucosides from Ajuga reptans flowers and the corresponding cell cultures. Phytochemistry 2001; 58: 493-500.
[http://dx.doi.org/10.1016/S0031-9422(01)00172-8]

[85]  Chandrasekhar J, Madhusudhan MC, Raghavarao KSMS. Extraction of anthocyanins from red cabbage and purification using adsorption. Food Bioprod Process 2012; 90: 615-23.
[http://dx.doi.org/10.1016/j.fbp.2012.07.004]

[86]  Buchweitz M, Brauch J, Carle R, Kammerer DR. Application of ferric anthocyanin chelates as natural blue food colorants in polysaccharide and gelatin based gels. Food Res Int 2013; 51: 274-82.
[http://dx.doi.org/10.1016/j.foodres.2012.11.030]

[87]  Srivastava J, Vankar PS. Canna indica flower: New source of anthocyanins. Plant Physiol Biochem 2010; 48: 1015-9.
[http://dx.doi.org/10.1016/j.plaphy.2010.08.011]

[88]   Prata ERBA, Oliveira LS. Fresh coffee husks as potential sources of anthocyanins. Lebensm Wiss Technol 2007; 40: 1555-60.
[http://dx.doi.org/10.1016/j.lwt.2006.10.003]

[89]   Assous MTM, Abdel-Hady MM, Medany GM. Evaluation of red pigment extracted from purple carrots and its utilization as antioxidant and natural food colorants. Ann Agric Sci 2014; 59: 1-7.
[http://dx.doi.org/10.1016/j.aoas.2014.06.001]

[90]   Coïsson JD, Travaglia F, Piana G, Capasso M, Arlorio M. Euterpe oleracea juice as a functional pigment for yogurt. Food Res Int 2005; 38: 893-7.
[http://dx.doi.org/10.1016/j.foodres.2005.03.009]

[91]   Mak YW, Chuah LO, Ahmad R, Bhat R. Antioxidant and antibacterial activities of hibiscus (Hibiscus rosa-sinensis L.) and Cassia (Senna bicapsularis L.) flower extracts. J King Saud Univ - Sci 2013; 25: 275-82.

[92]   Nitteranon V, Kittiwongwattana C, Vuttipongchaikij S, Sakulkoo J, Srijakkoat M, Chokratin P, *et al.* Evaluations of the mutagenicity of a pigment extract from bulb culture of Hippeastrum reticulatum. Food Chem Toxicol 2014; 69: 237-43.
[http://dx.doi.org/10.1016/j.fct.2014.04.007]

[93]   Cipriano PA, Ekici L, Barnes RC, Gomes C, Talcott ST. Pre-heating and polyphenol oxidase inhibition impact on extraction of purple sweet potato anthocyanins. Food Chem 2015; 180: 227-34.
[http://dx.doi.org/10.1016/j.foodchem.2015.02.020]

[94]   Pazmio-Durán EA, Giusti MM, Wrolstad RE, Glória MBA. Anthocyanins from banana bracts (Musa X paradisiaca) as potential food colorants. Food Chem 2001; 73: 327-32.
[http://dx.doi.org/10.1016/S0308-8146(00)00305-8]

[95]   Loypimai P, Moongngarm A, Chottanom P, Moontree T. Ohmic heating-assisted extraction of anthocyanins from black rice bran to prepare a natural food colourant. Innov Food Sci Emerg Technol 2015; 27: 102-10.
[http://dx.doi.org/10.1016/j.ifset.2014.12.009]

[96]   Pazmio-Durán EA, Giusti MM, Wrolstad RE, Glória MBA. Anthocyanins from Oxalis triangularis as potential food colorants. Food Chem 2001; 75: 211-6.
[http://dx.doi.org/10.1016/S0308-8146(01)00201-1]

[97]   Tan JBL, Lim YY, Lee SM. Rhoeo spathacea (Swartz) Stearn leaves, a potential natural food colorant. J Funct Foods 2014; 7: 443-51.
[http://dx.doi.org/10.1016/j.jff.2014.01.012]

[98]   Cerón IX, Higuita JC, Cardona CA. Design and analysis of antioxidant compounds from Andes Berry fruits (Rubus glaucus Benth) using an enhanced-fluidity liquid extraction process with CO2 and ethanol. J Supercrit Fluids 2012; 62: 96-101.
[http://dx.doi.org/10.1016/j.supflu.2011.12.007]

[99]   Smith MAL, Madhavi DL, Fang Y, Tomczak MM. Continuous cell culture and product recovery from wild Vaccinium pahalae germplasm. J Plant Physiol 1997; 150: 462-6.
[http://dx.doi.org/10.1016/S0176-1617(97)80099-5]

[100]  Vatai T, Škerget M, Knez Ž, Kareth S, Wehowski M, Weidner E. Extraction and formulation of anthocyanin-concentrates from grape residues. J Supercrit Fluids 2008; 45: 32-6.
[http://dx.doi.org/10.1016/j.supflu.2007.12.008]

[101]  Yang Z, Zhai W. Optimization of microwave-assisted extraction of anthocyanins from purple corn (Zea mays L.) cob and identification with HPLC–MS. Innov Food Sci Emerg Technol 2010; 11: 470-6.
[http://dx.doi.org/10.1016/j.ifset.2010.03.003]

[102]  Yang Z, Zhai W. Identification and antioxidant activity of anthocyanins extracted from the seed and cob of purple corn (Zea mays L.). Innov Food Sci Emerg Technol 2010; 11: 169-76.

[http://dx.doi.org/10.1016/j.ifset.2009.08.012]

[103]  Longo L, Scardino A, Vasapollo G. Identification and quantification of anthocyanins in the berries of Pistacia lentiscus L., Phillyrea latifolia L. and Rubia peregrina L. Innov Food Sci Emerg Technol 2007; 8: 360-4.
[http://dx.doi.org/10.1016/j.ifset.2007.03.010]

[104]  Harsha PSCS, Khan MI, Prabhakar P, Giridhar P. Cyanidin-3-glucoside, nutritionally important constituents and in vitro antioxidant activities of Santalum album L. berries. Food Res Int 2013; 50: 275-81.
[http://dx.doi.org/10.1016/j.foodres.2012.10.024]

[105]  Todaro A, Cimino F, Rapisarda P, Catalano AE, Barbagallo RN, Spagna G. Recovery of anthocyanins from eggplant peel. Food Chem 2009; 114: 434-9.
[http://dx.doi.org/10.1016/j.foodchem.2008.09.102]

[106]  Zhu Z, Wu N, Kuang M, Lamikanra O, Liu G, Li S, *et al.* Preparation and toxicological evaluation of methyl pyranoanthocyanin. Food Chem Toxicol 2015; 83: 125-32.
[http://dx.doi.org/10.1016/j.fct.2015.05.004]

[107]  Kapadia GJ, Balasubramanian V, Tokuda H, Iwashima A, Nishino H. Inhibition of 12--tetradecanoylphorbol-13-acetate induced Epstein-Barr virus early antigen activation by natural colorants. Cancer Lett 1997; 115: 173-8.
[http://dx.doi.org/10.1016/S0304-3835(97)04726-5]

[108]  Ravichandran K, Saw NMMT, Mohdaly AAA, Gabr AMM, Kastell A, Riedel H, *et al.* Impact of processing of red beet on betalain content and antioxidant activity. Food Res Int 2013; 50: 670-5.
[http://dx.doi.org/10.1016/j.foodres.2011.07.002]

[109]  Otálora MC, Carriazo JG, Iturriaga L, Nazareno MA, Osorio C. Microencapsulation of betalains obtained from cactus fruit (Opuntia ficus-indica) by spray drying using cactus cladode mucilage and maltodextrin as encapsulating agents. Food Chem 2015; 187: 174-81.
[http://dx.doi.org/10.1016/j.foodchem.2015.04.090]

[110]  Sun M, Temelli F. Supercritical carbon dioxide extraction of carotenoids from carrot using canola oil as a continuous co-solvent. J Supercrit Fluids 2006; 37: 397-408.
[http://dx.doi.org/10.1016/j.supflu.2006.01.008]

[111]  Martín A, Mattea F, Gutiérrez L, Miguel F, Cocero MJ. Co-precipitation of carotenoids and bio-polymers with the supercritical anti-solvent process. J Supercrit Fluids 2007; 41: 138-47.
[http://dx.doi.org/10.1016/j.supflu.2006.08.009]

[112]  Mejía EG, Loarca-Piña G, Ramos-Gómez M. Antimutagenicity of xanthophylls present in Aztec Marigold (Tagetes erecta) against 1-nitropyrene. Mutat Res 1997; 389: 219-26.
[http://dx.doi.org/10.1016/S1383-5718(96)00151-9]

[113]  Khalil M, Raila J, Ali M, Islam KMS, Schenk R, Krause J-P, *et al.* Stability and bioavailability of lutein ester supplements from Tagetes flower prepared under food processing conditions. J Funct Foods 2012; 4: 602-10.
[http://dx.doi.org/10.1016/j.jff.2012.03.006]

[114]  Fernandes TM, Gomes BB, Lanfer-Marquez UM. Apparent absorption of chlorophyll from spinach in an assay with dogs. Innov Food Sci Emerg Technol 2007; 8: 426-32.
[http://dx.doi.org/10.1016/j.ifset.2007.03.019]

[115]  Gómez-Estaca J, Gavara R, Hernández-Muñoz P. Encapsulation of curcumin in electrosprayed gelatin microspheres enhances its bioaccessibility and widens its uses in food applications. Innov Food Sci Emerg Technol 2015; 29: 302-7.
[http://dx.doi.org/10.1016/j.ifset.2015.03.004]

[116]  Silva LV, Nelson DL, Drummond MFB, Dufossé L. Glória MB a. Comparison of hydrodistillation methods for the deodorization of turmeric. Food Res Int 2005; 38: 1087-96.

[http://dx.doi.org/10.1016/j.foodres.2005.02.025]

[117]  Wang Y, Lu Z, Wu H, Lv F. Study on the antibiotic activity of microcapsule curcumin against foodborne pathogens. Int J Food Microbiol 2009; 136: 71-4.
[http://dx.doi.org/10.1016/j.ijfoodmicro.2009.09.001]

[118]  Maier E, Kurz K, Jenny M, Schennach H, Ueberall F, Fuchs D. Food preservatives sodium benzoate and propionic acid and colorant curcumin suppress Th1-type immune response in vitro. Food Chem Toxicol 2010; 48: 1950-6.
[http://dx.doi.org/10.1016/j.fct.2010.04.042]

[119]  Martins RM, Pereira SV, Siqueira S, Salomão WF, Freitas LAP. Curcuminoid content and antioxidant activity in spray dried microparticles containing turmeric extract. Food Res Int 2013; 50: 657-63.
[http://dx.doi.org/10.1016/j.foodres.2011.06.030]

[120]  Han S, Yang Y. Antimicrobial activity of wool fabric treated with curcumin. Dyes Pigments 2005; 64: 157-61.
[http://dx.doi.org/10.1016/j.dyepig.2004.05.008]

[121]  Xi L, Qian Z, Xu G, Zheng S, Sun S, Wen N, *et al.* Beneficial impact of crocetin, a carotenoid from saffron, on insulin sensitivity in fructose-fed rats. J Nutr Biochem 2007; 18: 64-72.
[http://dx.doi.org/10.1016/j.jnutbio.2006.03.010]

[122]  Li H-X, Han S-Y, Wang X-W, Ma X, Zhang K, Wang L, *et al.* Effect of the carthamins yellow from Carthamus tinctorius L. on hemorheological disorders of blood stasis in rats. Food Chem Toxicol 2009; 47: 1797-802.
[http://dx.doi.org/10.1016/j.fct.2009.04.026]

[123]  Guyot S, Serrand S, Le Quéré JM, Sanoner P, Renard CMGC. Enzymatic synthesis and physicochemical characterisation of phloridzin oxidation products (POP), a new water-soluble yellow dye deriving from apple. Innov Food Sci Emerg Technol 2007; 8: 443-50.
[http://dx.doi.org/10.1016/j.ifset.2007.03.021]

[124]  Tan M, Gan D, Wei L, Pan Y, Tang S, Wang H. Isolation and characterization of pigment from Cinnamomum burmannii' peel. Food Res Int 2011; 44: 2289-94.
[http://dx.doi.org/10.1016/j.foodres.2010.05.022]

[125]  Cerón IX, Ng RTL, El-Halwagi M, Cardona CA. Process synthesis for antioxidant polyphenolic compounds production from Matisia cordata Bonpl. (zapote) pulp. J Food Eng 2014; 134: 5-15.
[http://dx.doi.org/10.1016/j.jfoodeng.2014.02.010]

[126]  Li C-C, Hsiang C-Y, Lo H-Y, Pai F-T, Wu S-L, Ho T-Y. Genipin inhibits lipopolysaccharide-induced acute systemic inflammation in mice as evidenced by nuclear factor-kB bioluminescent imaging-guided transcriptomic analysis. Food Chem Toxicol 2012; 50: 2978-86.
[http://dx.doi.org/10.1016/j.fct.2012.05.054]

[127]  Inoue K, Shibutani M, Masutomi N, Toyoda K. One-year chronic toxicity of madder color in F344 rats--induction of preneoplastic/neoplastic lesions in the kidney and liver. Food Chem Toxicol 2008; 46: 3303-10.
[http://dx.doi.org/10.1016/j.fct.2008.07.025]

[128]  Inoue K, Shibutani M, Masutomi N, Toyoda K, Takagi H, Uneyama C, *et al.* A 13-week subchronic toxicity study of paprika color in F344 rats. Food Chem Toxicol 2008; 46: 241-52.
[http://dx.doi.org/10.1016/j.fct.2007.08.002]

[129]  Zou Y, Xie C, Fan G, Gu Z, Han Y. Optimization of ultrasound-assisted extraction of melanin from Auricularia auricula fruit bodies. Innov Food Sci Emerg Technol 2010; 11: 611-5.
[http://dx.doi.org/10.1016/j.ifset.2010.07.002]

[130]  EFSA. Scientific Opinion on the re-evaluation of Brilliant Black BN (E 151) as a food additive - EFSA Panel on Food Additives and Nutrient Sources added to Food (ANS). EFSA J 2010; 8: 1-30.

[131]  Kong C, Fodjo EK, Li D, Cai Y, Huang D, Wang Y, *et al.* Chitosan-based adsorption and freeze

deproteinization: Improved extraction and purification of synthetic colorants from protein-rich food samples. Food Chem 2015; 188: 240-7.
[http://dx.doi.org/10.1016/j.foodchem.2015.04.115]

[132] Ma K, Yang YN, Jiang XX, Zhao M, Cai YQ. Simultaneous determination of 20 food additives by high performance liquid chromatography with photo-diode array detector. Chin Chem Lett 2012; 23: 492-5.
[http://dx.doi.org/10.1016/j.cclet.2011.12.018]

[133] Liu F-J, Liu C-T, Li W, Tang A-N. Dispersive solid-phase microextraction and capillary electrophoresis separation of food colorants in beverages using diamino moiety functionalized silica nanoparticles as both extractant and pseudostationary phase. Talanta 2015; 132: 366-72.
[http://dx.doi.org/10.1016/j.talanta.2014.09.014]

[134] Medeiros RA, Lourencao BC, Rocha-Filho RC, Fatibello-Filho O. Simultaneous voltammetric determination of synthetic colorants in food using a cathodically pretreated boron-doped diamond electrode. Talanta 2012; 97: 291-7.
[http://dx.doi.org/10.1016/j.talanta.2012.04.033]

[135] Medeiros RA, Lourencao BC, Rocha-Filho RC, Fatibello-Filho O. Flow injection simultaneous determination of synthetic colorants in food using multiple pulse amperometric detection with a boron-doped diamond electrode. Talanta 2012; 99: 883-9.
[http://dx.doi.org/10.1016/j.talanta.2012.07.051]

[136] Minioti KS, Sakellariou CF, Thomaidis NS. Determination of 13 synthetic food colorants in water-soluble foods by reversed-phase high-performance liquid chromatography coupled with diode-array detector. Anal Chim Acta 2007; 583: 103-10.
[http://dx.doi.org/10.1016/j.aca.2006.10.002]

[137] Ni Y, Wang Y, Kokot S. Simultaneous kinetic spectrophotometric analysis of five synthetic food colorants with the aid of chemometrics. Talanta 2009; 78: 432-41.
[http://dx.doi.org/10.1016/j.talanta.2008.11.035]

[138] Pan X, Ushio H, Ohshima T. Effects of molecular configurations of food colorants on their efficacies as photosensitizers in lipid oxidation. Food Chem 2005; 92: 37-44.
[http://dx.doi.org/10.1016/j.foodchem.2004.07.017]

[139] Qi H, Takano H, Kato Y, Wu Q, Ogata C, Zhu B, *et al.* Hydrogen peroxide-dependent photocytotoxicity by phloxine B, a xanthene-type food colorant. Biochim Biophys Acta 2011; 1810: 704-12.
[http://dx.doi.org/10.1016/j.bbagen.2011.04.010]

[140] Vidotti EC, Costa WF, Oliveira CC. Development of a green chromatographic method for determination of colorants in food samples. Talanta 2006; 68: 516-21.
[http://dx.doi.org/10.1016/j.talanta.2005.01.059]

[141] Bonan S, Fedrizzi G, Menotta S, Elisabetta C. Simultaneous determination of synthetic dyes in foodstuffs and beverages by high-performance liquid chromatography coupled with diode-array detector. Dyes Pigments 2013; 99: 36-40.
[http://dx.doi.org/10.1016/j.dyepig.2013.03.029]

[142] Chen Q, Mou S, Hou X, Riviello J, Ni Z. Determination of eight synthetic food colorants in drinks by high-performance ion chromatography. J Chromatogr A 1998; 827: 73-81.
[http://dx.doi.org/10.1016/S0021-9673(98)00759-6]

[143] Berzas JJ, Flores JR, Llerena MJV, Fariñas NR. Spectrophotometric resolution of ternary mixtures of Tartrazine, Patent Blue V and Indigo Carmine in commercial products. Anal Chim Acta 1999; 391: 353-64.
[http://dx.doi.org/10.1016/S0003-2670(99)00215-9]

[144] Wang Y, Wei D, Yang H, Yang Y, Xing W, Li Y, *et al.* Development of a highly sensitive and specific monoclonal antibody-based enzyme-linked immunosorbent assay (ELISA) for detection of

Sudan I in food samples. Talanta 2009; 77: 1783-9.
[http://dx.doi.org/10.1016/j.talanta.2008.10.016]

[145]  EFSA. Scientific Opinion on the safety and efficacy of Patent Blue V (E 131) as feed additive for non food-producing animals - EFSA Panel on Additives and Products or Substances used in Animal Feed (FEEDAP). EFSA J 2013; 11: 1-13.

[146]  EFSA. Scientific Opinion on the re-evaluation of Brown FK (E 154) as a food additive - EFSA Panel on Food Additives and Nutrient Sources added to Food (ANS). EFSA J 2010; 8: 1-29.

[147]  EFSA. Scientific Opinion on the re-evaluation of Brown HT (E 155) as a food additive - EFSA Panel on Food Additives and Nutrient Sources (ANS). EFSA J 2010; 8: 1-31.

[148]  EFSA. Scientific Opinion on the re-evaluation of caramel colours (E 150 a,b,c,d) as food additives1 EFSA Panel on Food Additives and Nutrient Sources added to Food (ANS). EFSA J 2011; 9: 1-103.

[149]  Gandul-Rojas B, Roca M, Gallardo-Guerrero L. Detection of the color adulteration of green table olives with copper chlorophyllin complexes (E-141ii colorant). Lebensm Wiss Technol 2012; 46: 311-8.
[http://dx.doi.org/10.1016/j.lwt.2011.09.012]

[150]  Mortensen A, Geppel A. HPLC–MS analysis of the green food colorant sodium copper chlorophyllin. Innov Food Sci Emerg Technol 2007; 8: 419-25.
[http://dx.doi.org/10.1016/j.ifset.2007.03.018]

[151]  EFSA. Scientific Opinion on re-evaluation of copper complexes of chlorophylls (E 141(i)) and chlorophyllins (E 141(ii)) as food additives - EFSA Panel on Food Additives and Nutrient Sources added to food (ANS). EFSA J 2015; 13: 1-60.

[152]  EFSA. Scientific Opinion on the re-evaluation of Green S (E 142) as a food additive - EFSA Panel on Food Additives and Nutrient Sources added to Food (ANS). EFSA J 2010; 8: 1-32.

[153]  El-Sheikh AH, Al-Degs YS. Spectrophotometric determination of food dyes in soft drinks by second order multivariate calibration of the absorbance spectra-pH data matrices. Dyes Pigments 2013; 97: 330-9.
[http://dx.doi.org/10.1016/j.dyepig.2013.01.007]

[154]  Karanikolopoulos G, Gerakis A, Papadopoulou K, Mastrantoni I. Determination of synthetic food colorants in fish products by an HPLC-DAD method. Food Chem 2015; 177: 197-203.
[http://dx.doi.org/10.1016/j.foodchem.2015.01.026]

[155]  Obón JM, Castellar MR. Cascales J a.;Fernández-López JA. Assessment of the TEAC method for determining the antioxidant capacity of synthetic red food colorants. Food Res Int 2005; 38: 843-5.
[http://dx.doi.org/10.1016/j.foodres.2005.01.010]

[156]  Xie Y, Li Y, Niu L, Wang H, Qian H, Yao W. A novel surface-enhanced Raman scattering sensor to detect prohibited colorants in food by graphene/silver nanocomposite. Talanta 2012; 100: 32-7.
[http://dx.doi.org/10.1016/j.talanta.2012.07.080]

[157]  EFSA. Scientific Opinion on the re-evaluation of Allura Red AC (E 129) as a food additive - EFSA Panel on Food Additives and Nutrient Sources added to Food (ANS). EFSA J 2009; 7: 1-39.

[158]  Ryvolová M, Táborský P, Vrábel P, Krásenský P, Preisler J. Sensitive determination of erythrosine and other red food colorants using capillary electrophoresis with laser-induced fluorescence detection. J Chromatogr A 2007; 1141: 206-11.
[http://dx.doi.org/10.1016/j.chroma.2006.12.018]

[159]  Xing Y, Meng M, Xue H, Zhang T, Yin Y, Xi R. Development of a polyclonal antibody-based enzyme-linked immunosorbent assay (ELISA) for detection of Sunset Yellow FCF in food samples. Talanta 2012; 99: 125-31.
[http://dx.doi.org/10.1016/j.talanta.2012.05.029]

[160]  Ma M, Luo X, Chen B, Su S, Yao S. Simultaneous determination of water-soluble and fat-soluble

synthetic colorants in foodstuff by high-performance liquid chromatography-diode array detection-electrospray mass spectrometry. J Chromatogr A 2006; 1103: 170-6.
[http://dx.doi.org/10.1016/j.chroma.2005.11.061]

[161]   Daoud I, Mesmoudi M, Ghalem S. MM/QM study: Interactions of copper(II) and mercury(II) with food dyes in aqueous solutions. Int J Chem Anal Sci 2013; 4: 49-56.
[http://dx.doi.org/10.1016/j.ijcas.2013.04.003]

[162]   Mpountoukas P, Pantazaki A, Kostareli E, Christodoulou P, Kareli D, Poliliou S, *et al.* Cytogenetic evaluation and DNA interaction studies of the food colorants amaranth, erythrosine and tartrazine. Food Chem Toxicol 2010; 48: 2934-44.
[http://dx.doi.org/10.1016/j.fct.2010.07.030]

[163]   Basu A, Kumar GS. Interaction of toxic azo dyes with heme protein: Biophysical insights into the binding aspect of the food additive amaranth with human hemoglobin. J Hazard Mater 2015; 289: 204-9.
[http://dx.doi.org/10.1016/j.jhazmat.2015.02.044]

[164]   EFSA. Scientific Opinion on the re-evaluation of Amaranth (E 123) as a food additive - EFSA Panel on Food Additives and Nutrient Sources added to Food (ANS). EFSA J 2010; 8: 1-41.

[165]   Campardelli R, Adami R, Reverchon E. Preparation of stable aqueous nanodispersions of?? -carotene by supercritical assisted injection in a liquid antisolvent. Procedia Eng 2012; 42: 1493-501.
[http://dx.doi.org/10.1016/j.proeng.2012.07.542]

[166]   Fernandez A, Torres-Giner S, Lagaron JM. Novel route to stabilization of bioactive antioxidants by encapsulation in electrospun fibers of zein prolamine. Food Hydrocoll 2009; 23: 1427-32.
[http://dx.doi.org/10.1016/j.foodhyd.2008.10.011]

[167]   Paz E, Martín Á, Bartolomé A, Largo M, Cocero MJ. Development of water-soluble β-carotene formulations by high-temperature, high-pressure emulsification and antisolvent precipitation. Food Hydrocoll 2014; 37: 14-24.
[http://dx.doi.org/10.1016/j.foodhyd.2013.10.011]

[168]   EFSA. Scientific Opinion on the re-evaluation of mixed carotenes (E 160a (i)) and beta-carotene (E 160a (ii)) as a food additive - EFSA Panel on Food Additives and Nutrient Sources added to Food (ANS). EFSA J 2012; 10: 1-67.

[169]   Datta S, Mahapatra N, Halder M. pH-insensitive electrostatic interaction of carmoisine with two serum proteins: a possible caution on its uses in food and pharmaceutical industry. J Photochem Photobiol B 2013; 124: 50-62.
[http://dx.doi.org/10.1016/j.jphotobiol.2013.04.004]

[170]   Basu A, Kumar GS. Study on the interaction of the toxic food additive carmoisine with serum albumins: A microcalorimetric investigation. J Hazard Mater 2014; 273: 200-6.
[http://dx.doi.org/10.1016/j.jhazmat.2014.03.049]

[171]   Basu A, Kumar GS. Binding of carmoisine, a food colorant, with hemoglobin: Spectroscopic and calorimetric studies. Food Res Int 2015; 72: 54-61.
[http://dx.doi.org/10.1016/j.foodres.2015.03.015]

[172]   EFSA. Scientific Opinion on the re-evaluation of Azorubine/Carmoisine (E 122) as a food additive - EFSA Panel on Food Additives and Nutrient Sources added to Food (ANS). EFSA J 2009; 7: 1-40.

[173]   Chequer FMD, Venâncio VP, Bianchi MLP, Antunes LMG. Genotoxic and mutagenic effects of erythrosine B, a xanthene food dye, on HepG2 cells. Food Chem Toxicol 2012; 50: 3447-51.
[http://dx.doi.org/10.1016/j.fct.2012.07.042]

[174]   Ganesan L, Margolles-Clark E, Song Y, Buchwald P. The food colorant erythrosine is a promiscuous protein-protein interaction inhibitor. Biochem Pharmacol 2011; 81: 810-8.
[http://dx.doi.org/10.1016/j.bcp.2010.12.020]

[175]   EFSA. Scientific Opinion on the re-evaluation of Erythrosine (E 127) as a food additive - EFSA Panel

on Food Additives and Nutrient Sources added to Food (ANS). EFSA J 2011; 9: 1-46.

[176]  EFSA. Scientific Opinion on the re-evaluation of Litholrubine BK (E 180) as a food additive - EFSA Panel on Food Additives and Nutrient Sources added to Food (ANS). EFSA J 2010; 8: 1-26.

[177]  Capitán-Vallvey LF, Fernández MD, Orbe I, Avidad R. Simultaneous determination of the colorants tartrazine, ponceau 4R and sunset yellow FCF in foodstuffs by solid phase spectrophotometry using partial least squares multivariate calibration. Talanta 1998; 47: 861-8.
[http://dx.doi.org/10.1016/S0039-9140(98)00159-3]

[178]  EFSA. Scientific Opinion on the re-evaluation of Ponceau 4R (E 124) as a food additive - EFSA Panel on Food Additives and Nutrient Sources added to Food (ANS). EFSA J 2009; 7: 1-39.

[179]  Shahabadi N, Maghsudi M. Gel electrophoresis and DNA interaction studies of the food colorant quinoline yellow. Dyes Pigments 2013; 96: 377-82.
[http://dx.doi.org/10.1016/j.dyepig.2012.09.004]

[180]  EFSA. Scientific Opinion on the re-evaluation of Quinoline Yellow (E 104) as a food additive - EFSA Panel on Food Additives and Nutrient Sources added to Food (ANS). EFSA J 2009; 7: 1-40.

[181]  Liu XP, Fan SR, Bai FY, Li J, Liao QP. Antifungal susceptibility and genotypes of Candida albicans strains from patients with vulvovaginal candidiasis. Mycoses 2009; 52: 24-8.
[http://dx.doi.org/10.1111/j.1439-0507.2008.01539.x]

[182]  EFSA. Scientific Opinion on the re-evaluation of Sunset Yellow FCF (E 110) as a food additive - EFSA Panel on Food Additives and Nutrient Sources added to Food (ANS). EFSA J 2009; 7: 1-44.

[183]  Oancea P, Meltzer V. Photo-Fenton process for the degradation of Tartrazine (E102) in aqueous medium. J Taiwan Inst Chem Eng 2013; 44: 990-4.
[http://dx.doi.org/10.1016/j.jtice.2013.03.014]

[184]  Gu N, Hu H, Guo Q, Jin S, Wang C, Oh Y, *et al.* Effects of oral administration of titanium dioxide fine-sized particles on plasma glucose in mice. Food Chem Toxicol 2015; 86: 124-31.
[http://dx.doi.org/10.1016/j.fct.2015.10.003]

[185]  EFSA. Opinion of the Scientific Panel on Food Additives, Flavourings, Processing Aids and materials in Contact with Food on a request from the Commission related to the safety in use of rutile titanium dioxide as an alternative to the presently permitted anatas. EFSA J 2006; 390: 1-12.

# CHAPTER 8

# Flavour Enhancers

**Mahalingam Jeyakumar** and **Kasi Pandima Devi**[*]

*Department of Biotechnology, Alagappa University, Karaikudi 630 003, Tamil Nadu, India*

**Abstract:** Food flavors are chemicals that are added to food to enhance their smell and taste. Many of the food additives used by the food industries occur naturally in food that people consume each day. The flavors used by our ancestors were mostly isolated from the natural sources; however, since there was only limited supply, the food industries started using nature-identical and synthetic flavors as an alternative to the natural one. The sodium salt of glutamic acid, which is called Monosodium glutamate (MSG) is a flavor enhancer found naturally in tomato, parmesan cheese, and sardines in significant quantities and it is also produced synthetically. The synthetically produced MSG is one of the best food flavour enhancers used in many types of foods in the world, which are added during the different stages of foods for improving the taste, smell and shelf life. Though many flavor enhancers or food potentiators are considered to be safe, they are voluntarily discontinued to be used in baby foods, as a precaution. The current review discusses the types, uses and properties of the flavor enhancers commonly used in foods.

**Keywords:** Food additives, Food industry, Flavour enhancers, Health effects, Maximum usage level.

## INTRODUCTION

Every living cell needs nutrients to live, without food, they cannot survive in the human body [1]. Food has many nutrients, for example, carbohydrates, proteins, fats, vitamins and minerals which, when ingested, produce energy and motivate the growth and maintenance of life. For centuries, food additives which are chemical substances are added as flavors to enhance its taste, odor and coloring. Food loses its flavor due to many practices like storage for longer periods, physical treatment or premature harvesting, during which the addition of flavor enhancers becomes a necessity. One example of a flavor agent is vanilla, which is generally used as a flavoring agent in ice-creams [2]. People prefer to take fruit

[*] **Corresponding author Kasi Pandima Devi:** Department of Biotechnology, Alagappa University, Karaikudi 630 003, Tamil Nadu, India, E mail: devikasi@yahoo.com

**Seyed Mohammad Nabavi *et al.* (Eds.)**

and vegetable juices, which are stored in the freezer, mostly added with some food additives. Food additives are used during pasteurizing, freezing, boiling, dehydrating and pickling to store foods such as fruits, and vegetables. Sometimes sugar, acetic acid, honey, edible vegetable oils, salt, alcohol, and vinegar are also frequently used as food preservatives. Natural flavors are obtained from plants, spices, animals or microbial fermentation that enhance the food's taste and/or smell [3]. Most of the people prefer to eat ready-made foods available in the supermarket rather than preparing food at home. These foods contain some kinds of food additives that act as flavor enhancers and can also sometimes cause human health problems. Recently, it has been shown that a high amount of flavor enhancer intake may cause oxidative stress and lead to the cytotoxicity of the cells [4]. However, when they are used at lower concentrations, they cause only moderate health effects [5].

## TYPES OF FLAVOR ENHANCERS

### Natural Flavoring Substances

The flavoring substances which are obtained by enzymatic processes, physical extraction from natural sources and microbiological techniques, from plants and animal primary materials, are called natural flavors under the United States Code of Federal Regulations (1990). Natural flavor is usually described as "the essential oil, essence or extractive, protein hydrolysate, distillate of any invention of roasting, heating or enzymolysis, which contains the flavouring constituents derived from a spice, fruit juice, herb, vegetable or vegetable juice, eggs, edible yeast, meat, bark, root, leaf or similar plant material, seafood, poultry, dairy products or fermentation products thereof, whose significant function in food is imparting flavouring rather than nutrition' [6]. Examples of the natural flavor enhancers include natural citral, almond benzaldehyde, lemongrass, and butter [7]. The flavor enhancers obtained from natural sources are preferred by consumers over the synthetic flavor enhancers. Citral (3,7-dimethyl-2,6- octagenic) present in large amounts in lemon peel and lemongrass oil is used in Asian cuisine as a flavor enhancer. The combination of citral and capsaicin, the secondary metabolite present in chili is used in Thai cuisine [8]. Benzaldehyde, which is present in high amounts in almond oil, is the second most widely used flavor enhancer in the world. Although synthetic benzaldehyde is cheaper than natural benzaldehyde, the latter has a great preference as a flavor enhancer [9].

### Nature-identical Flavoring Substances

Nature-identical flavoring substances are flavoring agents which contain chemically synthesized products, but are identical to the natural compounds in their chemical aspects. Since the natural flavors are not available in the required amounts, most of the time they are quite expensive. Hence, these natural flavors are chemically synthesized which are called nature-identical flavoring agents. Since they are similar to the natural flavors, they are better accepted by consumers and not associated with adverse health effects. These flavors also have organoleptic properties, such as natural flavors that each person experiences through the senses, including taste, sight, smell, and touch. Examples of nature-identical flavor enhancers include vanillin, which is identical to vanilla obtained mainly from the pods of the Mexican species *Vanilla planifolia*, but has a slight change than the natural vanilla in flavor and taste [10]. Since they are chemically synthesized, they are less expensive than the natural flavors and they are also stable [11].

## Artificial Flavoring Substances

These flavoring substances are not identical to natural flavors, since they are made by chemical manipulation methods [12], for example, ethyl nitrite, ethyl benzoylacetate, diphenyl disulphide, and piperonyl acetate. According to the US Code of Federal Regulations, the term artificial flavor or artificial flavoring means "any substance, the function of which is to impart flavor, which is not derived from a spice, fruit or fruit juice, vegetable or vegetable juice, edible yeast, bark, bud, root, herb, leaf or similar plant material, eggs, meat, fish, poultry, dairy products, or fermentation products thereof". These flavoring agents are produced with varying molecular structures, however, the similarity of these molecules with the natural flavors on structure, flavor or the sensory properties differs among the different flavoring agents and they are not structure-dependent [13].

## PHYSICOCHEMICAL PROPERTIES OF FLAVOR ENHANCERS

Flavor enhancers are any substances which enhance the flavor of the food and are usually added at low quantities to food. Generally, the taste enhancement depends on the properties of the flavor enhancers to bind to the taste receptors or stimulation of the trigeminal receptors in the oropharyngeal cavity [14]. Improvement of odor is mainly contributed by the volatile compounds present in the flavors [15]. The physicochemical properties of flavor enhancers are shown in Table **1**.

**Table 1. Physicochemical properties of flavor enhancers.**

| Chemical Name | Cas No, MolWt and Molecular Formula | Synonyms | Form | Solubility |
|---|---|---|---|---|
| Monosodium glutamate | 142-47-2 <br><br> 187.13g·mol$^{-1}$ <br><br> C$_5$H$_8$NO$_4$Na | Glutamic acid, Monosodium glutamate anhydrous, Monosodium L-glutamate, Sodium hydrogen glutamate, Monosodioglutammato (Italian), Glutamic acid, monosodium salt, Natriumglutaminat(German), Sodium glutamate, MSG, Natrium L-hydrogenglutamat Natriumglutaminat, Glutammatomonosodico (Italian), Chinese seasoning | White crystalline powder | Freely soluble in water; practically insoluble in ethanol or ether |
| Calcium inosinate | 38966-29-9 <br><br> 386.27 g·mol$^{-1}$ <br><br> C$_{10}$H$_{11}$CaN$_4$O$_8$P | Calcium inosine-5'-monophosphate | Odourless, colourless or white crystals or powder | Sparingly soluble in water |
| Monopotassium glutamate | 540778-10-7 <br><br> 185.22 g·mol$^{-1}$ <br><br> C$_5$H$_8$KNO$_4$ | Potassium glutamate, Glutamic acid potassium salt, Monopotassium L-glutamate monohydrate, | crystalline powder or White, practically odourless crystals | Freely soluble in water; slightly soluble in ethanol |
| Inosinic Acid | 131-99-7 <br><br> 348.208 g·mol$^{-1}$ <br><br> C$_{10}$H$_{13}$N$_4$O$_8$P | Inosinate, Sodium Inosine Monophosphate Inosinic Acid Inosinic Acids Monophosphate, Inosine Monophosphate, Ribosylhypoxanthine Ribosylhypoxanthine Monophosphate Sodium Inosinate | Odourless, colourless or white crystals or powder | Soluble in water, slightly soluble in ethanol |
| Calcium diglutamate | 5996-22-5 <br><br> 332.32 g·mol$^{-1}$ <br><br> C$_{10}$H$_{16}$CaN$_2$O | Calcium glutamate, L-Glutamic acid calcium salt | crystals or crystalline powder | Freely soluble in water; practically insoluble in ethanol or ether |

# COMMONLY USED FLAVOR ENHANCERS

## Monosodium Glutamate (MSG)

Monosodium glutamate Fig. (**1**) is one of the natural flavors, a sodium salt which is made up of amino acid called glutamate. The Chinese have been adding seaweed to foods as flavor enhancers since nearly 2000 years ago and the identification of the chemical nature of the flavor enhancer revealed the presence of glutamate. Later on, companies started to commercialize it in the name of MSG [16]. Naturally, it is one of the neurotransmitters in the human brain. The food flavor MSG found in some protein-rich food such as meat, peas, soy sauces, cheese and mushrooms, increases the fifth taste called umami [17]. In 1958, MSG added to food was considered "generally accepted as safe" by the U.S. Food & Drug Administration (FDA), and they were used as food additives for many decades. Normally, it is made from gluten, but recently, it is made by bacterial fermentation from a starting material such as starch and molasses. On overusage of foods like dietary supplements, cosmetics, drugs, fertilizers and personal care products, it can cause multiple neuronal diseases, brain injuries as well as learning disabilities. It causes side effects such as headache, sweating, nausea, dizziness, chest pain, flushing, numbness and tingling in the mouth. Monosodium glutamate (E621) is traded in the name of Ajinomoto, Vetsin, and Accent [18]. Moreover, it is authorized in the European Union under Regulation (EC) 1333/2008 as additives for flavor modification in many processed foods [19].

## Monopotassium Glutamate

Monopotassium (E620) glutamate, which is a natural amino acid is produced commercially by bacterial molasses fermentation. The vegetable proteins like gluten and soy protein also act as a source. Almost all the proteins which have glutamic acid and glutamates and free glutamates are found in a large amount in ripened cheese, tomatoes, sardines and breast milk Fig. (**2**). Its E number is 622 and the compound has the formula $C_5H_8KNO_4$ [19].

## Neohesperidine (DC)

Neohesperidine DC (E959) (Neohesperidine dihydrochalcone) is one of the flavor enhancers authorized for use as additives up to 5 mg/kg under Regulation 1333/2008. Neohesperidine DC is also permitted for application at levels of up to 10 to 150 mg/kg as a sweetener in accordance with Regulation 1333/2008. It is added as a flavoring agent to food to improve the overall flavor of food and also has the property to reduce the bitterness in food. One of the most important properties is that it can be used as a flavor enhancer in foods which require pasteurization since it is heat stable [20].

## Inosinic Acid and Calcium Inosinate

Inosinic acid (E630) is a natural acid found primarily in animals and produced commercially from fish (sardines) or meat. Inosinic acid or inosine monophosphate has an important role in the metabolism and it is obtained from waste by-products of chicken and other meat industry [21] Fig. (**3**). It is a ribonucleotide of hypoxanthine, which is formed as the first nucleotide during the synthesis of purine. Inosinic acid and inosinates have no specific smell, but strongly enhance many other tastes, thus reducing the amount of salt or other flavor-enhancing agents needed by a product. Inosinic acid, calcium salt (E630) also contains natural acids that are mainly present in animals and are also produced through bacterial sugar fermentation. It is made from fish and meat and not from a vegetarian source Fig. (**4**). It is the disodium salt of inosinic acid and it is a flavor enhancer found in noodles, potato chips, and a variety of snacks, which provide umami taste to foods. Inosinic acid in combination with the other food enhancer, disodium guanylate, produces another flavor enhancer known as disodium 5-ribonucleotides (E-number is 633), which also creates the umami taste.

## Calcium Diglutamate (CDG)

CDG (E623) is a natural amino acid produced from bacterially fermented molasses. They are also produced from vegetable protein such as soy or gluten. The problem with flavor enhancers such as MSG is that the total sodium in the food is increased because MSG contains sodium. However, the use of the CDG will be free of sodium and is also an approved food additive by the regulatory authorities. Whereas care should be taken since the usage of CDG in soups could enhance the total calcium content [22].

## USES OF FLAVOR ENHANCERS AS FOOD ADDITIVES

### Herbs and Spices as a Flavor Enhancer

Herbs and spices when added to foods, not only enhance the flavor of food, but also increase the antioxidant capacity of the food, without adding extra calories [23]. Spices as powder or extracts of spices are added as a seasoning to food, before the food is served, for enhancing the flavor of food [24]. Examples of herbs used as flavor enhancers are Rosemary, Peppermint, Garlic, Aniseed, Horseradish, Borage, Cacao, Capers, Lemon, Melissa, Dill, Tarragon, Angelica, Hyssop, Juniper Berries, Caraway Seed, Chervil, Coffee, Cumin, Tea, Coriander, Mint, Lovage, Basil, Chives, and Summer Savory Parsley. Examples of spices used as flavor enhancers are Vanilla, Nutmeg, Pimento, Ginger and Yellow Root (Turmeric), Pepper, Cinnamon, Paprika, Mace, Star Aniseed, Bay Leaf Cardamom, Saffron, Cloves and Spanish Pepper [25].

## Condiments

Condiments are mostly processed spices, sauces, salt and pickles, which are added in small quantities to enhance the flavor of food. Since they are prepared food compounds, no cooking process is required for the condiment addition. Coriander is used as a condiment for making chutneys and sauces are added to enhance the flavor of soups and curries. Soy sauce is a condiment which is a mixture of soybeans (as a fermented paste), brine (mixture of salt and water), grains (roasted rice/barley/wheat) and moulds like, *Aspergillus oryzae* or *Aspergillus sojae* [24]. Examples of other condiments include MSG (Sodium Glutamate), yeast extracts, essences, Saltpeter (Sodium or potassium nitrate, a salt seasoning) and marmite (Vegetable Yeast Product). These flavours are used in sauces, soups or purees.

## Confectionery Products

Confectionery products include food items that are rich in carbohydrates, especially sugars. Examples of confectionery products are Jelly, Jam, Castor Sugar, Couverture, Marzipan, Lemon Rind, Honey and Syrup. One of the most important flavoring agents used in toffee and caramel production is milk, which gives a mild flavor [26].

## Soft Drinks, Fruit Juices and Beverages

Examples include wine, coffee, cognac, grappa, tomato juice, soy sauce, Madeira or whiskey [27]. In many soft drinks, lemon oil which is mixed in water is added as a flavoring agent [28].

# LEGISLATIVE FRAMEWORK OF FLAVOR ENHANCERS

## Commission Regulation No 1334/2008 of the European Parliament and of the Council of 16 December 2008

This European Commission (EC) Regulation applies to flavorings; Food ingredients with flavoring characteristics; food with flavoring properties and/or food ingredients; Source of flavoring materials and/or source materials for flavoring food ingredients. However: materials with a sweet, sour or salty taste, raw foods, non-compound foods and mixtures will not apply.

Article 3 of Regulation (EC) No 1334/2008 defines 'flavorings' as: 'Products added to food for the purpose of changing odor or taste, or made or consisting of the categories (like Flavoring materials, flavoring products, processing of thermal flavorings, smoke flavorings, flavor precursors or mixtures thereof) and not intended for consumption as such (EU Commission Regulation (2011). Flavoring substances refer to chemicals with flavoring characteristics. Though there is no definition for the flavorings properties, generally, these chemicals alter the taste or odor as interpreted in Article 32(a) (i). As per the regulation, these substances are not necessarily required to possess a flavor; therefore a flavored substance may be tasteless or odorless. A flavoring substance is defined as a chemical that is added to the food to modify its smell and/or flavor.

## Regulation (EC) No. 1333/2008

The meaning of 'flavor enhancer' according to paragraph 14 of Annex I of Regulation (EC) No 1333/2008 is: 'Flavor enhancer' is a substance that improves the existing taste and/or odor of food (EU Commission Regulation (2011). Article 3(2) (a) of the Regulation defines "food additive" as "any substance not usually used as a food in itself or as a food ingredient, without any nutritional value, deliberately added in the process of preparation, manufacture, processing, transportation or storage of food for a technical purposes. The substances that are not to be considered as food additives are further stated in Article 3 (2) (II) of the Regulations as "Foods, dried, or otherwise concentrated, including flavorings integrated into compound food production, due to their aromatic, sapid, or nutritional properties which gives a secondary coloring effect'. Furthermore, Article 5 of the Regulation provides details on when and when not a substance should be taken as a food additive. If the substances modify the taste or give flavor to food, such as salt replacers and minerals and vitamins, these substances should not be considered as food additives. Finally, the possible overlap between Regulations 1333/2008 and 1334/2008 is addressed in paragraph 2 of Regulation 1333/2008. As provided in Article 2, Paragraph 2 of Regulation 1333/2008: This

Regulation shall not apply to the following substance unless they are used as a food additive: Flavorings covered by Regulation (EC) No 1334/2008 relating to aromatic products and food ingredients with flavoring properties in and on foods. Since the name 'flavor enhancer' is specifically listed in Annex I as ' functional class of food additives, 'these should be considered as additions and the exclusion of Article 2 (2) (e) is not relevant to them. If a substance is defined as a flavor enhancer, the substance is not excluded from the additive regulations and should be authorized as a food additive. Article 19(c) of Regulation (EC) No 1333/2008 provides that a comitology procedure allows the Commission to decide whether a certain substance meets the definition of food additives referred to in Article 3.

## MAXIMUM USAGE LEVEL OF FLAVOR ENHANCERS

The flavoring products make a tasteless food more interesting to eat; hence they have a major role in imparting nutritive value to food. Foods that possess a high amount of amino acids have been used over many centuries by different cultures in food preparation to improve the flavors of foods [29]. The EFSA (European Food Safety Authority) Comprehensive European Food Consumption Database approves the assessment of exposure at the European level to food additives and additional food ingredients [30]. The toxicological reports available on the effect of the additives in the children, toddlers, infants and adult population of Europe are taken into consideration by the EFSA for assessing the risk factors of the food additives. There may be a possible risk factor for the consumers if the exposure rate is higher than the ADI (Acceptable Daily Intake). Hence, as per the Annex II Regulation 1333/2008, the food additives which are used in the foods may be used at a concentration of the MPL (Maximum Permitted Level) (EU Commission Regulation (2011). The maximum permitted usage levels of flavor enhancers are shown in Table **2** [31]. The naturally occurring glutamate in various foods is given in Table **3** [32, 33] and the free content of glutamates used for normal seasonings, different packaged foods and the meals served in the restaurants are shown in Table **4** [34].

Table 2. Maximum usage level of flavor enhancers.

| Flavor Enhancer | Food Name | Maximum Level mg/kg |
|---|---|---|
| Glutaraldehyde | Dairy products | 15 |
| | Fats and oils | 10 |
| | Confectionery | 20 |
| | Meat and meat products | 5 |
| | Alcoholic beverages | 20 |

*(Table 2) cont.....*

| | | |
|---|---|---|
| Dibutyl succinate | Bakery wares | 50 |
| | Salts, soups, sauces, spices, protein products, *etc.* | 25 |
| | Processed fruit | 35 |
| | Fish and fish products | 10 |
| Diethyl citrate | Dairy products | 35 |
| | Confectionery | 50 |
| | Meat and meat products | 10 |
| | Salts, spices, sauces, soups, protein products, *etc* | 25 |
| 4-Hydroxymethyl-2-methyl-1,3- dioxolane | Dairy products | 35 |
| | Cereals and cereal products | 25 |
| | Processed fruit | 35 |
| | Alcoholic beverages | 50 |
| Ethyl butyryl lactate | Dairy products | 35 |
| | Confectionery | 50 |
| | Bakery wares | 50 |
| | Fats and oils | 25 |
| 2-Ethyl-4-methyl-1,3-dioxolane | Dairy products | 35 |
| | Fats and oils | 25 |
| | Processed fruit | 35 |
| | Confectionery | 50 |
| Hexadecano-1,5-lactone | Dairy products, | 35 |
| | Alcoholic beverages | 50 |
| | Confectionery | 50 |
| | Fats and oils | 25 |
| Nonanedioic acid | Confectionery | 50 |
| | Processed fruit | 10 |
| | Dairy products | 15 |
| | Alcoholic beverages | 50 |
| Isobutyl lactate | Dairy products | 35 |
| | Processed fruit | 35 |
| | Fats and oils | 25 |
| | Bakery wares | 25 |
| Diethyl oxalate | Dairy products | 35 |
| | Processed fruit | 35 |

*(Table 2) cont.....*

|  | Confectionery | 50 |
|---|---|---|
|  | Alcoholic beverages | 50 |
| Butane-1,3-diol | Dairy products | 35 |
|  | Fats and oils | 25 |
|  | Confectionery | 50 |
|  | Meat and meat products | 10 |
| 2-Butoxyethan-1-ol | Dairy products | 35 |
|  | Fats and oils | 25 |
|  | Alcoholic beverages | 50 |
| 1,1,3-Triethoxypropane | Dairy products | 35 |
|  | Fats and oils | 25 |
|  | Alcoholic beverages | 50 |

Table 3. Naturally occurring glutamate in various foods.

| Food | Bound Glutamate (mg/100g) | Free Glutamate(mg/100g) |
|---|---|---|
| Poultry products: |  |  |
| Eggs | 1583 | 23 |
| Chicken | 3309 | 44 |
| Duck | 3636 | 69 |
| **Milk/dairy products:** |  |  |
| Cow's milk | 819 | 2 |
| Human milk | 229 | 22 |
| Parmesan cheese | 9847 | 1200 |
| **Fish**: |  |  |
| Cod | 2101 | 9 |
| Mackerel | 2382 | 36 |
| Salmon | 2216 | 20 |
| Meat: | 2846 | 2325 |
| Beef | 33 | 23 |
| **Pork** |  |  |
| Vegetables: | 5583 | 1765 |
| Peas | 218 | 289 |
| Corn | 238 | 280 |
| Carrots | 200 | 130 |
| Spinach | 33 | 39 |

*(Table 3) cont.....*

| Tomatoes | 140 | 180 |
|---|---|---|
| Potato | 5583 | 1765 |

**Table 4. Free glutamate content of usual seasonings, various packaged foods and restaurant meals.**

| Food Type | Free Glutamate Content (mg/100g) |
|---|---|
| **Soy sauce:** | |
| China | 926 |
| Japan | 782 |
| Korea | 1264 |
| Philippines | 412 |
| **Fish sauce:** | |
| Nam-pla | 950 |
| Nuoc-mam | 950 |
| Ishiru | 1383 |
| Bakasang | 727 |
| **Concentrated extracts:** | |
| Vegemite | 1431 |
| Marmite | 1960 |
| Oyster sauce | 900 |

## REPORTS ON TOXICOLOGICAL DATA OF FLAVOR ENHANCERS AND ITS ADVERSE HEALTH EFFECTS

Flavor enhancers are banned in foods for newborns in countries like America, Australia, and New Zealand since they cause severe damage to the brain and nervous system [35]. Monosodium glutamate is a common flavor enhancer used in Chinese food. The first report of MSG toxicity was termed as "Chinese restaurant syndrome", which was reported by Kowk in 1968. The toxicity of MSG after consuming the Chinese food was exhibited through numbness, tingling and tightness, which persisted even until 2 hours after eating the food. Consumption of MSG at higher concentrations without the intake of any solid food has been associated with headaches and other toxic symptoms [36]. Monosodium glutamate should not be permitted in foods for children <12 months and infants. MSG sometimes acts as an excitotoxin (which causes excessive brain receptor activation), leads to brain neuronal cell damage, and causes many of these neurodegenerative diseases such as Alzheimer's, Parkinson's and Huntington's disease [37]. High MSG dose may result in heart attack, asthma, irritability, restlessness, sleep disturbance, chest tightness, heart palpitations, heart arrhythmia, and anxiety. MSG symptom complex or Chinese restaurant syndrome usually refers to rapid and temporary responses such as asthma, headache, bruising, facial tightness, nausea and tingling [38]. Migraine, asthma, fatigue, depression, insomnia, shakes, dizziness, numbness, heart palpitations, dehydration and brain fog nausea are other harmful symptoms that are caused by flavor enhancers [39].

## REPORTS ON POSITIVE HEALTH EFFECTS OF FLAVOR ENHANCERS

Flavor enhancers are added to a large number of foods to improve the taste and smell of foods as well as to maintain nutritional quality. One of the common problems with the aged people is that they develop malnutrition and nutritional deficiencies due to poor dietary intake, which occurs due to the loss of taste and smell during aging. To determine whether the addition of flavor enhancers could increase the food consumption in the elderly people, they were subjected to a 16 weeks study in which the elderly people in a nursing home were fed with flavor enhancer added cooked meals. It was observed that the addition of flavor enhancers improved the daily dietary intake and increased the bodyweight with stable health status in the aged people [40]. Another report recommends that since flavor enhancers improve the food intake and body weight, it could be taken by older people who have less appetite [41].

## SAFETY ASSESSMENT AND PROHIBITED FLAVOR ENHANCERS

The FEMA GRAS program is one of the widely accepted food flavor safety assessment programmes. To evaluate the safety aspects of the flavor enhancers, in the year 1959, the FEMA (The US Association of Flavors and Extract Manufacturers) assessed the flavor enhancers and revealed their 'Generally Recognized as Safe' (GRAS) status. The safety of flavors was assessed using modern methods and since the year 1995, nearly 1000 flavoring substances were given the FEMA GRAS status. In 1997, the FDA also implemented the GRAS notification program in addition to the FEMA GRAS assessment programme. However, the FDA was in support of the regulatory tools of the GRAS assessment. In addition, the other programs which have added for analyzing the safety of flavors since the year 1995 include the Joint FAO/WHO Expert Committee on Food Additives (JECFA) and the European Union (currently *via* the European Authority for Food Safety – EFSA). The FDA prohibited the usage of calamus, cinnamyl anthranilate and safrole flavoring substances, based on its safety assessment [42]. The other prohibited flavoring substances include Santonin, Aloin, Hydrocyanic acid, Berberine, Beta-Azarone, Diethylene Glycol,

Hypericin, Sasafras Oil, Pyroligneous Acid, Cocaine, Cade Oil, Monoethyl Ether, Nitrobenzene, Safrole and Isosafrole [43].

Glutamate, which is a major component of many proteins and peptides in most tissues, is the most common amino acid present in nature. It is one of the most abundant amino acids, which is present in virtually all foods, with the highest levels in protein-rich foods. Since glutamate is also produced within the body, it plays an important role in human metabolism. Glutamate can occur in the body either as bounded to protein/peptide or as a free form of glutamate. Levels of free glutamate in foods of animal origin are generally quite low (*e.g.* beef 33 mg/100 g, cow's milk 2 mg/100 g). Higher levels are seen in vegetables (30-200 mg/100 g) and in seasonings, sauces and restaurant meals [25, 44]. The Joint FAO/WHO Food Additives Expert Committee (JECFA) has been constantly evaluating the safety of salts of glutamic acid, including MSG [45].

Due to the low toxic nature, the glutamate salts were not considered as agents that cause health hazards to humans. Hence, it was decided by the JEFCA that a numerical acceptable daily intake (ADI) is not necessary and therefore a status of 'group ADI not specified' was given for the glutamate salts [46]. The American Federation for Experimental Biology (FASEB) analyzed adverse MSG reactions to the FDA in 1995. The FASEB Expert Panel reported that 'there is a subgroup of apparently healthy individuals within the general population that responds, generally within one hour of exposure, with manifestations of the MSG Symptom Complex to an oral bolus of MSG ≥ 3 g in the absence of food'. The Panel also noted that there was a subgroup of people who reported asthmatic conditions in response to MSG [47]. The Food Standards Australia New Zealand (FSANZ) summarized the JECFA and FASEB reports and revealed the safety of MSG. The FSANZ evaluation concludes that 'no persuasive evidence exists that MSG causes systemic reactions that lead to severe disease or death'. The EFSA re-evaluated the safety of different flavor enhancers of glutamate and its salts, on request by the European Commission and published its report in the year 2017. Overall, the panel recommended that the EC should consider revising the maximum permitted levels of glutamic acid in foods [48].

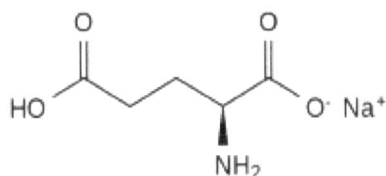

**Fig (1).** Monosodium glutamate (MSG).

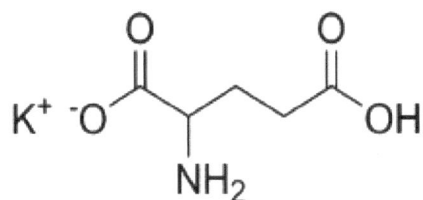

**Fig (2).** Monopotassium glutamate.

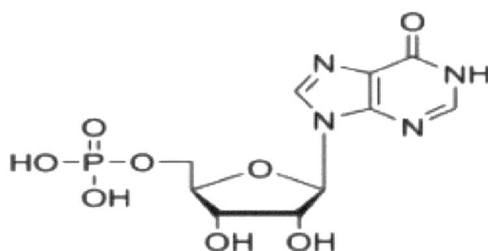

**Fig (3).** Inosinic acid.

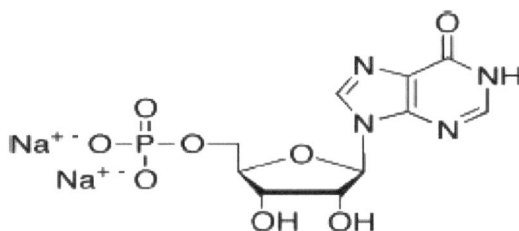

**Fig (4).** Calcium inosinate.

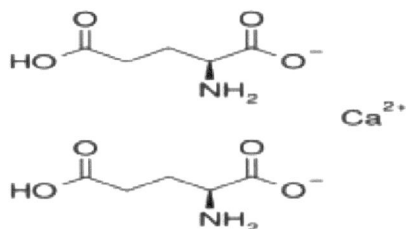

**Fig (5).** Calcium diglutamate (CDG).

## CONCLUSION

Food flavors are substances which are added in small quantities to food to add taste or smell to food. Flavoring substances have been used over thousands of years, and in the earlier days, people used simpler flavors like the herbs and spices available in their locality to improve the food taste. Mostly the flavoring substances were extracted from natural sources, but later, due to the unavailability of natural flavoring extracts, people started using natural identical and synthetic flavors. MSG, the sodium salt of glutamic acid or glutamate, is one of the most commonly used flavoring agents added to food to bring out the savory or umami taste. On December 16, 2008, the European Commission adopted the EC Regulation No 1334/2008 to enforce the safety of flavor enhancers and later, on October 1, 2012, the list of flavoring substances was approved to be used in foods. However, information about the flavoring agents used and their concentration should be mentioned in the food labels, so that the customers can make their choice in the purchase of the food ingredients.

## CONSENT FOR PUBLICATION

Not applicable.

## CONFLICTS OF INTEREST

The author confirms that this chapter contents have no conflict of interest.

## ACKNOWLEDGMENT

The authors wish to acknowledge the Computational and Bioinformatics facility provided by the Alagappa University Bioinformatics Infrastructure Facility (DBT, Government of India. BT/BI/25/012/2012, BIF) and the instrumentation facilities and grant provided by, DST-FIST (Grant No. SR/FST/LSI-639/2015(C)), UGC-SAP (Grant No. F.5-1/2018/DRS-II(SAP-II)), (DST-PURSE (Grant No. SR/PURSE Phase 2/38 (G)), RUSA 2.0 [F. 24-51/2014-U, Policy (TN Multi-Gen), Dept of Education, Government of India] and the University Science Instrumentation Centre (USIC), Alagappa University.

## REFERENCES

[1]    Sharma S. Food preservatives and their harmful effects. IJSRP 2015; 5: 1-2.

[2]    Mirza SK, Asema UK, Kasim SS. To study the harmful effects of food preservatives on human health. J Med Chem Drug Discov 2017; 2: 610-6.

[3]    Nwajei JC, Onuoha SC, Essien EB. Effects of Oral administration of selected food seasonings consumed in Nigeria on some sex hormones of Wistar albino rats. IOSR J Biotechnol Biochem 2015; 1(5): 15-21.

[4]    Sharma V, Deshmukh R. Ajimomoto (MSG) A fifth taste or a bio bomb. Eur J Pharm Med Res 2015; 2(2): 381-400.

[5]    Al-Shammari E, Bano R, Khan S, Shankity I. The effect of preservatives and flavour additive on the production of oxygen-free radicals by isolated human neutrophils. Int J Food Sci Nutr 2014; 3(3): 210-5.

[6]     Vandamme EJ, Soetaert W. Bioflavours and fragrances *via* fermentation and biocatalysis. J Chem Technol Biotechnol 2002; 77(12): 1323-32.
[http://dx.doi.org/10.1002/jctb.722]

[7]     Baines D, Seal R, Eds. Natural food additives, Ingredients and Flavourings. Elsevier 2012.
[http://dx.doi.org/10.1533/9780857095725]

[8]     Stotz SC, Vriens J, Martyn D, Clardy J, Clapham DE. Citral sensing by Transient receptor potential channels in dorsal root ganglion neurons. PLoS One 2008; 3(5)e2082
[http://dx.doi.org/10.1371/journal.pone.0002082] [PMID: 18461159]

[9]     Wolken WA, Tramper J, van der Werf MJ. Amino acid-catalysed retroaldol condensation: the production of natural benzaldehyde and other flavour compounds. Flavour Fragrance J 2004; 19(2): 115-20.
[http://dx.doi.org/10.1002/ffj.1326]

[10]    Esposito LJ, Formanek K, Kientz G, *et al.* Vanillin. In: Kirk-Othmer Encyclopedia of Chemical Technology John Wiley & Sons. 2001.

[11]    Christoph N, Bauer-Christoph C. Flavour of spirit drinks: Raw materials, fermentation, distillation, and ageing.Flavours and Fragrances. Berlin, Heidelberg: Springer 2007; pp. 219-39.
[http://dx.doi.org/10.1007/978-3-540-49339-6_10]

[12]    Bearth A, Cousin ME, Siegrist M. The consumer's perception of artificial food additives: Influences on acceptance, risk and benefit perceptions. Food Qual Prefer 2014; 38: 14-23.
[http://dx.doi.org/10.1016/j.foodqual.2014.05.008]

[13]    Wild D, King MT, Gocke E, Eckhardt K. Study of artificial flavouring substances for mutagenicity in the Salmonella/microsome, Basc and micronucleus tests. Food Chem Toxicol 1983; 21(6): 707-19.
[http://dx.doi.org/10.1016/0278-6915(83)90202-8] [PMID: 6420251]

[14]    Rowe D, Ed. Chemistry and technology of flavours and fragrances. John Wiley & Sons 2009. [February 12]

[15]    Taylor AJ. Modifying flavour in food. Elsevier 2007. [June 8]
[http://dx.doi.org/10.1201/9781439823842]

[16]    Samuels A. The toxicity/safety of processed free glutamic acid (MSG): a study in suppression of information. Account Res 1999; 6(4): 259-310.
[http://dx.doi.org/10.1080/08989629908573933] [PMID: 11657840]

[17]    Löliger J. Function and importance of glutamate for savory foods. J Nutr 2000; 130(4S) (Suppl.): 915S-20S.
[http://dx.doi.org/10.1093/jn/130.4.915S] [PMID: 10736352]

[18]    Sharma VK, Sharma P, Deshmukh R, Singh R. Age Associated Sleep Loss: A Trigger For Alzheimer's Disease. Klinik Psikofarmakol Bülteni 2015; 25(1): 78-88.
[http://dx.doi.org/10.5455/bcp.20140909070449]

[19]    EU Commission Regulation. Commission Regulation (EU) No 1129/2011 of 11 November 2011 amending Annex II to Regulation (EC) No 1333/2008 of the European Parliament and of the Council by establishing a Union list of food additives. Off J Eur Union L 2011; 295(4): 12-1.

[20]    Bassoli A, Merlini L. Sweeteners.Encyclopedia of Food Sciences and Nutrition. 2nd ed. 2003; pp. 5688-95.
[http://dx.doi.org/10.1016/B0-12-227055-X/01172-X]

[21]    Wang XF, Liu GH, Cai HY, *et al.* Attempts to increase inosinic acid in broiler meat by using feed additives. Poult Sci 2014; 93(11): 2802-8.
[http://dx.doi.org/10.3382/ps.2013-03815] [PMID: 25172930]

[22]    Ball P, Woodward D, Beard T, Shoobridge A, Ferrier M. Calcium diglutamate improves taste characteristics of lower-salt soup. Eur J Clin Nutr 2002; 56(6): 519-23.

[http://dx.doi.org/10.1038/sj.ejcn.1601343] [PMID: 12032651]

[23]    Collin H. Herbs, spices and cardiovascular disease. 2006.
        [http://dx.doi.org/10.1533/9781845691717.2.126]

[24]    Gadegbeku C, Tuffour MF, Katsekpor P, Atsu B. Herbs, spices, seasonings and condiments used by
        food vendors in Madina, accra. Caribb J Sci 2014; 2: 589-602.

[25]    Food Standards Australia New Zealand. Monosodium glutamate a safety assessment technical report
        series no. 20. 2003. Available from: https://www.foodstandards.gov.au/publications/documents/MS
        G%20Technical%20Report.pdf

[26]    NPCS Board of Food Technologists. Confectionery Products Handbook (Chocolate, Toffees, Chewing
        Gum & Sugar Free Confectionery). Asia Pacific Business Press Inc 2013.

[27]    Food Commodities. 2017. Available from: http://www.foodcommodities.nl/commodities/flavour
        enhancers.html

[28]    Taylor AJ, Mottram DS, Eds. Flavour Science: Recent Developments Royal Society of Chemistry:
        Special publication. Woodhead Publishing 1996.

[29]    Curtis RI. Umami and the foods of classical antiquity. Am J Clin Nutr 2009; 90(3): 712S-8S.
        [http://dx.doi.org/10.3945/ajcn.2009.27462C] [PMID: 19571231]

[30]    European Food Safety Authority. Use of the EFSA comprehensive European food consumption
        database in exposure assessment. EFSA J 2011; 9(3): 2097.
        [http://dx.doi.org/10.2903/j.efsa.2011.2097]

[31]    Flavouring Group Evaluation 10. Scientific Opinion of the Panel on Food Additives, Flavourings,
        Processing Aids and Materials in Contact with Food on a request from Commission on Flavouring
        Group Evaluation 10 Revision1 (FGE.10 Rev1). Aliphatic primary and secondary saturated and
        unsaturated alcohols, aldehydes, acetals, carboxylic acids and esters containing an additional
        oxygenated functional group and lactones from chemical groups 9, 13 and 30. EFSA 2009; 7(1): 934.

[32]    Yamaguchi S, Ninomiya K. What is umami? Food Rev Int 1998; 14(2-3): 123-38.
        [http://dx.doi.org/10.1080/87559129809541155]

[33]    Institute of Food Technologists'. Expert Panel on Food Safety and Nutrition. Monosodium Glutamate
        Food Technol 1987; 4: 143-5.

[34]    Nicholas PG, Jones S. Monosodium glutamate in Western Australian foods. Australia: Chemistry in
        Australia 1991.

[35]    FDA. FDA & Monosodium Glutamate 1995. Available from: http://www.cfsan.fda.gov/~lrd/msg.html

[36]    Bawaskar HS, Bawaskar PH, Bawaskar PH. Chinese restaurant syndrome. Indian J Crit Care Med
        2017; 21(1): 49-50.
        [http://dx.doi.org/10.4103/0972-5229.198327] [PMID: 28197052]

[37]    Olney JW. Excitotoxins in foods. Neurotoxicology 1994; 15(3): 535-44.
        [PMID: 7854587]

[38]    Geha RS, Beiser A, Ren C, *et al.* Review of alleged reaction to monosodium glutamate and outcome
        of a multicenter double-blind placebo-controlled study. J Nutr 2000; 130(4S) (Suppl.): 1058S-62S.
        [http://dx.doi.org/10.1093/jn/130.4.1058S] [PMID: 10736382]

[39]    Prescott J, Young O, O'neill L, Yau NJN, Stevens R. Motives for food choice: a comparison of
        consumers from Japan, Taiwan, Malaysia and New Zealand. Food Qual Prefer 2002; 13(7): 489-95.
        [http://dx.doi.org/10.1016/S0950-3293(02)00010-1]

[40]    Mathey MFA, Siebelink E, de Graaf C, Van Staveren WA. Flavor enhancement of food improves
        dietary intake and nutritional status of elderly nursing home residents. J Gerontol A Biol Sci Med Sci
        2001; 56(4): M200-5.
        [http://dx.doi.org/10.1093/gerona/56.4.M200] [PMID: 11283191]

[41]    Bautista EN, Tanchoco CC, Tajan MG, Magtibay EVJ. Effect of flavor enhancers on the nutritional status of older persons. J Nutr Health Aging 2013; 17(4): 390-2.
[http://dx.doi.org/10.1007/s12603-012-0438-9] [PMID: 23538664]

[42]    Hallagan JB, Hall RL. Under the conditions of intended use - New developments in the FEMA GRAS program and the safety assessment of flavor ingredients. Food Chem Toxicol 2009; 47(2): 267-78.
[http://dx.doi.org/10.1016/j.fct.2008.11.011] [PMID: 19041920]

[43]    Ziegler H, Ed. Flavourings: production, composition, applications, regulations. John Wiley & Sons 2007.
[http://dx.doi.org/10.1002/9783527611454]

[44]    Rhodes J, Titherley AC, Norman JA, Wood R, Lord DW. A survey of the monosodium glutamate content of foods and an estimation of the dietary intake of monosodium glutamate. Food Addit Contam 1991; 8(5): 663-72.
[http://dx.doi.org/10.1080/02652039109374021] [PMID: 1818840]

[45]    JECFA. J F L-glutamic acid and its ammonium, calcium, monosodium and potassium salts. Toxicological Evaluation of Certain Food Additives and Contaminants 1988; pp. 12-25.

[46]    SCF. Reports of the Scientific Committee for Food on a First Series of Food Additives of Various Technological Functions, Commission of the European Communities, Reports of the Scientific Committee for Food, 25th Series. Brussels, Belgium 1991.

[47]    Raiten DJ, Talbot J, Fisher KD. Executive summary from the report: analysis of adverse reactions to monosodium glutamate (MSG). J Nutr 1995; 125(11): 2891S-906S.
[http://dx.doi.org/10.1093/jn/125.11.2891S] [PMID: 7472671]

[48]    Mortensen A, Aguilar F, Crebelli R, *et al.* Re-evaluation of glutamic acid (E 620), sodium glutamate (E 621), potassium glutamate (E 622), calcium glutamate (E 623), ammonium glutamate (E 624) and magnesium glutamate (E 625) as food additives. EFSA J 2017; 15(7): 4910.

# CHAPTER 9

# Flavors (Including Umami Ingredients of Edible Mushrooms)

**Raees Khan[1,3,*], Faiz-ur- Rahman[1], Shehzad Mehmood[1], Saima Ali[1], Sheikh Zain Ul Abidin[1], Abdul Samad Mumtaz[1], Ejaz Aziz[1], Riffat Batool[1], Hussain Badshah[1] and Ömer Kiliç[2]**

[1] *Quaid-i-Azam University, Islamabad, 45320, Pakistan*

[2] *Faculty of Pharmacy, Adıyaman University, Turkey*

[3] *Zoological Survey of Pakistan, Ministry of Climate Change, Islamabad, Pakistan*

**Abstract:** Flavor is among the most essential factor for food selection and determines the taste, trigeminal and aroma of the food item. Currently, five main types of flavors are recognized *i.e.* sweet, sour, bitter, salty and umami. Umami flavor has a pleasant savory taste and is becoming popular in the food industry for the enhancement of food taste. Edible mushrooms are one of the major sources of umami flavor. Similarly different natural and synthetic flavorings and flavorants are added to enhance food products. These flavorings and flavorants also have health benefits and apprehensions to human health. The natural plant-based flavor products should be encouraged as they have health benefits and are being used for thousands of years as flavorings & flavorants and as traditional plant-based medicines. The food industry is looking for new plant-based flavoring agents to satisfy consumer demands.

**Keywords:** Flavorings and flavorants, Food additives, Synthetic flavorings agents, Umami flavor.

## INTRODUCTION

Flavor is the most significant factor that determines the selection of food in daily life. Flavor can be defined from the biological perception, such that, it is the sensation produced by a material taken in the mouth. The main targets of different flavors are taste receptors that produce stimulation to flavors [1]. Different chemical compounds are responsible for different types of flavors. According to estimates, 5,000 to 10,000 aromatic compounds are responsive to the human

---

\* **Corresponding author Raees Khan:** Quaid-i-Azam University Islamabad, 45320, Pakistan;
E-mail: raeeskhan@bs.qau.edu.pk

**Seyed Mohammad Nabavi *et al*. (Eds.)**

flavor sensory system, of which only 2,600 chemical compounds are known yet. Some compounds have few volatile compounds with characteristic essence, known as character impact compounds, which are responsible for a particular type of flavor. Flavor compounds are present naturally (*e.g.* in fruits, vegetables, meat and mushrooms) or added to different food derived from different sources [1]. These compounds have characteristic sensory stimulation and may be aldehydes (fruity, green oxidized and sweet), alcohols (bitter, medicinal piney and caramel), esters (fruity citrus), ketones (butter and caramel), Maillard reaction products (brown, burnt and caramel), phenolics (citrus, sweet), terpenoids (citrus), acids, sweet, sour and bitter) and flavonoids (astringent and bitter). Biotechnological techniques are now being used for the production of different flavor using microbes and enzymes [2].

## MAJOR FLAVOR TYPES

The flavors are classified into five main types based on three main different sensations: taste, trigeminal and aroma. Flavors are the sensations arising from the interplay/integration of signals, which are produced as a result of sensing aroma, taste and irritating stimuli originated from foods or beverages. Flavor perception is a complex process involving a sense of smell and taste and chemesthesis (a chemical sense that can recognize irritation or pungency). Once the visual inspection is done to identify whether the food is edible or not flavor analysis commences. During the eating process, the volatile components are released and transported from the mouth to the nasal cavity, while non-volatile components are facilitated by saliva to taste and irritant sensitive-regions of the oral cavity. Briefly, the flavor release is mainly controlled by the saliva, teeth and tongue [3].

### Sweet Flavor

The sweet taste is one of the basic gustatory sensations and is a product that comes due to the high contents of polyols and sugars [4]. Sugars are the main compounds in the development of sweet flavor in vegetables and fruits although some other components are also present which develop other flavors like saltiness, bitterness, or sourness [5]. The sweet flavors of vegetables like tomato and fruits like strawberry are due to a sweet and pleasant compound known as furanones [6], while the sweet flavor of mushroom is due to the contribution of soluble sugars [7]. The specific sweet flavor of the apple comes due to an alcoholic short chain compound called 1-butanol, which has a sweet aroma [8]. As far as the other fruits are concerned, their sweetness is due to the dissolved sugars like fructose, sucrose, sorbitol, glucose and several other components and they can be measured as total dissolved solids (TSSs). The sweetness increases as the sugar content increase from glucose to sucrose and from sucrose to fructose, comparatively. In fresh grape juice, the sweetness comes from glucose and fructose which are about 99% of the total sugar content and weigh from 12% to 27% of the total TSSs of a mature and fresh grape berry [9]. The sweetness in berries is a combined taste of glucose and fructose, where glucose accounts for about 85% of the total sugar content at initial stages, where it becomes equal with fructose when ripe, and fructose content exceeds glucose when the berries are over ripe [10, 11, 9]. The sweetness can be increased in the food items like fruits and vegetables through techniques like genetic engineering and recombinant DNA technology. The sweetness of tomato and lettuce has been increased by expressing a protein monellin that is the sweetness protein found in African berries. This protein enhances flavor and sweetness in fruits and vegetables to about 104 times by molar basis from that of sucrose. Due to the low cost and consumer demand, sucrose is the leading sweetener and food additive in the USA. This is also used in the manufacturing of adsorbent flavor carriers along with other simple sugars or sweeteners [13, 14].

We can identify many food products like lemons, oranges and apples solely due to their aroma, but when consuming beverages products or the fruit itself their fruity taste is more enhanced by the sourness or sweetness due to the organic acids or the sugars in it [15]. The sweetness of Texas sweet onions is defined by measuring the content of pyruvic acid. The unofficial industry standards state that Texas onion is sweet when the acid is below 5.0 levels [16]. To differentiate and value one product from other, this strategy has been developed for marketing purposes. A test has been developed which is called Brix test which measures the soluble solids contents or in other word, the sugars in a product. Although this test is not understood by the consumers but is widely applied in the wholesale market and is only adopted by growers and marketers. The buyers can only understand how much a product is sweet, so this test is applied and measures the sweetness of the product which is then mentioned on the product [17].

## Sour Flavor

The organic acids present in fruits or other food materials produce sour (acidic) flavor for example, citric acid in citrus fruits, quinic acid in pears, tartaric acid in grapes, malic acid in apples, and oxalic acid in bananas. These acids bring some bitterness to the fruits and other food substances. It has been studied that acid levels or sourness in tomatoes, along with its aroma affect the sweetness [18]. The flavor quality of a food is measured by the aroma it is produced and it is strongly recommended by the consumers while buying the products. It was reported by Baldwin *et al.* [19], highlighted that aroma and odor of the food items greatly affect the perception of sourness and sweetness in tomatoes [20]. The sourness/acidity in the meat comes from certain amino acids and other acids, such as orthophosphoric, succinic, inosinic and lactic acids [21]. It is a pre-set mechanism in the humans that we like or dislike the foods based on its flavors, if it has saltish, sweet, or umami flavor then consumers most probably will like food, but if it has sour or bitter flavor, consumers most probably won't eat it and they can avoid the toxic or harmful products in that way. This attraction towards some of the flavors and dislike for some others is based on the experience that starts from the womb [22]. The main taste that is detected by tongue receptors in fresh fruits is the sweet and sour sensation of the sugars and organic acids that are found abundantly, while some other minor substances also produce saltiness and bitterness. The sour flavor which can be called as bitterness and tartness is found in a raw nutshell, vegetables and more frequently in fruits [17].

Some people are sensitive to sour taste, while others prefer sour taste over sweet flavor, as we know that taste perception is linked to the ratio of acids to sugars. For example, in the United Kingdom, the consumers prefer sour taste apples over a sweet one. The sensitivity to sour taste has been found to be genetic and has been tested in twins who were sour taste sensitive using citric acid as a sour taste compound [17].

## Bitter Flavor

The bitter flavor in fruits is due to compounds like flavonoid glucosides (*e.g.*, naringin found in grapefruits) or terpenoid lactones (*e.g.*, limonene found in oranges) [20]. If we talk about meat, all four basic flavors (sour, salty, sweet and bitter) are found in meat irrespective of the animal species from which the meat is taken. These flavors can be found in different quantities and intensities where the compounds like hypoxanthine and peptides produce umami and bitter taste [23]. Although, for most of the common foods the odor identification is difficult to recognize, a basic perception is that sour and bitter odor of a product increases its rejection and therefore, the food industry tends not to use products that smell like that [24]. In all the amino acids, 8 amino acids, *i.e.*, phenylalanine, valine, arginine, methionine, tryptophan, leucine, histidine and isoleucine are considered to be bitter amino acids, but they are found to have no activity in taste [25]. Aqueous extract of the Brazilian mushroom *Agaricus blazei* Murril., which is also known as 'sun mushroom' or almond mushroom (due to its fragrance), is used as a food additive to bring bitter taste in the products [26]. The taste preferences of every individual are different for the four eminent flavors like sweet, sour, salty and bitter but one can find sweet and bitter taste mostly in vegetables and fruits [17].

## Salty Flavor

Various naturally found salts contribute to the saltiness of the food products. The different bitter taste components like, tannins, alkaloids, flavonoids and other such components in vegetables and fruits along with the salts react with each other and give a desirable flavor to the food which attracts the consumers [27, 20]. In meat, the sodium salts of aspartic acid and glutamic acid give it a salty taste which is easily detected by the receptors present on the surface of the tongue [28]. The US dietary guidelines recommend an average intake of sodium chloride to be about 6 grams which are needed for the normal function of the human body. This recommended amount of salt is taken in by the consumption of the salty food items [29]. World Health Organization (WHO) has also recommended < 5g/day, but global salt intake is estimated at more than 10g/day, which is well above the recommended intake [30]. The infants and children also have the perception of the salty flavor. It has been studied that infants of about 3-4 months preferred salty water over plain water. It is thought that the preferences of the infants for the salty water are a biologically unlearned response. This liking of the salty taste in water decreases as the infants enter the childhood, but then, they prefer the salty food instead of the salty water, so the overall liking of the salty flavor remains high [31].

## Umami Flavor

The presence of sodium salts of glutamic and aspartic amino acids and 5'-nucleotides give rise to a pleasant savory taste famously known as Umami flavor. Umami flavor occurs naturally in many edible foods including mushrooms, fish, meats and dairy products [32]. Today, umami flavor is recognized as the 5th basic taste and one of the most effective flavor enhancers in different food products. Different natural foods have umami taste including vegetables (*e.g.* tomato, potato, Chinese cabbage, carrot, soybean and green tea), edible mushrooms (*e.g.* *Agaricus*, *Volvariella* and *Morchella* species), seafoods (*e.g.* fish, kelp, seaweed, oyster, prawn, crab, sea urchin, clam and scallop), meats (*e.g.* beef and chicken) and cheeses [32, 33, 35]. Umami flavor is very important in the food industry and edible mushrooms are considered to be the most important in this regard with wider uses in different products. According to the Umami Information Center [65], the amount of Glutamate ranges from 2 to 3380mg per 100g in different food items (Table **1**).

**Table 1. Glutamate mg per 100g of different food items according to Umami Information Center 2019.**

| Ingredients | Glutamate |
|---|---|
| Seaweed | |
| Rausu kombu | 2290?3380 |
| Ma kombu | 1610?3200 |

*(Table 1) contd.....*

| Ingredients | Glutamate |
|---|---|
| Rishiri kombu | 1490?1980 |
| Hidaka kombu | 1260?1340 |
| Naga kombu | 240?1400 |
| Nori | 550~1350 |
| Wakame | 2~50 |
| **Green tea** | 220?670 |
| **Vegetables, Beans and Potatoes** | |
| Tomatoes | 150?250 |
| Dried Tomatoes | 650? 1140 |
| Green peas | 110 |
| Lotus root | 100 |
| Garlic | 100 |
| Corn | 70?110 |
| Shungiku | 80 |
| Soy Beans | 70?80 |
| Fava beans | 60?80 |
| Chinese Cabbage | 40?90 |
| Potatoes | 30?100 |
| Sweet Potato | 60 |
| Spinach | 50?70 |
| Carrot | 40?80 |
| Bamboo shoots | 14?90 |
| Asparagus | 30?50 |
| Daikon | 30?70 |
| Cabbage | 30?50 |
| Onion | 20?50 |
| Green Onion | 20?50 |
| Broccoli | 30?60 |
| Celery | 20?30 |
| Burdock root | 20 |
| Ginger | 20 |
| **Mushrooms** | |
| Dried shiitake mushroom | 1060 |
| Shiitake mushroom | 70 |

*(Table 1) contd.....*

| Ingredients | Glutamate |
|---|---|
| Shimeji mushroom | 140 |
| Enoki Mushroom | 90 |
| Common Mushroom | 40~110 |
| Truffles | 60~80 |
| **Seafood** | |
| Scallop | 140 |
| Shrimp/Prawn | 120 |
| Uni(sea urchin) | 100 |
| Japanese littleneck clam | 90 |
| Niboshi | 40?50 |
| Katsuobushi | 30?40 |
| Frozen shelled shrimp | 15?30 |
| Squid | 20~30 |
| Octopus | 20~30 |
| Hamachi | 5~9 |
| Sardine | 10~20 |
| Tuna | 1~10 |
| Sea Bream | 10 |
| Aji(Horse mackerel) | 4~13 |
| Bonito | 1~10 |
| Sawara | 3~11 |
| Mackerel | 10~30 |
| Cod | 5~10 |
| Oyster | 40~150 |
| Clam | 210 |
| Mussel | 110 |
| Dried shirasu(Whitebait) | 40 |
| Anchovies | 630 |
| Salted squid | 620 |
| Caviar | 80 |
| Ikura | 20 |
| **Egg and Meats** | |
| Chicken eggs | 20 |
| Pork | 10 |

(Table 1) contd.....

| Ingredients | Glutamate |
|---|---|
| Chicken | 20?50 |
| Beef | 10 |
| Dry-Cured Hams | 340 |

## UMAMI INGREDIENTS OF EDIBLE MUSHROOMS

Mushrooms belonging to Basidiomycota are the macro-fungi used historically as a source of food, medicine and income. The edible mushrooms are a good source of nutrients and minerals and considered as healthy food [35]. Umami flavor represents savory, broth-like or meaty flavor present in edible mushrooms makes it one of the best foods and also used in the preparation of different food products [32] and now cultivated on large scale and available in local markets Fig. (**1**). The phytochemical evaluations of mushrooms with umami flavor show the presence of amino acids (aspartic acid and glutamic acid) and flavor 5$'$-nucleotides (5$'$-guanosine monophosphate, 5$'$-inosine monophosphate and 5$'$-xanthosine monophosphate) [36]. The umami taste of edible mushrooms is heat sensitive and requires low heat to avoid loosing of amino acids [37]. The use of edible mushrooms for umami taste is common in the food industry now and it is increasing day by day. Different species are also dried and processed sold out in cans. The edible mushrooms with umami taste are important from a health point of view including a reduction in weight gain, gastrointestinal disorders and control of hypertension due to their nutritional and mineral contents [32].

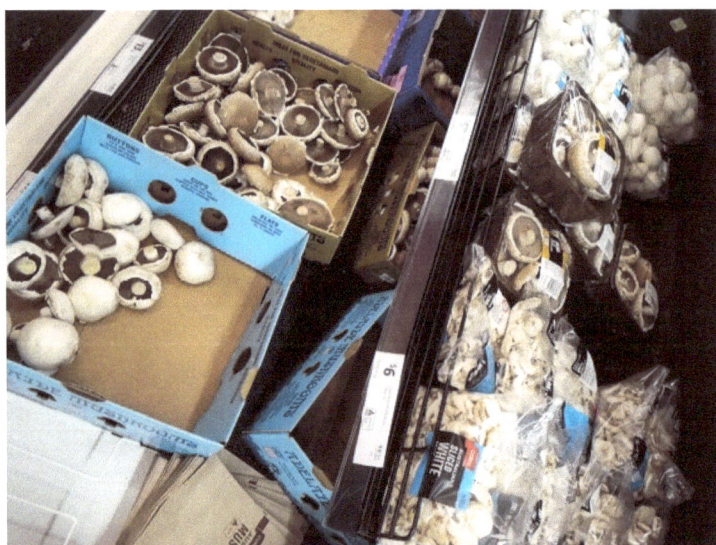

**Fig. (1).** Availability of cultivated mushrooms in the local markets of Adelaide, Australia.

## FLAVORINGS AND FLAVORANTS

Flavorings are substances used to enhance or impart taste, smell, sensory characteristics which are important in the assessment of nutritious value and freshness of food. A flavoring substance is defined as naturally occurring or chemically synthesized substance with flavoring characteristics [38]. The use of flavor to enhance food quality is an ancient practice. Food has been treated using many techniques including the use of salt as a preservative and flavor enhancer, the use of heat to cook food has to make it more digestible. Today, the food production pattern has been changed over the past ten to twenty years with the trends of cooking food with basic ingredients and simply reheating the food that has been produced at industrial scale. Flavor is very important as compared to other ingredients, for part of the world which has an adequate food supply [39].

Food technologists have the job to develop healthy food products while keeping their flavor profile at a specific level to meet consumers' demands. Huge advancement has brought about the identification and characterization of volatile organic compounds in foods dating back to 1960. Today, the number of volatile organic compounds characterized in foods is 7670 as recorded in the Nutrition and Food Research Institute of the Netherlands [40]. So, this high number of flavors in the food makes it difficult for food technologist to identify which volatile organic compound is creating flavor. Some of the flavors don't have a distinct aroma, some of the flavors have higher odor threshold and cannot be detected and others have an unwanted aroma. The first flavor used at commercial scale is vanillin (I) which is produced from vanilla beans and it was further synthesized by Tiemann and Haarmann [41]. This advancement led to the start of modern flavor understanding, the discovery of different and interesting flavoring elements using organic synthesis and the world's first industrial unit for the synthesis of artificial flavor and fragrance was founded in 1874 [41].

### Natural Flavoring Agents

The United States Code of Federal Regulations defined naturally occurring flavorings as "the essence, essential oil, extracts, protein hydrolysate, product of roasting of natural substance, oleoresin, cooking or enzymatic reaction, which may contain the flavoring ingredients obtained from a spice, vegetables or vegetable juice, fruit or fruit juice, edible yeast and yeast extract, herbal extract and any other edible part of a plant, meat of animal seafood and other dairy products, poultry, eggs, as well as fermentation products whose main purpose in food is flavoring rather than nutritional [42]. The European Parliament and of the Council of the European Union in 2008 formulated rules for the regulation of flavorings and certain food ingredients with flavoring properties to be used in food [43]. As food flavoring strongly influences food assessment as well as consumer satisfaction, which has always received great consideration from the food industries. As far as the records can be traced to historic civilizations, societies have attempted to obtain flavors and perfumes from natural sources using various methods and at that time plant tissues were the only sources of flavor compounds. Naturally occurring flavors usually have very simple structures with low toxicity and are efficient at very low concentrations. This aspect has become an increasingly significant demand for the food market since the 1980s. Today, more than 65% of all flavoring ingredients used in Europe and the United States are labelled as natural [38].

Natural flavoring substances are extracted from various sources including plants, herbs, spices, animals, or microbial products. Herbs, spices, and sweetness are all natural flavorings. The natural element of flavorings can be either used directly without processing in natural form or it can be processed for human consumption but the natural flavoring is not amended with any synthetic flavoring substances. Enzymatic mechanisms and microorganisms technologies yield complex volatiles similar to plant extracts including terpenes, aliphatic esters, carbonyls and lactones which are used for flavor synthesis [44, 45]. On the other hand, some fungi also have remarkable metabolic mechanisms diversity which is used to produce industrially important volatile compounds [46].

Many methods are used to extract flavors from natural sources including conventional extraction procedures for flavors as well as essential oils, but they have certain drawbacks such as they are time-consuming, labour-intensive, expensive as well as they cause thermal decomposition of the target compound which led to a partial loss of volatiles. But certain hindrances have been recorded in extracting and using natural flavoring. The main difficulties encountered in isolating natural flavoring compounds are: the target compound may be present in low quantities or in a bound form; the chemical complexity of the source may require to elaborate procedures of extraction; and, finally, the natural source material may be seasonal or not easily available [40].

## Synthetic Flavorings Agents

The term synthetic flavor means any constituent added to food whose purpose is to impart flavor and it is not derived from any natural source like a spice, fruits, vegetables, edible yeast, plants, bark of plants, leaf or any other material derived from plant or animal source like meat, fish, eggs, dairy products, or any fermentation and enzymolysis products. Chemistry of synthetic flavoring agents is similar to natural flavorings and is more easily accessible and is cost effective. But one disadvantage is that synthetic flavoring may not be a particular copy of the natural flavorings. Synthetic flavoring agents are composed of purely chemical constituents obtained through chemical processes. The chemical composition of synthetic flavorings is similar to their natural counterpart but are prepared chemically in the laboratory.

Synthetic flavoring started in the nineteenth century when modern consumerism increased and population as well. Before that only flavorings available at that time were some natural extracts and essential oils with limited availability and quality. Then, the advancement of synthetic organic chemistry gave many nature-identical and artificial flavors which allowed improved fidelity to the original materials and greater flavor intensity, stability and reproducibility. This is reflected in a comparison of modern and traditional flavor formulations for cherry [47].

## FLAVORANTS FOR MODIFYING FLAVORS

The use of different flavorants for modification of food flavors is an ancient practice from a very long time. Salt is the most commonly used flavorant as well as a preservative [48]. Spices and condiments are frequently used as a flavoring component in cooked foods. The use of flavorants is increased significantly in the modern era and due to which it became a major industry. The marketability of different food items depends upon the presentation of different flavors. Flavorings are added to different food items (beverages, cakes, biscuits, rice, meat, cereals, salads, vegetables and many cooked and uncooked food items) as an essential component.

## HEALTH BENEFITS AND CONCERNS OF FLAVORS

Flavors or flavoring agents are normally added to foods for imparting aroma or taste, but their usage should not cause a risk to human health by either misleading the consumers or causing health problems. Similar to other food additives, they must be of appropriate food-grade quality and prepared in the same way as any food ingredient is prepared. Moreover, the quantities of flavors added must be minimal so as to achieve only the intended flavoring effect [49]. Essential oils extracted from various parts of the plant have gained popularity as flavoring antimicrobial and antioxidant agents, capable of improving the nutritional value, as well as the shelf-life of foods. The essential oil is extracted from fruits which are sweet; having pleasant textures and flavors and can be consumed as dessert or snack-foods. A related example is the oil extracted from pulp and skin of feijoa fruit, which is highly volatile and has excellent potential as food-flavoring material. The oil exhibits antimicrobial and antioxidant capabilities due to high polyphenolic content present [50]. Another example is the aromatic oil extracted from lemongrass, which is widely utilized in flavoring, medicinal, therapeutic and perfumery applications. Though there are many lemongrass species, *Cymbopogon citratus* having a lemony flavor is the most recommended variety for various medicinal and food ingredients [51]. The bulk of volatile oils (essential oils) are made up of two compound classes; phenylpropenes and terpenoids. The major peppermint constituent comprises a terpenoid; menthol, which is responsible for the herbs cool, peppery-aroma and flavor. Similarly, cinnamon leaves comprise significant amounts of eugenol which is responsible for its distinctive pungent aroma [52]. A number of factors are responsible for the modification of flavor, texture and overall appearance of foods. The qualitative and quantitative nature of flavor depends upon various intrinsic and extrinsic parameters including physiological, genotypic, abiotic and biotic factors [53]. Temperature changes and food processing ranging from the knife cutting to processing the foods *via* heating or freezing also affect the nature of the flavor. Food processing alters the cell wall structure due to both enzymatic and non-enzymatic reactions. A simple example of this involves the cruciferous vegetables such as broccoli, which upon cutting/trimming liberates the enzyme "myrosinase". Myrosinase is responsible for converting glucosinolates to isothiocyanates when the cells are damaged, which in turn are accountable for the pungency and flavor of cruciferous vegetables [54].

Plant and plant-products, as well as mushrooms, are considered as healthy and balanced diet. Despite the fact that these plants and mushrooms are being reported for thousands of years, but recently mushrooms are gaining more popularity based on their texture, aroma and flavor and stand as the first choice for consumption due to their high nutritional value and uncountable medicinal properties [55].

## THE SIGNIFICANCE OF FLAVORS IN FOOD INDUSTRY AND CURRENT TRENDS

Flavors can either act in enhancement, taste modification, or aroma production in natural foods or they can completely create flavors in food that is likable to the consumers. From this point of view, flavors can be natural including seafood, nuts, spice-blends, wine and vegetables, among others, or they can be artificial including those chemicals that imitate natural flavors. Examples of artificial flavoring chemicals include alcohol having bitter and medicinal taste, esters having fruity, terpenoids having pine/citrus, phenols having smoke flavors and pyrazines and ketones imparting flavors to caramel. Natural flavoring gains advantage over artificial flavoring in many aspects, as one of the disadvantages of artificial flavoring agents, is that they may not completely imitate natural flavors and replace them to be their exact copy. Such examples of artificial flavoring agents are amyl acetate and ethyl butyrate used for imparting banana flavor and pineapple flavor respectively [56].

Consumers select their food based upon various factors of which the most important factor is flavor. Enhancing the flavor of vegetables and legumes *via* preparation and cooking methods can facilitate their consumption, especially among the children [49]. Children develop preferences in their initial developmental years when exposed to the food supply. As a result, certain flavors appear for well-liked food in society at certain concentrations; however, individual preferences may also yet exist based on health, age and food neophobia. This consumer segmentation patterns may also explain the abundant food supply in western countries [56].

Herbal teas are highly accepted based upon many factors of which flavors are considered the most important. High-quality herbal teas, therefore, need to have superior flavor. Flavors of tea are strongly connected to the chemical components they retains, such as volatile components contributing to aroma properties and non-volatile components contributing to taste [57]. Both volatile and non-volatile components are involved in flavor perception mechanisms. Volatile components are sensed as the aroma in the nose, whereas non-volatile components are sensed as taste in tongue along with the texture of other compounds. The overall flavor can be effectively determined by aroma rather than taste, as well demonstrated in studies involving subjects facing difficulties in identifying flavored drinks when air flow through their nose was prevented by clipping their nostrils [58]. Moreover, the volatile components have received considerable importance in determining the overall flavor of foods as well as being effectively and easily analyzed *via* instrumental for *e.g.* GC/MS (Gas-chromatography/mass spectroscopy), GC, GC×GC, as compared to non-volatile components having extreme difficulties in identifying. This acquired scientific knowledge *via* technological processes is further required for the improvement of flavoring as well as inhibition of off-flavoring [51, 59].

Edible mushrooms have long been used in soups and sauces as traditional seasoning materials, owing to their unique and subtle flavors [25]. Most mushrooms are believed to have umami taste, characterized by pleasant-savory flavor. This umami taste has been attributed to the manifestation of mono-sodium glutamate (MSG), free amino acids (FAAs), 5′–mononucleotides, and 5′-xanthosine monophosphate (XMP), which are found to act synergistically on taste-enhancement in several studies [60]. One of the most widely used potent flavor-enhancer is maltol (3-hydroxy, 2-methyl, 4H-pyran, 4-one). Its sources include beverages, coffee, bread crusts, baked cereals, sucrose pyrolysis, caramelized foods or starch thermal degradation. When used at high concentrations or upon interaction with different components, it can enhance/modify the flavor of food products, thereby depicting its wide use as a flavor enhancer of food products mostly in cakes, breads, beers, malt beverages and chocolate milk [61]. Another widely used flavor in almost every food component is salt. In the case of mayonnaise, salt acts as the most significant component acting both as a flavor as well as in the preparation of the emulsion and its stabilization. It may also influence auto-oxidation rate; however, this is not a major consideration as this can easily be overcome by the flavor imparting and emulsion stabilization properties of salt itself. New formulations are in demand towards developing low-fat containing mayonnaise, which will meet customer requirements keeping in mind its oxidative, physical, and flavor stability [62].

A world-wide challenge is a re-formulation of foods in order to achieve healthy eating, but this, in turn, is related to the reduction of salt, sugar, and fat which will modify the flavor profiles of foods completely. For the consumers to accept the food products, scientists are embedded with the task to deliver healthy foods while at the same time also maintaining their flavors. The tools available to optimize the flavor profile of food products is therefore of great interest. New discoveries from basic flavor-research will, therefore, play significant roles in the future of the food industry. First being that the whole industry will benefit when new food categories are discovered *e.g.* the development and the widespread acceptance of calorie-free beverages. Secondly, the individuals and companies readily investing in this long-term endeavor would have a competitive advantage and surely benefit themselves [63].

An important advancement in this field is the development of nano-sized additives. Most of them are natural-occurring substances used for food, animal-feed applications and health food supplements. They possess greater advantages as a small amount is used for the taste and flavor enhancement due to their large surface area compared to bulk forms. They have also been claimed as having enhanced adsorption and increased bioavailability inside the body as well as better dispersibility of water-insoluble additives in food products without needing additional emulsifiers or fats. In addition to this, nano-sized or nano-encapsulated supplements or food additives can improve food taste, hygienic food storage, reduced use of sugar, salt, fat, and preservatives and ineffective uptake and bioavailability of supplements and nutrients. Current examples of this category comprise antioxidants, vitamins, flavors, colors, and preservatives [64].

## CONCLUSION

Flavors have a critical role in the selection and acceptance of food in daily life and they are an important tool for food industries in the preparation of different food products. Different types of natural and synthetic flavoring agents are available in the market in five flavors, in which umami flavor is gaining market due to its use in fast food. Some health concerns are also associated with the use of synthetic flavoring agents and proper legislation is needed in this regard to ensure food safety. Therefore, the food industry demands new flavoring agents from natural origin to satisfy the consumers and to replace the current flavor system.

## CONSENT FOR PUBLICATION

Not applicable.

## CONFLICT OF INTEREST

The author confirms that this chapter contents have no conflict of interest.

## ACKNOWLEDGEMENTS

We acknowledge Ana Sanches Silva and Seyed Mohammad Nabavi for proofreading the chapter.

## REFERENCES

[1]     Fisher C, Scott TR. Food flavors: biology and chemistry. Royal Society of chemistry 2007 Oct; 31

[2]     Chen J. Food oral processing—A review. Food Hydrocoll 2009; 23(1): 1-25.
[http://dx.doi.org/10.1016/j.foodhyd.2007.11.013]

[3]     Laing DG, Jinks A. Flavor perception mechanisms. Trends Food Sci Technol 1996; 7(12): 387-9.
[http://dx.doi.org/10.1016/S0924-2244(96)10049-2]

[4]     Tsai SY, Huang SJ, Lo SH, Wu TP, Lian PY, Mau JL. Flavor components and antioxidant properties of several cultivated mushrooms. Food Chem 2009; 113(2): 578-84.
[http://dx.doi.org/10.1016/j.foodchem.2008.08.034]

[5]     Perez AG, Rios JJ, Sanz C, Olias JM. Aroma components and free amino acids in strawberry variety Chandler during ripening. J Agric Food Chem 1992; 40(11): 2232-5.
[http://dx.doi.org/10.1021/jf00023a036]

[6]     Gutiérrez-Rosales FG. History and principles of flavor analysis. Handbook of Fruit and Vegetable Flavors. 2010; 159.
[http://dx.doi.org/10.1002/9780470622834.ch10]

[7]     Beluhan S, Ranogajec A. Chemical composition and non-volatile components of Croatian wild edible mushrooms. Food Chem 2011; 124(3): 1076-82.
[http://dx.doi.org/10.1016/j.foodchem.2010.07.081]

[8]     Mehinagic E, Royer G, Symoneaux R, Jourjon F, Prost C. Characterization of odor-active volatiles in apples: influence of cultivars and maturity stage. J Agric Food Chem 2006; 54(7): 2678-87.
[http://dx.doi.org/10.1021/jf052288n]

[9]     Unwin T. Wine and the vine: an historical geography of viticulture and the wine trade. Routledge 2005.Jul12

[10]    Peynaud E, Ribéreau-Gayon P. The grape.The Biochemistry of Fruits and their Products. 171-205.

[11]    Coombe BG. BOVIO M, SCHNEIDER A. Solute accumulation by grape pericarp cells: v. relationship to berry size and the effects of defoliation. J Exp Bot 1987; 38(11): 1789-98.
[http://dx.doi.org/10.1093/jxb/38.11.1789]

[12]    Penarrubia L, Aguilar M, Margossian L, Fischer RL. An antisense gene stimulates ethylene hormone production during tomato fruit ripening. Plant Cell 1992; 4(6): 681-7.

[http://dx.doi.org/10.2307/3869526]

[13]　Nicol WM. Sucrose in food systems. Carbohydrate Sweeteners in Foods and Nutrition 1980; pp. 151-62.

[14]　Zeller BL, Saleeb FZ, Ludescher RD. Trends in development of porous carbohydrate food ingredients for use in flavor encapsulation. Trends Food Sci Technol 1998; 9(11-12): 389-94.
[http://dx.doi.org/10.1016/S0924-2244(99)00007-2]

[15]　Noble AC. Taste-aroma interactions. Trends Food Sci Technol 1996; 7(12): 439-44.
[http://dx.doi.org/10.1016/S0924-2244(96)10044-3]

[16]　Lee SL. Texas Sweet Onions. Produce Business 2007; 23(3): 70.

[17]　Brückner B, Wyllie SG, Eds. Fruit and vegetable flavor: recent advances and future prospects. Elsevier 2008.
[http://dx.doi.org/10.1533/9781845694296]

[18]　Malundo TM, Shewfelt RL, Scott JW. Flavor quality of fresh tomato (Lycopersicon esculentum Mill.) as affected by sugar and acid levels. Postharvest Biol Technol 1995; 6(1-2): 103-10.
[http://dx.doi.org/10.1016/0925-5214(94)00052-T]

[19]　Baldwin EA, Scott JW, Einstein MA, *et al.* Relationship between sensory and instrumental analysis for tomato flavor. J Am Soc Hortic Sci 1998; 123(5): 906-15.
[http://dx.doi.org/10.21273/JASHS.123.5.906]

[20]　Hui YH. Handbook of fruit and vegetable flavors Science Technology System. Hoboken, New Jersey: John Wiley & Sons, Inc. 2010.
[http://dx.doi.org/10.1002/9780470622834]

[21]　Wong E, Johnson CB, Nixon LN. The contribution of 4-methyloctanoic (hircinoic) acid to mutton and goat meat flavor. N Z J Agric Res 1975; 18(3): 261-6.
[http://dx.doi.org/10.1080/00288233.1975.10423642]

[22]　Mennella JA, Jagnow CP, Beauchamp GK. Prenatal and postnatal flavor learning by human infants. Pediatrics 2001; 107(6): e88-8.
[http://dx.doi.org/10.1542/peds.107.6.e88]

[23]　Imafidon GI, Spanier AM. Unraveling the secret of meat flavor. Trends Food Sci Technol 1994; 5(10): 315-21.
[http://dx.doi.org/10.1016/0924-2244(94)90182-1]

[24]　Lawless H, Engen T. Associations to odors: interference, mnemonics, and verbal labeling. J Exp Psychol Hum Learn 1977; 3(1): 52.
[http://dx.doi.org/10.1037/0278-7393.3.1.52]

[25]　Li W, Gu Z, Yang Y, Zhou S, Liu Y, Zhang J. Non-volatile taste components of several cultivated mushrooms. Food Chem 2014; 143: 427-31.
[http://dx.doi.org/10.1016/j.foodchem.2013.08.006]

[26]　Kuroiwa Y, Nishikawa A, Imazawa T, *et al.* Lack of subchronic toxicity of an aqueous extract of Agaricus blazei Murrill in F344 rats. Food Chem Toxicol 2005; 43(7): 1047-53.
[http://dx.doi.org/10.1016/j.fct.2005.02.007]

[27]　Baldwin EA. Fruit flavor, volatile metabolism and consumer perceptions. Fruit quality and its biological basis 2002 May; 189-106.

[28]　Mottram DS. Meat.Volatile compounds in food and beverages. New York: Marcel Dekker 1991; pp. 107-77.

[29]　Drake SL, Lopetcharat K, Drake MA. Salty taste in dairy foods: Can we reduce the salt? J Dairy Sci 2011; 94(2): 636-45.
[http://dx.doi.org/10.3168/jds.2010-3509]

[30]    Sookram C, Munodawafa D, Phori PM, Varenne B, Alisalad A. WHO's supported interventions on salt intake reduction in the sub-Saharan Africa region. Cardiovasc Diagn Ther 2015; 5(3): 186.

[31]    Liem D. Infants' and Children's Salt Taste Perception and Liking: A Review. Nutrients 2017; 9(9): 1011.
[http://dx.doi.org/10.3390/nu9091011]

[32]    Zhang Y, Venkitasamy C, Pan Z, Wang W. Recent developments on umami ingredients of edible mushrooms–A review. Trends Food Sci Technol 2013; 33(2): 78-92.
[http://dx.doi.org/10.1016/j.tifs.2013.08.002]

[33]    Chandrashekar J, Hoon MA, Ryba NJ, Zuker CS. The receptors and cells for mammalian taste. Nature 2006; 444(7117): 288.
[http://dx.doi.org/10.1038/nature05401]

[34]    Rotzoll N, Dunkel A, Hofmann T. Quantitative studies, taste reconstitution, and omission experiments on the key taste compounds in morel mushrooms (Morchella deliciosa Fr.). J Agric Food Chem 2006; 54(7): 2705-11.
[http://dx.doi.org/10.1021/jf053131y]

[35]    Musa H, Abolude DS, Andong FA. Utilization of Wild Edible Mushrooms for Rural Livelihood in Zaria and its Environs. Journal of Advanced Laboratory Research in Biology 2013; 4(3): 93-5.

[36]    Sommer I. Effect of gamma irradiation on selected compounds of fresh mushrooms (Doctoral dissertation, uniwien)

[37]    Li Q, Zhang HH, Claver IP, Zhu KX, Peng W, Zhou HM. Effect of different cooking methods on the flavor constituents of mushroom (Agaricus bisporus (Lange) Sing) soup. Int J Food Sci Technol 2011; 46(5): 1100-8.
[http://dx.doi.org/10.1111/j.1365-2621.2011.02592.x]

[38]    Baines D, Seal R, Eds. Natural food additives, ingredients and flavorings. Elsevier 2012.
[http://dx.doi.org/10.1533/9780857095725]

[39]    Cravotto G, Cintas P. Extraction of flavorings from natural sources.Modifying flavor in food. Woodhead Publishing 2007; pp. 41-63.
[http://dx.doi.org/10.1533/9781845693367.41]

[40]    Cuevas FJ, Moreno-Rojas JM, Ruiz-Moreno MJ. Assessing a traceability technique in fresh oranges (Citrus sinensis L. Osbeck) with an HS-SPME-GC-MS method. Towards a volatile characterisation of organic oranges. Food Chem 2017; 221: 1930-8.
[http://dx.doi.org/10.1016/j.foodchem.2016.11.156]

[41]    Tiemann F, Haarmann W. Ueber das Coniferin und seine Umwandlung in das aromatische Princip der Vanille. Ber Dtsch Chem Ges 1874; 7(1): 608-23.
[http://dx.doi.org/10.1002/cber.187400701193]

[42]    Pan BS, Chung-May Wu, Jen-Min Kuo, Bonnie Sun Pan. Chemical and Functional Properties of Food Components 2002 Jun; 27231

[43]    Tiemann F, Haarmann W. Ueber das Coniferin und seine Umwandlung in das aromatische Princip der Vanille. Ber Dtsch Chem Ges 1874; 7(1): 608-23.
[http://dx.doi.org/10.1002/cber.187400701193]

[44]    Speiser W. Enzymes and the fruit juice industry-a love affair? Fruit processing (Germany) 1993; 2: 8-39.

[45]    Dufosse L, Perrin CB, Souchon I, Feron G. Microbial production of flavors for the food industry. A case study on the production of gamma-decalactone, the key compound of peach flavor, by the yeasts Sporidiobolus sp. Food Sci Biotechnol 2002; 11(2): 192-202.

[46]    Feron G, Bonnarme P, Durand A. Prospects for the microbial production of food flavors. Trends Food Sci Technol 1996; 7(9): 285-93.

[http://dx.doi.org/10.1016/0924-2244(96)10032-7]

[47]    Cheetham PS. Natural sources of flavors. 2nd ed. Food Flavor Technology 2002; pp. 127-77.

[48]    Taylor AJ. 2007.

[49]    Poelman AA, Delahunty CM, de Graaf C. Cooking time but not cooking method affects children's acceptance of Brassica vegetables. Food Qual Prefer 2013; 28(2): 441-8.
[http://dx.doi.org/10.1016/j.foodqual.2012.12.003]

[50]    Weston RJ. Bioactive products from fruit of the feijoa (Feijoa sellowiana, Myrtaceae): A review. Food Chem 2010; 121(4): 923-6.
[http://dx.doi.org/10.1016/j.foodchem.2010.01.047]

[51]    Lasekan O, Lasekan A. Flavor chemistry of mate and some common herbal teas. Trends Food Sci Technol 2012; 27(1): 37-46.

[52]    Gang DR, Wang J, Dudareva N, *et al.* An investigation of the storage and biosynthesis of phenylpropenes in sweet basil. Plant Physiol 2001; 125(2): 539-55.
[http://dx.doi.org/10.1104/pp.125.2.539]

[53]    Kulkarni RS, Chidley HG, Pujari KH, Giri AP, Gupta VS. Geographic variation in the flavor volatiles of Alphonso mango. Food Chem 2012; 130(1): 58-66.
[http://dx.doi.org/10.1016/j.foodchem.2011.06.053]

[54]    Fabbri AD, Crosby GA. A review of the impact of preparation and cooking on the nutritional quality of vegetables and legumes. International Journal of Gastronomy and Food Science 2016; 3: 2-11.

[55]    Reis FS, Martins A, Vasconcelos MH, Morales P, Ferreira IC. Functional foods based on extracts or compounds derived from mushrooms. Trends Food Sci Technol 2017; 66: 48-62.
[http://dx.doi.org/10.1016/j.tifs.2017.05.010]

[56]    Tuorila H. Hedonic responses to flavor and their implications for food acceptance. Trends Food Sci Technol 1996; 7(12): 453-6.
[http://dx.doi.org/10.1016/S0924-2244(96)10048-0]

[57]    Scharbert S, Hofmann T. Molecular definition of black tea taste by means of quantitative studies, taste reconstitution, and omission experiments. J Agric Food Chem 2005; 53(13): 5377-84.

[58]    Jackson RS. Wine tasting: a professional handbook 2016 Dec; 22

[59]    Taylor AJ, Linforth RS. Flavor release in the mouth. Trends Food Sci Technol 1996; 7(12): 444-8.
[http://dx.doi.org/10.1016/S0924-2244(96)10046-7]

[60]    Poojary MM, Orlien V, Passamonti P, Olsen K. Improved extraction methods for simultaneous recovery of umami compounds from six different mushrooms. J Food Compos Anal 2017; 63: 171-83.
[http://dx.doi.org/10.1016/j.jfca.2017.08.004]

[61]    Altunay N, Gürkan R, Orhan U. Indirect determination of the flavor enhancer maltol in foods and beverages through flame atomic absorption spectrometry after ultrasound assisted-cloud point extraction. Food Chem 2017; 235: 308-17.

[62]    Depree JA, Savage GP. Physical and flavor stability of mayonnaise. Trends Food Sci Technol 2001; 12(5-6): 157-63.
[http://dx.doi.org/10.1016/S0924-2244(01)00079-6]

[63]    Beauchamp GK. Basic flavor research and the food industry. Trends Food Sci Technol 1996; 12(7): 457-8.
[http://dx.doi.org/10.1016/S0924-2244(96)20011-1]

[64]    Chaudhry Q, Castle L. Food applications of nanotechnologies: an overview of opportunities and challenges for developing countries. Trends Food Sci Technol 2011; 22(11): 595-603.

[65]    Publications [Umami Information Center [Internet]. 2019 Apr; 8 Available from: https://www.umami info.com/publications/

# CHAPTER 10

# Sweeteners

**Francesca Aiello**[*]

*Department of Pharmacy, Health and Nutritional Sciences, University of Calabria, Edificio Polifunzionale, Arcavacata di Rende (CS) 87036, Italy*

**Abstract:** A sweetener is a molecule that gives a food, or a drink, a sweet taste, thus activating the areas of taste used to perceive this as flavor. Sweeteners, as they increase the palatability of food, are widely used in the production, including industrial, of foodstuffs. In this regard, it is a common practice to add quantities of sugar to the recipes in order to gain consensus on the food market, since the sweetest products are most welcome among consumers. The need to use sweeteners has increased significantly in recent decades, due to the increased sensitivity to problems caused by excess sucrose (the common kitchen sugar) in human nutrition. It is clear that a diet rich in sugars, which exceeds 5% of daily caloric needs, can lead to very important pathologies ranging from common caries to diabetes. For this reason, it is preferred to adopt different "safer" solutions. In this chapter, the most commonly used sweeteners have been described, highlighting their chemical structure, their safe amount, and utilizable and toxic effects, where applicable. To guarantee an easy reading, the chapter includes three categories, natural sweeteners, sugar alcohols and intense sweeteners, which collect all the similar sweeteners.

**Keywords:** Food additive, Intense sweeteners, Natural sweeteners, Sugars.

## INTRODUCTION

Delivering food and guaranteeing the optimal conditions include huge efforts, not only regarding the refrigeration procedures, but also the selection of useful packaging, "smart packaging", or the application of additives to preserve the food and reduce drying, dehydrating and other processes [1]. In a global market defined as competitive, the least expensive method of food preservation is to employ food additives and select the appropriate preservative for each kind of food. Additionally, food additives are used to assist the food industry in making food pleasant to eat [2]. There are six groups of molecules used in food additives and are labeled according to the EU regulation division as follows:

[*] **Corresponding author Francesca Aiello:** Department of Pharmacy, Health and Nutritional Sciences, University of Calabria, Edificio Polifunzionale, Arcavacata di Rende (CS) 87036, Italy; E-mail: francesca.aiello@unical.it

**Seyed Mohammad Nabavi** *et al.* **(Eds.)**

- Coloring agents, E100-E199;
- Preservatives, E200-E285 and E1105,
- Antioxidants, E300-316, E319-321, E392, E586;
- Sweeteners, E420, 421, E950-969;
- Emulsifiers, stabilisers, thickeners, and gelling agents, E322, E400- 495, E1103;
- Others, E260-385, E422-1521.

Among these, the preservatives are classified into antimicrobials, antioxidants and anti-browning agents. At the same time, the coloring agents encompass the azo compounds, the chinophthalon derivatives, the triarylmethane compounds, the xanthenes and the indigos. Regarding the flavoring agents including the sweeteners, the natural and synthetic flavors, flavor enhancers, and the texturizing agents can be divided into emulsifiers and stabilizers [3].

Among the sweeteners, mainly the "intensive sweeteners", such as saccharine, aspartame, sucralose and acesulfame K are the most commonly used in the food industry, mainly in low caloric food products. All of them provide the sweetening power at low doses. Saccharine and sucralose as regarded as safe to consume with a restrictive maximum level (EU Reg. 1129/2011), regarding aspartame there are still divisive effects [4, 5]. Acesulfame K has been demonstrated to have clastogenic effects in mice and to induce allergies in humans (doses between 15 and 2250 mg acesulfame kg/body weight) [6, 7]. The correct determination of the ADI relatively for synthetic additives has always been of great importance for the governing bodies. In fact, in 2001, the EU published a report informing the consumption of additives in relation to their ADI. In general, we can say that high sugar consumption is not consistent with a healthy diet. Consumers should intake sugar in the diet and reach a healthy balance between nutrients and sugar intake. This is very difficult; even regarding the foods defined "ready to eat". Recently, there is an intense demand for low-sugar food that encourages weight loss or even erroneous dietetic programs that aims to eliminate all sugar, even the natural sugars found in fruit. A balanced diet that includes food from all five-food groups (listed below) is a basic starting point to healthy eating.

- Vegetables and legumes/beans;
- Fruits;
- Grain (cereal) foods, mostly wholegrain and/or high cereal fibre varieties;
- Lean meats and poultry, fish, eggs, tofu, nuts and seeds and legumes/beans;
- Milk, yogurt cheese and/or alternatives, mostly reduced fat.

*Sweeteners,* often called "alternative sweeteners", are substances with a sweet taste used in foodstuff as substitute to sucrose. Usually, to distinguish the sweeteners the relative sweetness potency is used compared to sucrose, and consequentially, it is possible to classify them in:

- "intense" sweeteners due to their intense property to produce the required effect in small quantities, also called "artificial" sweeteners to outline that most of them are produced by chemical synthesis;
- "natural" sweeteners such as sugars naturally present in plants.

Sweeteners do the following things: enhance bulk to ice cream, give sweet flavor, retain the freshness, afford fermentation, are preservative in several products, and enrich the flavor.

The "bulk" sweeteners group includes substances with sweetness similar to that of sucrose that are fillers (providing or improving consistency). Bulk sweeteners are hydrogenated carbohydrates, well known as sugar alcohols or polyols, some of them are natural. Their use as sweeteners is legalized in desserts, ice-cream, breakfast cereals, and sauces due to certain functional advantages (*e.g.* lowering the freezing point of an ice-cream mix, reducing caramelization) or dietetic advantages (*e.g.* in being more slowly assimilated, being non-cariogenic or not creating a demand for insulin). Bulk sweeteners do not provide a significant reduction of energy content in food products; in fact, their energy value is approximately 10 kJ/g, while that of sucrose is 17 kJ/g [8]. The European Food Safety Authority is a scientific guarantor for the safety of food additives (including sweeteners).

The safety of food additives is well documented by the results of several *in vitro* and *in vivo* animal studies, tests in humans, and epidemiological studies. The correspondent organization in the USA is the FDA. Sometimes there are little differences in order to define "permitted" or "no" relative to each sweetener used as food additive, in different countries. The sweetener defined "permitted" have been allocated an acceptable daily intake (ADI), "which is the amount of a food additive, expressed as milligrams per kilograms of body weight that can be ingested daily over a lifetime without incurring any appreciable health risk". Any sweetener with an "acceptable" ADI relative to a food additive, means that the levels used can guarantee the safe technological effects for the consumers. Fig. (**1**) depicts the molecular structure of all sweeteners reported and Table **1** summarizes interesting properties of each one.

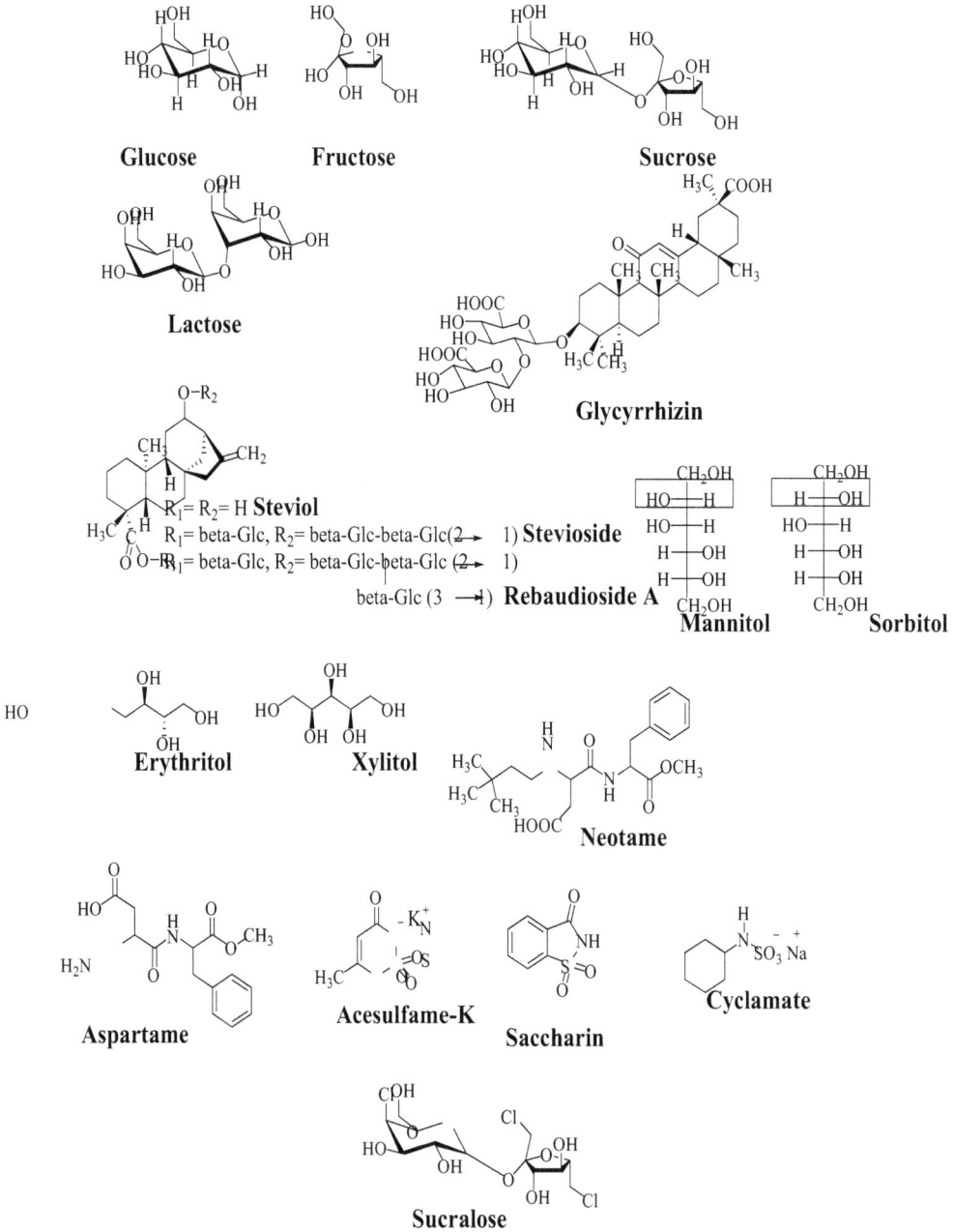

**Fig. (1).** Molecular structures of sweeteners described in this chapter.

**Table 1. Interesting aspects of described sweeteners.**

| Name | Chemical formula | RS | ADI | GI | Energy Cal/g | Sweetness^ |
|---|---|---|---|---|---|---|
| Glucose | $C_6H_{12}O_6$ | A | - | 100 | 4 | 0.6 |
| Fructose | $C_6H_{12}O_6$ | A | - | 25 | 4 | 1.5 |
| Sucrose | $C_{12}H_{22}O_{11}$ | A | - | 65 | 4 (16 calories *per* teaspoon) | 1 |
| Lactose | $C_{12}H_{22}O_{11}$ | A | - | 45 | 4 | |
| Glycyrrhizin | $C_{42}H_{62}O_{16}$ | A | 100 mg/day | 0 | - | 50 |
| Stevia | - | A* | 4 g/day | 0 | - | 300 |
| Sorbitol | $C_6H_{14}O_6$ | A | 50 g/day Accetable (UE) | 4 | 75† | 0.5-1 |
| Mannitol | $C_6H_{14}O_6$ | A | 20 g/day Accetable (UE) | 2 | 1.6 (USA) 2.4 (UE) 50† | 0.7 |
| Erythritol | $C_4H_{10}O_4$ | A | Not Specified (US) Accetable (UE) | 1 | 0.2 10† | 0.6-0.8 |
| Xylitol | $C_5H_{12}O_5$ | A | Not Specified (US) Accetable (UE) | 8 | 2.4 100† | 1 |
| Aspartame | $C_{14}H_{18}N_2O_5$ | A | 50 g/day (US) 0-40 (UE) | 0 | 4 | 180-200 |
| Acesulfame K | $C_4H_4KNO_4S$ | A | 15 mg/kg/bw/d (USA) 0-9 (UE) | 0 | 0 | 200 |
| Saccharin | $C_7H_5NO_3S$ (saccharic acid) $C_7H_4NNaO_3S$ (sodium saccharin) | A** | 0-5 mg/kg/bw/d | 0 | 0 | 200-700 |
| Neotame | $C_{20}H_{24}N_2O_5$ | A*** | 18 mg/person/day (US) | 0 | 0 | 8000 |
| Cyclamate | $C_6H_{13}NO_3S$ (cyclamic acid) $C_6H_{12}NNaO_3S$ (sodium cyclamate) $C_{12}H_{24}CaN_2O_6S_2$ (calcium cyclamate) | A | 11 g/day (US) 0-7 g/day (UE) | 0 | 0 | 30 |
| Sucralose | $C_{12}H19Cl_3O_8$ | A | 5 mg/kg/d (US) 0-15 mg/kg/d (UE) | 0 | 0 | 600 |

A: approved; ADI: Acceptable Daily Intake; RS: Regulatory Status; GI: Glycaemic Index; ^compared to sucrose. * ≥ 95% pure glycosides Subject of GRAS notices for specific conditions of use GRAS Notice Inventory; ** Approved as a sweetener only in certain special dietary foods and as an additive used for certain technological purposes 21 CFR 180.37; *** Approved as a sweetener and flavor enhancer in foods generally (except in meat and poultry) 21 CFR 172.829; † available energy (% of sucrose).

## NATURAL SWEETENERS

The sweeteners are frequently defined as SUGARS, using this term to describe a wide range of compounds, such as glucose, fructose, galactose, sucrose, lactose, and maltose. Sugars are naturally present in fruits and milk derivatives, and in honey as well, where there is a combination of fructose, glucose, and water. Some sweeteners are made by processing sugar compounds. In a number of any foods stuff, the processed sugars are added sugars, which can only improve the calories and not the nutrients. These kind of foods and drinks are titled as "empty" calories. Sucrose is made from a low-sugar beet juice or sugar cane, which includes raw sugar and granulated sugar. The well-known brown sugar is made from sugar crystals that come from molasses syrup. The powdered sugar, also known as confectioner's sugar is a finely ground sucrose. Sugar provides calories and no other nutrients. Other commonly natural used sugars are:

- Fructose is the naturally occurring sugar in all fruits, also called levulose or fruit sugar;
- Honey is a combination of fructose, glucose, and water;
- High fructose corn syrup (HFCS) and corn syrup are made from corn;
- Dextrose is glucose combined with water;
- Agave nectar is a highly processed type of sugar from the Agave tequilana (tequila) plant.
- Glucose is found in fruits in small amounts. It is also a syrup made from corn starch.
- Lactose (milk sugar) is the carbohydrate that is in milk. It is made up of glucose and galactose.
- Maltose (malt sugar) is produced during fermentation usually found in beer and breads.
- Maple sugar comes from the sap of maple trees. It is made up of sucrose, fructose, and glucose.
- Molasses is taken from the residue of sugar cane processing.

The main adverse effects due to sugar intake and its use as a sweetener are that it leads to tooth decay and obesity in children and adults. Among this, the obese people are at much higher risk for type 2 diabetes, metabolic syndrome, and high blood pressure [8]. Sugar is listed as safe foods [8 - 11], and containing 16 calories per teaspoon but must be used in moderation. In fact, it is indispensable to limit the amount of added sugars in your diet, not more than 10% of your calories per day, and this limit is true for all types of added sugars. Regarding the gender differences, women should get no more than 100 calories per day from sugar (about 6 teaspoons of sugar); men should get no more than 150 calories per day from sugar (about 9 teaspoons of sugar).

In addition, regarding diabetics, they can eat limited amounts of foods containing natural sweeteners, in place of other carbohydrates, or prefer foods that contain sugar alcohols. The sugars affect blood glucose control in the same manner as other carbohydrates. The American Diabetes Association nutrition guidelines suggest one should not avoid all sugar but just reduce the quantity, and balance the sources of it.

## SUGARS

### Glucose

Glucose, (2R,3S,4R,5R)-2,3,4,5,6-Pentahydroxyhexanal, it is categorized as a hexose, a sub-category of monosaccharides. D-glucose is one of the 16 aldohexose stereoisomers. The D-isomer (D-glucose), also known as dextrose, occurs widely in nature, but the L-isomer (L-glucose) does not. It is the primary product of photosynthesis in plants; furthermore, it is a component of sucrose, starch, glycogen, and cellulose. Chemically, it is a monosaccharide, the open-chain form is thermodynamically unstable, and it spontaneously isomerizes to the cyclic forms. All forms of glucose are colorless and easily soluble in water, acetic acid, and several other solvents. In liquid solutions at room temperature, the four cyclic isomers interconvert over a time scale of hours, in a process called mutarotation.

They are only sparingly soluble in methanol and ethanol and still considered an important nutrient, being the major energy source for brain cells. The human body stores it as glycogen, and converts the excess to fat. Glucose provides approximately 4 calories per gram. Insulin is a hormone that regulates glucose levels, allowing the body's cells to absorb and use glucose. Without it, glucose cannot enter the cell and therefore cannot be used as fuel for the body's functions. Glucose is produced commercially via the enzymatic hydrolysis of starch. Many crops are used as the source of starch. Maize, rice, wheat, cassava, corn husk and sago are all used in various parts of the world. In the United States, corn starch (from maize) is used exclusively in food products and is responsible for bulk and binds moisture [12].

### Fructose

Fructose, 1,3,4,5,6-Pentahydroxy-2-hexanone, is a monosaccharide found in most fruits, in honey and is a component of sucrose, which provides 4 calories per gram and is very water-soluble. Commercially, fructose is frequently derived from sugar cane, sugar beets, and corn. The name "fructose" was coined in 1857 by the

English chemist, William Miller. Pure and dry fructose is a very sweet, white, odorless crystalline solid and is the most water-soluble of all the sugars [13].

Fructose shows a high hygroscopic behavior. This property enables it to bind water in food products, and preserve them from drying. Fructose is an important ingredient of the human diet from prehistoric times, and more awareness should be raised regarding the difference between fructose and high fructose corn syrup (HFCS). In fact, HFCS is produced by enzymatically converting corn starch to glucose, and then adding a second enzyme that converts part of the glucose to fructose. Numerous suppositions suggested that excessive fructose consumption is a cause of negative effects, such as insulin resistance, obesity [14], elevated LDL cholesterol and triglycerides, and finally leading to metabolic syndrome [15 - 17], type 2 diabetes and cardiovascular disease [18]. However, the European Food Safety Authority stated that fructose is preferred over sucrose and glucose in sugar-sweetened foods and beverages because of its lower effect on post-prandial blood glucose levels. Further, the UK's Scientific Advisory Committee on Nutrition in 2015 disputed the claims of fructose causing metabolic disorders, stating that "there is insufficient evidence to demonstrate that fructose intake... leads to adverse health outcomes independent of any effects related to its presence as a component of total and free sugars" [19].

## Sucrose

Sucrose, (2R,3R,4S,5S,6R)- 2 -[(2S,3S,4S,5R)- 3, 4 -dihydroxy-2,5-bis(hydroxy-methyl)oxolan-2-yl]oxy-6-(hydroxymethyl)oxane-3,4,5-triol, is a disaccharide, water soluble, composed of two sugar molecules, glucose and a fructose, linked together. It takes place naturally in sugar cane, sugar beets, and most fruits. Modern industrial sugar refinement processes often involve bleaching and crystallization, producing a white, odorless, crystalline powder with a sweet taste of pure sucrose, devoid of vitamins and minerals. This refined form of sucrose is commonly referred to as table sugar or simply sugar. It plays a central role as an additive in food production and food consumption all over the world. After ingestion, the body quickly digests it, release glucose and fructose, and metabolizes both monomers for energy production. In food products, sucrose provides bulk and binds moisture. Before the 1700s, sucrose was consumed in diet, mainly as a component of plant products. Only when the crystalline form becomes available it contributed to extensive obesity and dental caries. Overconsumption of sucrose has been linked with adverse health effects.

Dental caries or tooth decay may be caused by oral bacteria converting sugars, including sucrose, from food into acids that corrode tooth enamel. When large amounts of refined foods that contain high percentages of sucrose are consumed, essential nutrients can be eliminated from the diet, which can contribute to an increased risk for chronic disease. The rapidity with which sucrose raises blood glucose can cause problems for people suffering from defective glucose metabolism, such as persons with hypoglycaemia or diabetes mellitus.

Sucrose can contribute to the development of metabolic syndrome [20]. In an experiment with rats that were fed a diet one-third of which was sucrose, the sucrose first elevated blood levels of triglycerides, which induced visceral fat and ultimately resulted in insulin resistance [21]. Another study found that rats fed sucrose-rich diets developed high triglycerides, hyperglycaemia, and insulin resistance [22]. A 2004 study recommended that the consumption of sucrose-containing drinks should be limited due to the growing number of people with obesity and insulin resistance [23].

## Lactose

Lactose, $\beta$-D-galactopyranosyl-$(1\rightarrow4)$-D-glucose, is a disaccharide formed by galactose and glucose and naturally occurs in milk. To digest it, the intestinal villi secrete an enzyme called lactase ($\beta$-D-galactosidase), responsible to the cleavage in two monomers, sugars glucose and galactose, which can be easily absorbed. Lactose intolerance is a common digestive problem where the body is unable to digest lactose. Symptoms of this intolerance are flatulence (wind), diarrhea, bloated stomach, stomach cramps and pains, stomach rumbling, and feeling sick.

All the lactose presents in milk comes from the cow, where no sugar is added. The lactose in milk and its derivatives do not increase the risk of type 2 diabetes. Diversely, it may play a protective role against type 2 diabetes, particularly in those who consume low-fat dairy products. On the other hand, milk components, such as whey, calcium, vitamin D, fatty acids and/or lactose are thought to help with sugar metabolism.

Several epidemiologic evaluations confirmed that children who drink flavored milk, drink more milk and have higher intakes of added sugar or total fat [24, 25]. Food industry applications have markedly increased since the 1960s. Lactose is not added directly to many foods, because its solubility is less than that of other sugars commonly used in food. Infant formula is a notable exception, where the addition of lactose is necessary to match the composition of human milk. Lactose is not fermented by most yeast during brewing, which may be used as an advantage [26]. For example, lactose may be used to sweeten the stout beer; the resulting beer is usually called a milk stout or a cream stout.

## Glycyrrhizin E958

Chemically, (3β,20β)-20-carboxy-11-oxo-30-norolean-12-en-3-yl 2-O-β-D-gluco-pyranuronosyl-α-D-glucopyranosiduronic acid, is a triterpene glycoside extracted from licorice roots. This compound is the chief sweet-tasting constituent of *Glycyrrhiza glabra* (licorice) roots. Structurally, it is a saponin and has been used as an emulsifier and gel-forming agent in foodstuff and cosmetics and has a sweet taste with a characteristic licorice taste sometimes defined as "cooling" sensation. Regarding the sweetener potency, it is about 50 times to that of sucrose. The perceptions of the sweet taste come slow but remain for a long time, and an important characteristic is that it does not provide calories, but at high consumption levels, there is considerable risk of adverse effects. After oral ingestion, glycyrrhizin is first hydrolyzed to 18β-glycyrrhetinic acid by intestinal bacteria. After complete absorption from the gut, β-glycyrrhetinic acid is metabolized to 3β-monoglucuronyl-18β-glycyrrhetinic acid in the liver. This metabolite then circulates in the bloodstream. Consequently, its oral bioavailability is poor. The main part is eliminated by bile and only a minor part (0.31-0.67%) by urine [27]. Many studies have demonstrated that glycyrrhizin inhibits an enzyme that normally inactivates cortisol, so that excessive consumption of licorice or glycyrrhizin can increase the level of cortisol in the body. Cortisol has anti-inflammatory properties, but high levels of it can lead to water retention, hypertension, and loss of potassium and calcium. Furthermore, an excess of cortisol during pregnancy correlates with low birth weight, so glycyrrhizin and licorice consumption are discouraged during pregnancy.

Taking into consideration these scientific evidences, the European Union's Scientific Committee on Food recommended an upper limit of 100 mg/day, which corresponds to about two ounces per day of licorice candy. The Food and Drug Administration stated that, for persons over 40 years of age, eating two ounces of black licorice a day for two weeks could cause serious health problems. A similar limit is suggested in Japan.

## Stevia e rebaudioside E960

*Stevia rebaudiana* is a plant native to Paraguay used as a sweetener. This plant contains a number of diterpene glycosides that taste sweet; the main ones are stevioside and rebaudioside A. The leaves of *S. rebaudiana* can be used directly for sweetening, but the taste quality is not as good as the purified glycosides. Stevioside is about 200 times as sweet as sucrose, with significant bitter taste and licorice-like taste at higher concentrations. Rebaudioside A is about 300 times as sweet as sucrose, with less bitter and licorice off-tastes than stevioside. Both sweeteners are non-caloric. Bacteria in the colon remove the sugars from stevioside and rebaudioside, and the remaining steviol is absorbed by the body. It is conjugated in the liver (glucuronic acid is attached to make it more water-soluble) and then excreted in the urine.

## SUGAR ALCOHOLS

Polyols (also known as sugar alcohols) are often used to replace sugar in foods. Polyols provide fewer calories per gram than carbohydrates because they are not efficiently absorbed and metabolized by humans. When polyols are consumed in large quantities, the unabsorbed materials can have several adverse effects. There have been clinical studies performed to determine the "laxative threshold values" (LTV) for many of the polyols. The LTV is the amount that may cause a laxative effect if consumed in a single meal by a normal adult. Sugar alcohols include mannitol, sorbitol, and xylitol. These sweeteners are used as an ingredient in many food products that are labeled as "sugarfree", "diabetic", or "low carb". They should not be confused with sugar substitutes that are calorie free. Sugar alcohol may cause stomach cramps and diarrhea in some people. Erythritol is a naturally occurring sugar alcohol found in fruit and fermented foods. It is 60 to 70% as sweet as table sugar, but has fewer calories. In addition, it does not improve the level of sugar in blood after meals or cause tooth decay.

### Sorbitol E420

Sorbitol, (2S,3R,4R,5R)-hexane-1,2,3,4,5,6-hexol, shows humectant activity and when is used in food systems produces appropriate texture. The body only partly and slowly absorbs sorbitol, and converts absorbed sorbitol into glucose. Its caloric value depends on how much is consumed, and individual variation in the absorption rate. In the European Union, it is registered at 2.4 calories per gram, and in the United States, 2.6 calories per gram. Sorbitol is the most common ingredient in sugar-free chewing gum. For several polyols, the Joint FAO/WHO Expert Committee on Food Additives (JECFA) has determined the "Laxative Threshold Value" (LTV), and sorbitol resulted in the more laxative polyols with an LTV of 23 grams per meal. For this reason, the FDA needs the following tag: "Excess consumption may have a laxative effect" for any food that may result in the daily ingestion of 50 grams of sorbitol.

### Mannitol E421

The isomer of sorbitol, that differ in the stereochemistry at carbon atom 2, is named mannitol. Mannitol, 2R,3R,4R,5R)-Hexane-1,2,3,4,5,6-hexol, is obtained by hydrogenation of fructose, but also occurs naturally in mushrooms, algae, and trees, and was first isolated from the sap of a flowering ash tree found in southern Europe and Asia. Likely, to other polyols, the body does not efficiently absorb mannitol, and it is eliminated to be partly metabolized. The pleasant taste, stability to hot temperatures and mouthfeel of mannitol also makes it a popular excipient to be used as a dusting powder on chewing gums and in chocolate flavored coatings. The LTV for mannitol should be between 10 and 20 grams per meal.

## Erythritol E968

Erythritol, (2R,3S)-butane-1,2,3,4-tetraol, is a polyol naturally present in many fruits, mushrooms, and fermented foods. When it is ingested, it produces a cooling effect in the mouth, similar to xylitol, but the real advantage is that bacteria in the mouth cannot utilize Erythritol, so it does not contribute to tooth decay.

Erythritol is occasionally used in combination with a high potency sweetener. In Japan, its use is permitted since 1990 and has Generally Recognized as Safe (GRAS) status in the USA since 1996, however, in 2008, it received full approval from the European Union.

## Xylitol E967

Xylitol, (2R,3r,4S)-Pentane-1,2,3,4,5-pentol, is a polyol present naturally in small amount, in raspberries, plums, and some other fruits. Xylitol has sweetness similar to sucrose but diversely produces a cooling feeling in the mouth, frequently used in chewing gums and confections. Xylitol is stable over the range of pH found in foods, it is heat-stable, moderately soluble in water, and presents LTV of 20 grams per meal. The result shows that it partly absorbed in the human body, in fact, in the colon which may ferment with a consequential production of gas and acids. These acids osmotically draw water into the colon, leading to diarrhea. A positive feature is that xylitol reduces dental caries [28]. In fact, bacteria in the mouth does not use this polyol, and furthermore, when used in chewing gum, it stimulates saliva flow, and increased saliva flow, thus inhibiting caries formation. In several studies, it has been reported that xylitol may even help in remineralization of teeth, and then a combination of calcium source with xylitol in a chewing gum can deliverhealthier effects than the xylitol alone [29].

## INTENSE SWEETENERS

Obesity and diabetes are the major problems consequential from an improper diet, and to overcome these "side effects" of the modern lifestyle, the people choose to eat sugar-free foods, because of their less calorie content. Therefore, this trend, led the food industry to discover several forms of alternative intense sweeteners, which have made it possible to deal with the sweet taste without the calories.

The food industry uses numerous artificial sweeteners, which are low in calorie content instead of high calorie sugar. The sweeteners of this type currently approved to be used in the United States are Aspartame, Acesulfame-K, Neotame, Saccharin, Sucralose, Cyclamate and Alitame [30]. However, it is important to take into consideration that these sweeteners have also controversial health and metabolic effects [31]. This type of intense sweetener cannot simply replace sugar without considering the quality, quality, intensity of sweetness and physical characteristics. Considering to all these features, sporadic sugars are appropriate for low calorie, as well as bulk sweetener. Very frequently, these sugars required sweetness but are not easily metabolized in the human body and therefore do not provide calorie intake.

High-intensity sweeteners are extensively used in foods and beverages marketed as "sugar-free" or "diet" comprising baked goods, soft drinks, powdered drink mixes, candy, puddings, canned foods, jams and jellies, dairy products, and scores of other foods and beverages. The presence of high-intensity sweeteners is highlighted by its name in the ingredient list. In this way, the consumers also with phenylketonuria (PKU) should avoid to eat foods containing these sweeteners. The term 'Intense sweeteners' (IS) refers to various substances of plant origin or obtained by chemical synthesis, used for their high sweetening power and their low caloric value. The intense sweeteners currently authorized in Europe comprise ten compounds of various chemical natures. They are used in the formulation of foods and beverages, both for their sweetening role and technological properties, such as stabilizers and texturizers. Their sweetening power is hundred (*e.g.* acesulfame K, aspartame) to several thousand (*e.g.* neotame) times higher than that of sucrose. Their overall use has sharply risen in the last 20 years [32].

The IS authorized in Europe, after scientific review are; aspartame, acesulfame potassium (K), cyclamic acid and its salts, steviol glycosides, neohesperidin dihydrochalcone, neotame, saccharin and its salts, sucralose, aspartame-acesulfame salt and thaumatin. Before their authorization, the potential risks of each intense sweetener are assessed, on the other hand, any general assessment of the overall nutritional risks and benefits of these products has been conducted at the European level up to now [33 - 35]. Despite a large number of studies conducted, the data are insufficient to determine any long-term nutritional benefits related to the consumption of products containing IS as sugar substitutes. However, due to the limited number of studies, it is not possible to rule out potential long-term risks related to IS consumption in specific populations, particularly adult daily consumers and children. In fact, the consumption of intense sweeteners has not shown any beneficial effects on the prevention of type 2 diabetes; similarly, their regular consumption as a sugar substitute does not have any beneficial effect on regulating blood glucose concentrations.

For the risks of developing cancer, type 2 diabetes, or premature births, the data available to date do not enable a link to be documented between the onset of these risks and the consumption of intense sweeteners. Lastly, in a nutritional policy context aimed to suggest the reduction of sugar intake in the consumers, as pointed out in 2015 by WHO guidelines on sugar intake, this review points out that no important data exist that justify or even encourage the substitution of sugars by intense sweeteners. This objective of reduction of sugar intake levels should be reached generally at an early age by reducing the consumption of sweet tasting foods. It should, therefore, be suggested that artificially-sweetened and sugar-sweetened soft drinks should not be consumed as a replacement for water [36]. Higher intake, >1500 milligrams per kilograms of body weight/day, of saccharin, have been documented by JECFA using in vivo assays in rats. Several toxic effects, such as swelling of renal glomeruli, growth depression, and carcinoma appear to be associated with this large amount. The data are then extrapolated for humans by applying a safety factor of 100 to reach at the ADI values, as studies in humans are lacking.

A number of studies have observed the intake of artificial sweeteners, such as saccharin, aspartame, cyclamate, stevioside, and sorbitol, and the chemical analysis was done in most studies to monitor sweetener concentration in foods [37, 38]. All the studies showed that the intake was found to be below the ADI, except a study that showed that the intake of saccharin exceeded the ADI when sweetened crushed ice and ice candy were consumed by children and when sweetened betel leaf was consumed by adults [39]. Therefore, studies on the intake of artificial sweeteners should focus on population groups who are likely to consume more artificial sweeteners, such as diabetics or those trying to lose/maintain weight.

**Aspartame E951**

Aspartame, L-aspartyl-L-phenylalanine methyl ester, is composed of two natural amino acids, aspartic acid and phenylalanine, esterified with methanol, two amino acids that are building blocks of proteins. When used in foods it is completely digested. Aspartame digested is converted to three components: aspartic acid, phenylalanine, and methanol [12] both amino acids provide calories, in general, about 4 calories per gram. Methanol is present in a lot of fruits and fruit juices, partly in the form of methyl esters, including pectin. The stability of aspartame is pH-and- temperature-dependent and this limits the aspartame's use in baked goods. The FDA, the European Food Safety Authority, and several other regulatory agencies revised efficiently the safety of aspartame and accomplished that aspartame is nontoxic. The exception is for people with the rare genetic disorder phenylketonuria (PKU).

## Acesulfame K E950

A chemist, Karl Clauss, discovered Acesulfame in 1967. He noticed a sweet taste when he licked his finger to pick up a piece of paper in the laboratory [40]. Acesulfame, 6-metil-1,2,3-oxathiazin-4(3H)-one-2,2-dioxyde, is chemically very similar to saccharin structure. The presence of hydrogen on the nitrogen is responsible for the moderately acidic behavioral (pKa ~2) and for this, it can readily form salts; in fact, the sweetener is the potassium salt. Acesulfame has numerous positive aspects, such as good heat stability; good water solubility is quite good and sweet in taste.

## Saccharin E954

Saccharin, $2H$-$1\lambda^6$, 2-Benzothiazole-1,1,3-trione, is a cyclic sulfimide, and the sodium or calcium salts, water soluble, are used as sweeteners in the foods. Discovered in 1879, saccharin was the first synthetic sweetener used commercially. When it is ingested, the stomach adsorbs it by neutralizing the salt to the free acid form and quickly excreted in the kidneys. Several studies showed that saccharin produces urinary bladder tumors in rats, and fact leads to prohibition of its use in some countries and especially a proposed ban in the US. However, to better understand how saccharin drives these dangerous effects, the International Agency for Research on Cancer has found that a combination of sodium saccharin with high pH, high calcium phosphate concentration, and high protein concentration, are those conditions that are exclusive in the rats, and lead to the formation of solid material in the rat bladder. This material provokes overactive regrowth of bladder cells. This phenomenon has not been observed in mice or in any other species, including humans. Thus, it is likely that saccharin is carcinogenic only in rats, and that it is reasonably safe for humans. In a study aimed to review saccharine's genotoxicity and carcinogenicity [41] it is reported that it is not metabolized in the gastrointestinal (GI) tract and, therefore, does not affect blood insulin levels. Saccharine is 500 times sweeter than sucrose which is commonly used in many foods like soft drinks, baked goods, jams, canned fruits, candy, salad dressings, dessert *etc*. Because saccharine is consumed by millions of people, including children and even pregnant women, it draws a significant interest of the public about its safety.

A number of studies have been conducted for the safety of saccharine, and all literature between 1975 and 2014 reviewed about saccharine's safety. However, among all these, the genotoxicity and carcinogenicity of saccharine are still confusing. Therefore, consumers should be careful about the consumption of this artificial sweetener. There are many studies about saccharin about its effects on health. Some studies found that the use of saccharin is associated with an intense feeling of hunger [42 - 44]. A study conducted on rats showed that when their diets were sweetened with saccharin for over 5 weeks, they gained weight and adiposity, as well as a decrease in the central body temperature when compared to glucose supplementation [45]. Calorie predictive relations in energy regulation by rats. In another study, it was found that when taken together, the use of aspartame, acesulfame, cyclamate and saccharin in foods might be considered as safe, with regard to no effects on CYP1A1 induction and activation of AhR and GR receptors. A few epidemiological studies also found some relationships between saccharin and bladder cancer risk in humans [46 - 49] but most – and the largest – studies found no association [50, 51].

**Neotame E961**

Neotame, (3S)-3-(3,3-Dimethylbutylamino)-4-[[(2S)-1-methoxy-1-oxo-3-phenyl-propan-2-yl]amino]-4-oxobutanoic acid, is produced by adding a neo-hexyl group to the amine nitrogen of aspartame. Neotame is sweet, with a potency about 8000 times sucrose, but the taste quality of neotame limits its usefulness as a sole sweetener, and so it is used in combination with one or more other sweeteners, to reach a sweet taste. This compound does not provide any calory, it has a slight licorice-like cooling effect in the mouth, does not produce phenylalanine when metabolized it is considered safe to be used during pregnancy. Like aspartame, its stability is pH-dependent, with optimum stability at about pH 4.5. Its stability is also temperature-dependent, but it is sufficiently heat-stable to work in baking applications. Neotame was approved by the FDA in 2002 to be used in the United States. JECFA approved neotame in 2003. Nowadays, it is approved in Australia and New Zealand, and a number of countries in Europe and South America.

**Cyclamate E952**

Cyclamate, sodium N-cyclohexylsulfamate, is a sulfamic acid, usually used as the sodium or calcium salt, though it has a sweet taste sweet, at high concentrations its salty taste may be detectable. Cyclamate provides no calories and its free acid is scarcely soluble in water, and is slowly hydrolyzed in hot water, in fact, it is used such as calcium or sodium cyclamate. Cyclamate was eliminated from the United States market in 1969, consequentially to a study in which it was indicated that rats consuming large quantities of a cyclamate-saccharin blend developed bladder tumors. Now, present evidence indicates that cyclamate is not carcinogenic, but it is still banned in the United States, although the rest of the world has approved it. Relatively to other high potency sweeteners, cyclamate is not very potent, therefore it usually used in blends with one or more other sweeteners, to minimize the off-tastes of individual sweeteners.

## Sucralose E955

Sucralose, 1,6-Dichloro-1,6-dideoxy-β-D-fructofuranosyl-4-chloro-4-deoxy-α- D-galactopyranoside, is a sucrose molecule in which three of the -OH groups have been replaced by chlorine atoms. In the course of the chlorination, the stereochemistry results at position 4 of the glucose ring are inverted, so it becomes a derivative of galacto-sucrose. It is a non-nutritive sweetener. The body does not break down the majority of ingested sucralose, so it is non-caloric, and is efficiently used in baking applications. In the European Union, it is also known under the E number E955. Sucralose is about 320 to 1,000 times sweeter than sucrose, three times as sweet as aspartame and twice as sweet as saccharin. The story of sucralose is reported in an interesting document, the Sweetener Book" is written by D. Eric Walters [12]. Tate & Lyle, a British sugar company, aimed to to use sucrose as a chemical intermediate. In collaboration with Prof. Leslie Hough's laboratory at King's College in London, halogenated sugars were being synthesized and tested. A foreign graduate student, Shashikant Phadnis, misunderstood a request for "testing" of a chlorinated sugar as a request for "tasting" leading to the discovery that many chlorinated sugars are sweet with potencies of some hundreds or thousands of times as great as sucrose. The FDA, EFSA, and JECFA have approved the use of sucralose in the food industry.

## CONCLUDING REMARKS

Sweeteners represent a versatile category of food additives, whether using natural or synthetic ones. Most of the sweeteners showed a safe profile, when used as a food additive. It is possible to obtain the desired sweet effect associatedwith the merchandise of the final products. The reported side effects on the human health of the registered sweeteners are attributable to a no-reasonable and responsible consumption of sweetened drinks and foods.

## CONSENT FOR PUBLICATION

Not applicable.

## CONFLICT OF INTEREST

The authors declare that there are no conflicts of interest.

## ACKNOWLEDGEMENTS

The authors are grateful to the Foundation for Science and Technology (FCT, Portugal) for financial support to CIMO (UID/AGR/00690/2013) research centre.

# REFERENCES

[1]     Carocho M, Morales P, Ferreira ICFR. Natural food additives: Quo vadis? Trends Food Sci Technol 2015; 45(2): 284-95.
[http://dx.doi.org/10.1016/j.tifs.2015.06.007]

[2]     Saltmarsh M. Essential guide to food additives. 4th ed., Cambridge, UK: RSC Publishing 2013.
[http://dx.doi.org/10.1039/9781849734981]

[3]     Carocho M, Barreiro MF, Morales P. Ferreira ICFR. Adding molecules to Food, pros and cons: a review of synthetic and natural food additives. Compr Rev Food Sci Food Saf 2014; 13: 377-99.
[http://dx.doi.org/10.1111/1541-4337.12065]

[4]     Choudhary AK, Rathinasamy SD. Effect of long intake of aspartame on ionic imbalance in immune organs of immunized wistar albino rats. Biomed Pharmacother 2014; (4): 243-9.

[5]     von Poser Toigo E, Huffell AP, Mota CS, Bertolini D, Pettenuzzo LF, Dalmaz C. Metabolic and feeding behavior alterations provoked by prenatal exposure to aspartame. Appetite 2015; 87: 168-74.
[http://dx.doi.org/10.1016/j.appet.2014.12.213] [PMID: 25543075]

[6]     Mukherjee A, Chakrabarti J. In vivo cytogenetic studies on mice exposed to acesulfame-K--a non-nutritive sweetener. Food Chem Toxicol 1997; 35(12): 1177-9.
[http://dx.doi.org/10.1016/S0278-6915(97)85469-5] [PMID: 9449223]

[7]     Stohs SJ, Miller MJS. A case study involving allergic reactions to sulfur-containing compounds including, sulfite, taurine, acesulfame potassium and sulfonamides. Food Chem Toxicol 2014; 63(63): 240-3.
[http://dx.doi.org/10.1016/j.fct.2013.11.008] [PMID: 24262485]

[8]     Evert AB, Boucher JL, Cypress M, *et al.* American Diabetes Association. Nutrition therapy recommendations for the management of adults with diabetes. Diabetes Care 2013; 36(11): 3821-42.
[http://dx.doi.org/10.2337/dc13-2042] [PMID: 24107659]

[9]     Gardner C, Wylie-Rosett J, Gidding SS, *et al.* American Heart Association Nutrition Committee of the Council on Nutrition, Physical Activity and Metabolism, Council on Arteriosclerosis, Thrombosis and Vascular Biology, Council on Cardiovascular Disease in the Young; American Diabetes Association. Nonnutritive sweeteners: current use and health perspectives: a scientific statement from the American Heart Association and the American Diabetes Association. Diabetes Care 2012; 35(8): 1798-808.
[http://dx.doi.org/10.2337/dc12-9002] [PMID: 22778165]

[10]    Johnson RK, Appel LJ, Brands M, *et al.* American Heart Association Nutrition Committee of the Council on Nutrition, Physical Activity, and Metabolism and the Council on Epidemiology and Prevention. Dietary sugars intake and cardiovascular health: a scientific statement from the American Heart Association. Circulation 2009; 120(11): 1011-20.
[http://dx.doi.org/10.1161/CIRCULATIONAHA.109.192627] [PMID: 19704096]

[11]    U.S. Department of Health and Human Services and U.S. Department of Agriculture. 2015-2020 Dietary Guidelines for Americans 2015 December; health.gov/dietaryguidelines/2015/guidelines/

[12]    Eric Walters D. The Sweetener Book. Eric Walters 2013; Vol. D.

[13]    Hyvonen L, Koivistoinen P. Fructose in Food Systems.Nutritive Sweeteners. London, New Jersey: Applied Science Publishers 1982; pp. 133-44.

[14]    Elliott SS, Keim NL, Stern JS, Teff K, Havel PJ. Fructose, weight gain, and the insulin resistance syndrome. Am J Clin Nutr 2002; 76(5): 911-22.
[http://dx.doi.org/10.1093/ajcn/76.5.911] [PMID: 12399260]

[15]    Basciano H, Federico L, Adeli K. Fructose, insulin resistance, and metabolic dyslipidemia. Nutr Metab (Lond) 2005; 2(1): 5.
[http://dx.doi.org/10.1186/1743-7075-2-5] [PMID: 15723702]

[16]    Isganaitis E, Lustig RH. Fast food, central nervous system insulin resistance, and obesity. Arterioscler

Thromb Vasc Biol 2005; 25(12): 2451-62.
[http://dx.doi.org/10.1161/01.ATV.0000186208.06964.91] [PMID: 16166564]

[17]   Malik VS, Hu FB. Fructose and Cardiometabolic Health: What the Evidence From Sugar-Sweetened Beverages Tells Us. J Am Coll Cardiol 2015; 66(14): 1615-24.
[http://dx.doi.org/10.1016/j.jacc.2015.08.025] [PMID: 26429086]

[18]   Rippe JM, Angelopoulos TJ. Fructose-containing sugars and cardiovascular disease. Adv Nutr 2015; 6(4): 430-9.
[http://dx.doi.org/10.3945/an.114.008177] [PMID: 26178027]

[19]   Williams L. Carbohydrates and Health UK Scientific Advisory Committee on Nutrition, Public Health England. Norwich, UK: TSO 2015.

[20]   Aguilera AA, Díaz GH, Barcelata ML, Guerrero OA, Ros RM. Effects of fish oil on hypertension, plasma lipids, and tumor necrosis factor-alpha in rats with sucrose-induced metabolic syndrome. J Nutr Biochem 2004; 15(6): 350-7.
[http://dx.doi.org/10.1016/j.jnutbio.2003.12.008] [PMID: 15157941]

[21]   Fukuchi S, Hamaguchi K, Seike M, Himeno K, Sakata T, Yoshimatsu H. Role of fatty acid composition in the development of metabolic disorders in sucrose-induced obese rats. Exp Biol Med (Maywood) 2004; 229(6): 486-93.
[http://dx.doi.org/10.1177/153537020422900606] [PMID: 15169967]

[22]   Lombardo YB, Drago S, Chicco A, *et al.* Long-term administration of a sucrose-rich diet to normal rats: relationship between metabolic and hormonal profiles and morphological changes in the endocrine pancreas. Metabolism 1996; 45(12): 1527-32.
[http://dx.doi.org/10.1016/S0026-0495(96)90183-3] [PMID: 8969287]

[23]   Ten S, Maclaren N. Insulin resistance syndrome in children. J Clin Endocrinol Metab 2004; 89(6): 2526-39.
[http://dx.doi.org/10.1210/jc.2004-0276] [PMID: 15181020]

[24]   Frary CD, Johnson RK, Wang MQ. Children and adolescents' choices of foods and beverages high in added sugars are associated with intakes of key nutrients and food groups. J Adolesc Health 2004; 34(1): 56-63.
[http://dx.doi.org/10.1016/S1054-139X(03)00248-9] [PMID: 14706406]

[25]   Murphy MM, Douglass JS, Johnson RK, Spence LA. Drinking flavored or plain milk is positively associated with nutrient intake and is not associated with adverse effects on weight status in US children and adolescents. J Am Diet Assoc 2008; 108(4): 631-9.
[http://dx.doi.org/10.1016/j.jada.2008.01.004] [PMID: 18375219]

[26]   Linko P. Lactose and Lactitol.Birch, GG, Parker, KJ, Natural Sweeteners. London, New Jersey: Applied Science Publishers 1982; pp. 109-32.

[27]   Kočevar Glavač N, Kreft S. Excretion profile of glycyrrhizin metabolite in human urine. Food Chem 2012; 131: 305-8.
[http://dx.doi.org/10.1016/j.foodchem.2011.08.081]

[28]   Maguire A, Rugg-Gunn AJ. Xylitol and caries prevention--is it a magic bullet? Br Dent J 2003; 194(8): 429-36.
[http://dx.doi.org/10.1038/sj.bdj.4810022] [PMID: 12778091]

[29]   Suda R, Suzuki T, Takiguchi R, Egawa K, Sano T, Hasegawa K. The effect of adding calcium lactate to xylitol chewing gum on remineralization of enamel lesions. Caries Res 2006; 40(1): 43-6.
[http://dx.doi.org/10.1159/000088905] [PMID: 16352880]

[30]   Godshall MA. The Expanding World of Nutritive and Non-Nutritive Sweeteners. Sugar J 2007; (69): 12-20.

[31]   Chattopadhyay S, Raychaudhuri U, Chakraborty R. Artificial sweeteners - a review. J Food Sci Technol 2014; 51(4): 611-21.

[http://dx.doi.org/10.1007/s13197-011-0571-1] [PMID: 24741154]

[32] Olivier B, Serge AH, Catherine A, *et al.* Review of the nutritional benefits and risks related to intense sweeteners. Arch Public Health 2015; 73: 41.
[http://dx.doi.org/10.1186/s13690-015-0092-x] [PMID: 26430511]

[33] VKM. Risk assessments of cyclamate, saccharin, neohesperidine DC, steviol glycosides and neotame from soft drinks, "saft" and nectar Opinion of the Panel on Food Additives, Flavorings, Processing Aids, Materials in Contact with Foods and Cosmetics of the Norvegian Scientific Committee for Food Safety 2014. Doc.no. 13-406-2_endeling

[34] ANSES. Evaluation des bénéfices et des risques nutritionnels des édulcorants intenses.Avis de l'Anses et rapport d'expertise collective. 2015.

[35] WIV-ISP. Studie van de tafelzoetstoffen en de schatting van de totale inname van geselecteerde zoetstoffen door de volwassen Belgische bevolking. Brussel, Belgium: Wetenschappelijk Instituut Volksgezondheid 2010.

[36] Arushi J, Mathur P. Estimation of Food Additive Intake-Overview of the Methodology. Food Rev Int 2015; 31(4): 355-84.
[http://dx.doi.org/10.1080/87559129.2015.1022830]

[37] Singhal P, Mathur P. Availability and consumption pattern of artificial sweeteners among diabetics, overweight individuals and college girls in Delhi. Ind. J Nutr Diet 2008; (45): 26-33.

[38] Husøy T, Mangschou B, Fotland TO, *et al.* Reducing added sugar intake in Norway by replacing sugar sweetened beverages with beverages containing intense sweeteners - a risk benefit assessment. Food Chem Toxicol 2008; 46(9): 3099-105.
[http://dx.doi.org/10.1016/j.fct.2008.06.013] [PMID: 18639604]

[39] Tripathi M, Khanna SK, Das M. Usage of saccharin in food products and its intake by the population of Lucknow, India. Food Addit Contam 2006; 23(12): 1265-75.
[http://dx.doi.org/10.1080/02652030600944395] [PMID: 17118869]

[40] Clauss K, Jensen H. Oxathiazinone Dioxides--A New Group of Sweetening Agents. Angew Chem. Internat lth Ed. Engl. 1973; 12: pp. 869-76.

[41] Uçar A, Yilmaz S. Saccharin Genotoxicity And Carcinogenicity: A Review. AFS 2015; 37(3): 138-42.

[42] Appleton KM, Blundell JE. Habitual high and low consumers of artificially-sweetened beverages: effects of sweet taste and energy on short-term appetite. Physiol Behav 2007; 92(3): 479-86.
[http://dx.doi.org/10.1016/j.physbeh.2007.04.027] [PMID: 17540414]

[43] Blundell JE, Green SM. Effect of sucrose and sweeteners on appetite and energy intake. Int J Obes Relat Metab Disord 1996; 20 (Suppl. 2): S12-7.
[PMID: 8646266]

[44] Lavin JH, French SJ, Read NW. The effect of sucrose- and aspartame-sweetened drinks on energy intake, hunger and food choice of female, moderately restrained eaters. Int J Obes Relat Metab Disord 1997; 21(1): 37-42.
[http://dx.doi.org/10.1038/sj.ijo.0800360] [PMID: 9023599]

[45] Swithers SE, Davidson TL. A role for sweet taste: calorie predictive relations in energy regulation by rats. Behav Neurosci 2008; 122(1): 161-73.
[http://dx.doi.org/10.1037/0735-7044.122.1.161] [PMID: 18298259]

[46] Howe GR, Burch JD, Miller AB, *et al.* Artificial sweeteners and human bladder cancer. Lancet 1977; 2(8038): 578-81.
[http://dx.doi.org/10.1016/S0140-6736(77)91428-3] [PMID: 71398]

[47] Bravo MP, Del Rey-Calero J, Conde M. Risk factors of bladder cancer in Spain. Neoplasma 1987; 34(5): 633-7.
[PMID: 3696304]

[48]   Sturgeon SR, Hartge P, Silverman DT, *et al.* Associations between bladder cancer risk factors and tumor stage and grade at diagnosis. Epidemiology 1994; 5(2): 218-25.
[http://dx.doi.org/10.1097/00001648-199403000-00012] [PMID: 8172997]

[49]   Andreatta MM, Muñoz SE, Lantieri MJ, Eynard AR, Navarro A. Artificial sweetener consumption and urinary tract tumors in Cordoba, Argentina. Prev Med 2008; 47(1): 136-9.
[http://dx.doi.org/10.1016/j.ypmed.2008.03.015] [PMID: 18495230]

[50]   Hoover RN, Strasser PH. Artificial sweeteners and human bladder cancer. Preliminary results. Lancet 1980; 1(8173): 837-40.
[http://dx.doi.org/10.1016/S0140-6736(80)91350-1] [PMID: 6103207]

[51]   Walker AM, Dreyer NA, Friedlander E, Loughlin J, Rothman KJ, Kohn HI. An independent analysis of the National Cancer Institute study on non-nutritive sweeteners and bladder cancer. Am J Public Health 1982; 72(4): 376-81.
[http://dx.doi.org/10.2105/AJPH.72.4.376] [PMID: 7065315]

# CHAPTER 11

# Emulsifiers

**Devasahayam Jaya Balan** and **Kasi Pandima Devi**[*]

*Department of Biotechnology, Alagappa University, Karaikudi 630 003, Tamil Nadu, India*

**Abstract:** Emulsifiers are high molecular weight surface-active agents that facilitate the formation and stabilization of emulsions. They are used in food products to obtain uniform quality with improved texture and long shelf life. They are commonly found in packaged and prepared foods, such as baked goods, soft drinks, candies, gums, whipped creams, biscuits, breads, ice creams and margarines. Emulsifiers, in food products, allow uniform blending by reducing the interfacial tension between different phases like water, oil and gases. Their wide applications have established the presence of emulsifiers in nearly all food products and have also advanced the food processing techniques. However, the stability of emulsifiers can be affected by the salt content and pH variations in food emulsions. Emulsifiers, produced by biological systems, such as microorganisms and yeast, are called bio-emulsifiers which are also used in various food products. The synthetic emulsifiers pass through the body without being metabolized, whereas naturally occurring molecules are metabolized in the body. Worldwide, about 500,000 metric tons of emulsifiers are produced and sold. The legislation on emulsifiers governs their safety assessment, authorisation, use and labelling. The food legislation community aims to establish the right balance between the risks and benefits of substances that are used intentionally and to reduce the contaminants in accordance with consumer protection. In the food industry, many emulsifiers are used without any evidence of harmful effects that were confirmed by various safety analyses. The current review focuses on the food emulsifiers which play an indispensable role in the production of food products with the highest quality.

**Keywords:** Bio-emulsifiers, Emulsifiers, Food additives, Health effects, Legislation.

## INTRODUCTION

Emulsifiers are ingredients that facilitate the formation and stabilization of emulsions. In general, the mixing of water and oil causes the dispersion of oil droplets in water, but it starts to separate when the shaking stops. However, the surface-active agents like emulsifiers, which consist of a "water-loving" hydroph-

---

[*] **Corresponding author Kasi Pandima Devi:** Department of Biotechnology, Alagappa University, Karaikudi 630 003, Tamil Nadu, India; E-mail: devikasi@yahoo.com

**Seyed Mohammad Nabavi** *et al.* **(Eds.)**

ilic head and an "oil-loving" hydrophobic tail, make the droplets remain dispersed and lead to the formation of a stable emulsion [1]. The emulsifiers provide different benefits to food which include acting as lubricants, emulsifying oil or fat in butters, building structure, aerating, improving eating quality, extending shelf life, modifying crystallization, preventing sticking and retaining moisture [2]. They are one of the important ingredients in packaged and prepared food, such as baked goods, soft drinks, candies, gums, whipped creams, biscuits, breads, ice creams and margarines.

Emulsifiers can be natural and synthetically produced. Natural emulsifiers are produced by biological systems, such as plant or animal tissue. For instance, the surface-active compounds (SACs) produced by microorganisms are amphiphilic metabolites containing both hydrophobic and hydrophilic moieties and are known as bio-emulsifiers. Whereas, the synthetic ones are manufactured by industries [3]. Based on the molecular weight, the SACs are classified into two main groups, low molecular weight and high molecular weight SACs. The primary activity of the low molecular weight molecules, which are called as biosurfactants, is to cause a reduction in the surface tension. The molecular weight of the biosurfactants ranges from 500 to 1500 Da [4]. Whereas, the high molecular weight SACs, which are called bioemulsifiers, are amphiphilic biomolecules produced by a wide range of microorganisms, such as bacteria [5, 6] yeasts [7] and filamentous fungi [8]. The composition of bioemulsifiers includes heteropolysaccharides, lipopolysaccharides, lipoproteins and proteins [9, 10]. Emulsifiers play a role in the formation and stabilization of emulsions and do not have any effect on surface tension, whereas the surfactants are mainly involved in the reduction of surface tension. The major characteristic features of bioemulsifiers are non-toxicity, biodegradability, bio-compatibility, efficiency at low concentrations and their synthesis from natural substrates. The protein and polysaccharide composition of the bioemulsifiers is mainly involved in the emulsifying activity. The hydrophobic amino acid which is present in the protein of bioemulsifiers reversibly binds with hydrocarbons and the polysaccharides covalently attach to the protein to stabilize the emulsion [11, 12].

The emulsification activities of bioemulsifiers with different hydrocarbons are identified through the emulsification index test [13]. The identification of emulsifiers producing microorganisms can be identified by the bacterial adhesion to hydrocarbon assay (BATH). If low surface hydrophobicity is exhibited by any microorganism, it indicates the extracellular release of emulsifying agents in the production media, which can be determined by bacterial adhesion to hydrocarbon assay. Irrespective of the source, both synthetic and natural emulsifiers allow the formation of partition at the interface between fluid phases with varied polarity and play a vital role in maintaining the quality of food products. They are used to keep the food fresh, increase the shelf life, and improve the texture and other qualities of food products.

## TYPES OF FOOD EMULSIFIERS

Food is a complex colloidal system that needs surface-active lipids like emulsifiers to attain uniform quality with improved texture and long shelf life. Various types of emulsifiers are used in the food industry. These are discussed below.

### Mono and Diglycerides

Mono and diglycerides are fatty acids that are used as emulsifiers in food products to combine ingredients, such as fat and water. Usually, glycerides consist of a glycerol molecule and one or more fatty acid chains. Here, as the name implies, the monoglycerides contain one fatty acid and diglycerides contain two fatty acids [14]. The mono and diglyceride emulsifiers were first used in the 1930s for margarine production. The inter-esterification of edible fats with glycerol results in the production of monoglycerides. This reaction occurs at high temperature (200-260°C) and under alkaline conditions [15]. This process is called glycerolysis, by which the production of mono and diglycerides takes place. It also occurs naturally in various seed oils. Mono and diglycerides are commonly found in packaged and prepared foods, such as baked goods, soft drinks, candies, gums, whipped creams, ice creams and margarines.

### Di-Acetyltartaric Esters of Monoglycerides (DATEM)

Diacetyl tartaric acid ester of mono- and diglyceride (DATEM) is a food emulsifier used in making biscuits, breads, coffee whiteners, ice creams, and salad dressings. It forms a strong gluten network in the dough to make bakery products with good quality [16]. It is used to make breads with a crusty, springy and chewy texture. It is produced by a chemical reaction in the presence of tartaric acid in which mono and di-glycerides react with acetic anhydride in order to produce DATEM [17].

### Polyglycerol Esters

Polyglycerol esters are synthetic and non-ionic surfactants. They are produced by the addition of esters to the hydroxy groups of polyglycerol. Polyglycerol results from alkaline-catalyzed random polymerization of glycerol [18]. Due to its amphiphilic properties, it is used in food, pharmaceutical, and cosmetic industries. In food, it is used as an emulsifying agent in the production of baked goods, chewing gums and in place of fats [19]. The bakery products which are produced with the ingredients, oil, water and flour, are not soluble in each other. Some interfaces hinder the solubility of water, oil, gases (air bubbles), solid substances (flour components), air and water. Whereas, polyglycerol esters allow uniform blending by reducing the interfacial tension among different phases [20].

## Lactylates

Lactylate esters include sodium stearoyl-2-lactylate (SSL), calcium stearoyl-2-lactylate (CSL) [2] and lactylic esters of fatty acids. SSL has various applications in the food industry including its applications in diversified food products, such as cakes, biscuits, chocolates, meats, gravies and pet foods. It improves the volume of processed foods and is approved by the FDA due to its non-toxicity and biodegradability [21 - 23]. Stearic acid esterification with lactic acid followed by sodium carbonate neutralization is the manufacturing procedure for SSL. CSL is also a commercially available and an FDA approved food additive. It is used in yeast-leavened bakery products. Stearic acid esterification with lactic acid, followed by calcium hydroxide neutralization, is the manufacturing procedure for CSL [24]. Though CSL is also available in the market, SSL is mainly used in many applications. This is because of the more significant crumb softening effects of SSL used in the bakery products.

## Sucrose Esters

Sucrose esters are used as food emulsifiers in almost all food products, including bakery, confectionery, cereals, dairy, ice creams and sauces [25]. They are emulsifiers with some unique characteristics, such as they boost other emulsifiers to improve the air bubble structure, prevent protein browning, early starch staling and fat bloom in chocolate, speed up crystallization in fine-grained confectioners' sugar and improve the texture and flavor of ice cream [26]. Apart from their application as an emulsifier, they have other notable applications, such as starch interaction, protein protection, sugar crystallization and aeration. These wide applications show the presence of sucrose esters in nearly all the food products. The sucrose esters are manufactured by the process of esterification of sucrose with fatty acids [14].

## Propylene Glycol Fatty Acid Esters

Normally, fats consist of glycerol and fatty acids, whereas in Propylene Glycol Fatty Acid Esters (PGFAE), glycerol is replaced by propanediol. The fats can be taken from plant or animal origin for the production of PGFAE [14]. PGFAE is a lipophilic, oil-soluble emulsifier with some specific crystalline properties. Apart from the industrial food applications, PGFAE is also used in many cosmetic products, including creams and lotions. The specific crystalline property of PGFAE is beneficial in many aerated products, such as non-dairy desserts, whipping creams, powdered toppings and cake emulsifiers [27].

## Lecithins

The emulsifiers with the composition of phospholipids and phosphatidylcholine are known as lecithins which are used as food emulsifiers. The sources of lecithins are soybeans, rapeseeds, sunflower seeds, egg yolk, milk and brain tissue [28]. Lecithin is a molecule with a hydrophilic and a hydrophobic end. This emulsifier is very well suited to be used in very thin or liquid emulsions where other emulsifiers fail [29]. Lecithin emulsifier is suited to water in oil or oil in water emulsions depending upon temperature and ratio. One of the characteristics of lecithin is its suitability to both oil and water, thus making it a choice for a variety of emulsion applications. It is valued due to the fact that it can be completely metabolized by the body and it has an excellent non-toxic profile. Lecithins are obtained by the extraction and purification of phospholipids from naturally occurring products, such as soybeans, eggs, sunflower and canola seeds [30]. Lecithins make the chocolate and powdered baby formula smooth since it dissolves easily in water. Cooking spray is a spray form of oil in which lecithin is used to avoid the sticking of food in frying pans [14].

## PHYSICOCHEMICAL PROPERTIES OF EMULSIFIERS

Understanding the physicochemical properties of emulsifiers, such as colour, shape, odour, mass, boiling point, density, viscosity, solubility, stability and solid-state properties, is essential so that the emulsification process can be rational and streamlined. By integrating this knowledge, one can make decisions regarding emulsifier usage in food products. Emulsifiers with standard physiochemical properties exhibit good performance in food production. This knowledge also provides valuable insight into the manufacturing of emulsifiers (Table **1**).

## ORIGIN OF EMULSIFIERS

Initially, emulsifiers were naturally originated, and they were developed with advances in food processing techniques. For example, the solid fat is dispersed into the aqueous phase by the influence of milk. Hence, milk is traditionally being used as a natural emulsifier and major food formulation to make butter, cheese, whipped cream and ice cream [2]. In France, egg lipoproteins and phospholipids are utilized to disperse oil into an acidified aqueous phase. These lipoproteins have a standard emulsifying property which causes up to 80% oil dispersion. Margarine is a low-cost substitute for butter invented by the French chemist, Hippolyte Mege-Mouries, in 1889. The stability of emulsion in food must be taken into account for long time storage and consumption. During the second half of the twentieth century, people started to use synthetic emulsifiers for commercial usage [31]. The processed food industries started to use synthetic emulsifiers to maintain the stability of the products for distribution through mass-market channels. The stability could be affected by the salt content and pH variations in food emulsions. Depending on the manufacturers, the composition of the natural or commercial emulsifiers varies. Surface active particles and processing conditions can alter the characteristics of the emulsions [1].

The formulation of food emulsions has become an art because of the complex relationship with surface-active agents, composition, and processing conditions, among others. The analytical instruments, such as electron microscopy, nuclear magnetic resonance and chromatography/mass spectrometry, were employed to find the scientific dimension of the emulsifiers [32]. Food emulsifiers play an indispensable role in the production of bakery products. Worldwide, about 500,000 metric tons of emulsifiers are produced and sold. The emulsifiers sales in the European Union and the United States are about 200–300 million EUR and 225–275 million USD, respectively. However, the trade of emulsifiers is low or yet to be developed globally [33]. In the near future, the necessity of food emulsifiers for making high-quality bakery products will increase their global trade.

## USES OF EMULSIFIERS AS FOOD ADDITIVES

Emulsifiers play a prominent role in the production of food products with high quality. Their major functions in the production of bakery products are ingredients emulsification, properties of shortening enhancement, interaction with the components of flour and other ingredients in the mix, creaming, conditioning the dough and crumb softening [1].

## Halva Preparation

Halva is a sweetened sesame paste and a familiar sweet food in northern Africa, southern Europe and the Middle East [34, 35]. It is prepared by adding the composition of sesame paste, that is obtained by grinding roasted sesame seeds, to sugar syrup and citric acid. To satisfy consumer preferences, flavouring agents, almond or pistachio nuts, chocolate and dehydrated fruits can also be added. A major problem in making halva is the release of some quantity of sesame oil from the food matrix to the surface, which affects the stability of the product during storage. This causes the halva to toughen, thus reducing their marketability and contaminating the packaging [36]. The surface-active agents like emulsifiers can form and stabilize the emulsion in oil-rich foods [37]. Commercial emulsifiers, such as lecithins and monoglycerides, reduce the oil exudation in halva by stabilizing the oil holding fibers [38, 39]. Monoglycerides (MGs), emulsifiers with two free hydroxyl groups produced by the chemical hydrolysis of triacylglycerols, are used for the industrial production of food [40, 41]. They exhibit stronger surface activity than diglycerides [37]. Halva oil retention can be improved by increasing the concentration of the emulsifier. This will increase the viscosity of the oil phase and homogenous dispersion of the oil droplets and water phase. The concentration of monoglycerides can be increased up to 2.25% to get the optimum oil retention capacity in halva without causing any change in the texture and colour of the product.

## Cheese Making

Sodium aluminium phosphates (SALPs) are FDA-approved food additives generally recognized as safe (GRAS) that provide a high amount of oral aluminium (Al) to the diet [42, 43]. To process the cheese, emulsifying salts are needed to be added. SALP is one of the emulsifying salts which are used in cheese processing. The protein which is present in cheese reacts with SALP and produces a smooth, uniform film around each fat droplet. This withholds the fat and prevents the bleeding of fat from the cheese. The soft texture, easy melting characteristics and desirable slicing properties are the advantages of using basic SALP as an emulsifying salt [44]. Basic SALP has been permitted up to 3% by the FDA (Food and Drugs Administration) in the pasteurization process of cheese [45].

## Cake Baking

Cakes are a baked food with the following major ingredients: eggs, wheat flour, sugar and fat. Of these ingredients, egg, is an important source of cholesterol but it is expensive [46]. However, eggs play a vital role in baking, such as in emulsification, coagulation, foaming and flavour enhancement [47, 48]. This makes it difficult to reduce the usage of eggs in cake production [46]. The applications of emulsifiers in the baking process can significantly reduce or substitute the use of eggs in cake production since they provide the necessary aeration and gas bubble stability [49]. The quality of cakes is shown by the high volume, uniform crumb structure, tenderness, shelf life and tolerance to staling which can be achieved by using different types of emulsifiers [50]. A mixture of polar lipids called lecithin is extracted from crude vegetable oils which can be used as an emulsifier to provide enhanced aeration in cake production [51 - 53]. Researchers have confirmed that a combination of lecithin emulsifiers with soy milk can make a completely eggless cake.

### Gluten-free Cookies Preparation

The patients who have serious autoimmune disorders, such as *Celiac disease,* are highly allergic to protein gluten. The intake of gluten-containing foods causes severe damage to the small intestine [54]. Due to the prevalence of *celiac disease*, the interest in gluten-free (GF) products is increasing. Cookies are one of the favourite snacks, the major composition of which is wheat flour. However, the *Celiac disease* patients are allergic to gluten-rich wheat flour. Many non-wheat flours are used to make gluten-free cookies which possess baked and sensory characteristics [55]. Rice flour cookies with emulsifiers, such as glycerol monostearate (GMS), SSL and lecithin, were tested for improved characteristics. Among these, the emulsifier GMS significantly improved the textural characteristics of the cookie dough with rice flour, as shown by the decrease in the hardness, adhesiveness, gumminess and increase in the cohesiveness and springiness similar to gluten proteins [56]. Moreover, the emulsifiers in the production of cookies decrease the redness of the cookies with whey protein concentrate (WPC). The crumb color from yellowish-white to creamish white, and from medium-size islands to slightly bigger islands were also significantly improved by the addition of GMS. Among different emulsifiers tried, GMS brought about significant improvement in crust color, island formation, texture, mouthfeel and overall quality. With respect to the quality of the wheat flour cookies, the acceptable quality could be exhibited by GF cookies without any allergic symptoms to the people with gluten allergy [57].

### Rice Products

Rice is a staple food in Asia. It is a desirable grain because of its unique functional properties, such as flavor carrying capability, hypoallergenicity and bland flavor [58]. The quality of extrudate rice or broken rice cooked foods can be improved by the addition of some additives [59]. The extrusion-cooked instant rice was prepared by optimizing the formulation with thickeners and emulsifiers, such as GMS, soybean lecithin (LC) and SSL. The addition of these emulsifiers improves the texture, reduces adhesiveness and retains the extrudate's final shape after hydration [60]. In combination with emulsifiers, thickeners can also be used to improve the quality of the extruded instant rice. The unique physicochemical properties, acceptable texture and rehydration properties can be provided by the combination of emulsifiers and thickeners. The emulsifiers are thus effectively used to enhance the economic value of broken rice [61].

## LEGISLATION ON FOOD EMULSIFIERS

Emulsifiers are one of the important food additives which play a vital role in food production and distribution. Emulsifiers prolong the shelf life of foods, colours and flavourings which may make the food more attractive. Food additives are substances that are not normally consumed as a food in itself or as a characteristic ingredient of food, whether or not it has nutritive value. The intentional addition of food additives to food for a technological purpose in the manufacture, processing, preparation, treatment, packaging, transport or storage of such food results or may be reasonably expected to result in it or its by-products, becoming directly or indirectly a component of such foods. There are two types of emulsifiers used in food production, natural or synthetic emulsifiers, which have very similar structures to natural products. Like other food additives, emulsifiers are subject to stringent EU legislation governing their safety assessment, authorisation, use and labelling. These legislations require all the added emulsifiers to be declared on food packaging with either their name or E-number Table **2**. The legislation is the procedure to authorise the use of this additive in particular foods. An emulsifier can be legislated after the evaluation for their safety. Moreover, these emulsifiers remain under continuous evaluation during their use in order to remain approved [2]. The legislation on food additives states that only additives that are explicitly authorised may be used, often in limited quantities, in specific foodstuffs. The food legislation community aims to establish the right balance between risks and benefits of substances that are used intentionally and to reduce the contaminants in accordance with consumer protection that is required in Article 152 of the Treaty established by the European Community. The usage of emulsifiers is under some legislation rules. The emulsifier can be used after the approval of the legislation committee which determines the dosages specified for each application based on the safety evaluation report [62]. The emulsifiers at European level are under regulation (EC) No 1333/2008 on food additives other than colours and sweeteners and subsequent amendments. European Commission (EC) has developed a regulatory measure related to food additive safety on scientific basis. All the scientific assessments linked to the safety of food emulsifiers are provided by the European Food Safety Authority's (EFSA) scientific panel on Additives and Nutrient Sources (ANS). The authorized food emulsifiers must fulfil the purity criteria specifications. In 2011, the European Union adopted Regulation No 1169 on the provision of food information to the consumer which sets out all the EU labelling rules in one piece of legislation [63].

## MAXIMUM USAGE LEVEL OF FOOD EMULSIFIERS

The maximum usage level of emulsifiers is strictly regulated based on the toxicological reports. A concentration above the maximum limit causes undesirable health effects. Depending on the type of food emulsifiers, their usage level varies Table **3**.

**Table 1. Physicochemical Properties of food emulsifiers.**

| S.NO | Types of emulsifier | Physicochemical Properties | | | | |
|------|---------------------|-----------------------------|------------|--------|----------------------|-----------|
| | | Solubility | Appearance | Source | Melting temperature | Reference |
| 1 | Mono and diglycerides | oil | White coloured waxy | Animal fats or vegetable oils, glycerin | 105°C | [1, 14] |
| 2 | Di-Acetyltartaric Esters Of Monoglycerides (DATEM) | Methanol/ ethanol/acetone | Cream white fluid powder | soybean oil | 45 - 50 °C | [1, 17] |
| 3 | Polyglycerol Esters | water or oil | white and odorless powder | Cotton seed oil, castor oil | 58 °C | [2, 19] |
| 4 | Calcium stearoyl--lactylate (CSL) | hot water | Cream colored non-hygroscopic powder | Whole Foods | 45 °C | [2] |
| 5 | Sodium stearoyl-2-lactylate (SSL) | Ethanol | White or cream-colored powder with a caramel odor | Biorenewable feedstocks | 49 °C | [2] |
| 6 | Sucrose Esters | Water | White to yellow-brown powdery | Beet and cane | 40°C and 60°C | [14, 25] |
| 7 | Propylene Glycol Fatty Acid Esters | oil | Yellowish white beads | Vegetable oil | <100°C | [27, 70] |
| 8 | Lecithins | Water / oil | Amber Viscous Liquid | Soy, sunflower oil | 236 °C | [29] |

Table 2. Legislation E Number for food emulsifiers.

| Sl.NO | Type of emulsifier | E- Number |
|---|---|---|
| 1 | Mono and diglycerides | E471 |
| 2 | Di-Acetyltartaric Esters Of Monoglycerides (DATEM) | E472 |
| 3 | Polyglycerol Esters | E475 |
| 4 | Calcium stearoyl-2-lactylate | E482 |
| 5 | Sodium stearoyl-2-lactylate | E 481 |
| 6 | Sucrose Esters | E473 |
| 7 | Propylene Glycol Fatty Acid Esters | E477 |
| 8 | Lecithins | E322 |

Table 3. Maximum usage levels of food emulsifiers.

| S.No | Type of emulsifier | Maximum usage level per kg of body weight |
|---|---|---|
| 1 | Mono and diglycerides | 0.25 mg/kg bw/day |
| 2 | Di-Acetyltartaric Esters Of Monoglycerides (DATEM) | 30 mg/kg bw/day |
| 3 | Polyglycerol Esters | 14.2 mg/kg bw/day |
| 4 | Lactylates | 22.1 mg/kg bw/day |
| 5 | Sucrose Esters | 40 mg/kg bw/day |
| 6 | Propylene Glycol Fatty Acid Esters | 25 mg/kg bw/day |
| 7 | Lecithins | 450 mg/kg bw/day |

## REPORTS ON TOXICOLOGICAL DATA OF FOOD EMULSIFIERS AND THEIR ADVERSE HEALTH EFFECTS

In the food industry, many synthetic emulsifiers are used without any evidence of harmful effects. The synthetic emulsifiers are chemically modified fats and oils [64]. They can be designed on the basis of naturally occurring molecules or non-naturally occurring molecules. The non-naturally occurring molecules developed as synthetic emulsifiers pass through the body without being metabolized [65], whereas the naturally occurring molecules are metabolized in the body.

At practicable dosage levels, monoglycerides and diglycerides do not exhibit any `toxic effects. Five male hamsters treated with the emulsifier glyceryl monostearate at a level ranging from 5 to 15% for 28 weeks showed enlarged livers without any significant histopathological changes, with normal reproductive performance and lactation [66]. In our body, the digestion of meal containing fat, such as triglycerides, results in the generation of monoglycerides and diglycerides. This confirmed that monoglycerides and diglycerides are not associated with any harmful effects [67].

Lipases hydrolyse the mono- and di-glycerides into glycerol and fatty acids in the gastrointestinal tract. Toxicological studies on mono- and di-glycerides do not show any evidence of adverse effects. No reports have been observed on mono- and di-glycerides and on their potential to initiate or promote carcinogenicity. This was confirmed after various studies, such as sub-chronic studies, chronic, reproductive and developmental toxicity studies [68]. *In vitro* experiments on lipase digestion of polyglycerol esters showed a slower rate of digestion than that of olive oil. The digestibility was calculated to be 92 per cent. Rats fed with polyglycerol ester for 54 days as 9% of the diet showed no difference in the composition of carcass fat, liver fat, free fatty acids and phosphorus when compared with the groups fed with 1 or 10% ground-nut oil in the diet [69]. The polyglycerol ester was shown to be absorbed by intestinal lymphatics and the chylomicron counts showed normal lipaemia. Rats given single doses of 7, 14 and 29 g/kg body weight of polyglycerol ester by incubation also showed no signs of any toxic effect. Metabolic studies highlight the hydrolysis of these polyglycerol esters in the gastrointestinal tract and the utilization and digestibility studies justify the assumption that the fatty acid moiety is metabolized in a normal manner [70]. Analytical studies have produced no evidence of the accumulation of polyglycerol moiety in the body tissues. No adverse effects were identified during the safety assessment of polyglycerol esters in Colworth Wistar rats which were fed with polyglycerol ester (2,500 mg/kg bwt per day) for two years. 5% groundnut oil was used as a control. The results showed no side effects or changes in body weight, food consumption, haematological parameters, and survival rate. This confirmed the non toxicity of polyglycerol esters [71].

The emulsifier, DATEM, has the digestibility coefficient of >90%. It is digested into mono- and diglycerides and acetylated tartaric acid, accelerated by pancreatic lipase in the gastrointestinal tract [72]. The formed mono and diglycerides are subjected to natural digestion and absorption processes as they are a natural dietary constituent. DATEM, with a concentration of 10%, was exposed to rats for long and short term studies. Long-term exposure caused depletion in food consumption and body weight loss, hereas short-term exposure did not show any significant effect in both the sexes. It has been reported that DATEM is digested into acetic and tartaric acids [73].

The evaluation of the emulsifier, lactylate, for its safety to be used as a food additive showed its non-toxic nature leading to FDA approval in April 1961 [74]. An *in vitro* study showed that lactylates are broken down into stearic acid and lactic acid by the action of lipase. The efficiency of excretion was studied by feeding rats with [14]C labelled calcium stearoyl-2-lactylate. The results confirmed the 60% of excretion within the time period of 24 hours [75]. Two percent of lactylates consumption in rats did not show any observable side effects. However, at high concentration, it showed growth retardation and caused an increase in liver weight. However, when the lactylates-tested rats were brought back to normal diet, it caused recovery in the normal growth. The rats subjected to 0-5% of sodium stearoyl-2-lactylate treatment showed that 0-5% levels were tolerated by rats without causing any significant adverse effects [76]. Sucrose fatty acid ester primarily consists of monoesters with lesser amounts of diesters and triesters. The intestinal cells completely hydrolyse the monoesters prior to absorption, however, the higher esters are not hydrolyzed completely and thus are not absorbed and are excreted in the faeces [77]. The toxicological studies conducted on human showed that physiological effects, such as soft stools, were observed when these esters were administered at doses of 2 grams or greater per day. Sucrose fatty acid esters were subjected to Ames assay and chromosome aberration assay. No mutagenic effects or chromosomal aberrations were observed following exposure to up to 5.0 mg/plate and 0.036 mg/mL, respectively [78].

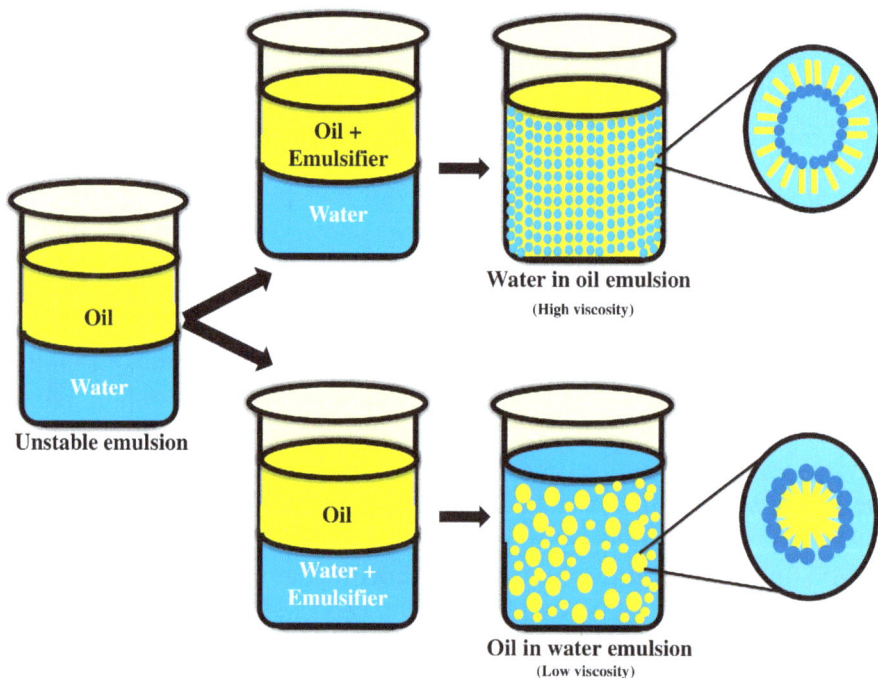

**Fig. (1).** Emulsification of water and oil.

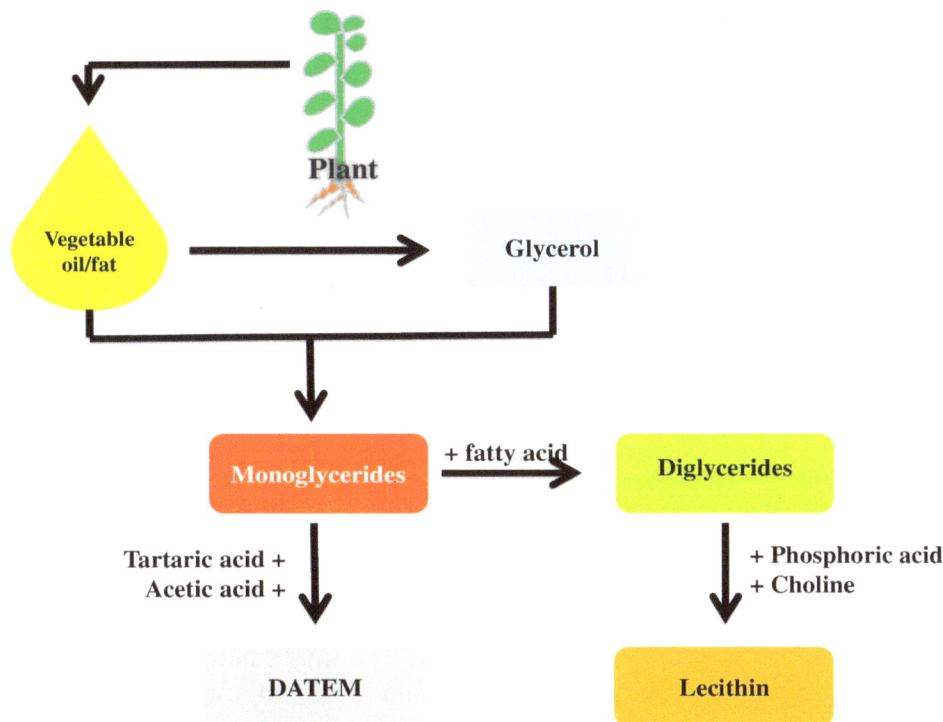

**Fig. (2).** Production of emulsifiers.

Both male and female Wistar rats were fed with 0-5% of sodium stearoyl lactylate (SSL) for one year. The long term treatment results did not show any adverse effects which were confirmed by the absence of toxicity [79]. The administration of various dietary concentrations of DAG (diacylglycerol) and TG (triacylglycerol used as a control for comparison), such as 0% DAG/9.5% TG, 1.5% DAG/8.0% TG, 5.5% DAG/4.0% TG, and 9.5% DAG/0% TG, daily for a week revealed that the clinical parameters and the animal's body weight, food consumption, hematology and urinalysis were unaffected [80]. However, excessive consumption of food additives leads to the incidence of autoimmune diseases. Generally, the intercellular tight junction in the intestinal epithelial barrier maintains the equilibrium between tolerance and immunity to non-self-antigens. The dysfunction of the tight junction leads to autoimmune diseases. The increased food additive consumption causes autoimmune diseases by the destabilization of tight junctions and, therefore, intestinal leakage [81].

Propylene glycol esters are normally present in the body. Hence, they are metabolised in the normal way. In sensitive individuals, it can cause eczema at high concentrations. It was evidenced that the propylene glycol esters of fatty acids are hydrolyzed to propylene and fatty acids [82]. More than 70% of propylene glycol monostearate are hydrolysed by pancreatic lipase under *in vitro* conditions at 40 °C in 15 hours [83]. Likewise, steapsin hydrolyses 70 percent of propylene glycol di-stearate (PGDS) *in vitro* at 30 °C in 18 hours. By using isotopically labelled compounds, the absorption, metabolism and hydrolysis of PGDS were studied in rats which was found to be non-toxic in nature [82].

## REPORTS ON POSITIVE HEALTH EFFECTS OF FOOD EMULSIFIERS

Generally, the oil and fat get separated in low fat spreads and causes the formation of moulds. However, the use of emulsifiers prevents mould formation by producing oil and fat emulsion. In our body, mono- and diglycerides are easily absorbed by the intestinal cells and hydrolysed into triglycerides. Triglycerides play an important role in heart's health [84]. In order to reduce calorie consumption, polyglycerol esters have been used to replace fats. The polyglycerol esters were known to resist the digestive enzyme hydrolysis, leading to reduced calorie consumption to avoid obesity [85, 86].

Lecithin, which is a fatty substance, forms the hydrophobic walls of cell membranes in all the cells in nature. Lecithin helps to transport fat-soluble essential nutrients, such as vitamins A, D, E and K, all over the body and plays an important role in brain function. Lecithin is a medically effective emulsifier that helps to treat many diseases, such as multiple sclerosis, bipolar disorder and Alzheimer's diseases [87]. Traditionally, lecithin is used to reduce high cholesterol level and prevents the accumulation of fats or lipids in arterial walls. This helps in preventing the risk of cardiovascular diseases [88, 89]. Alcohol consumption causes chronic inflammation of the liver called cirrhosis. This leads to an extensive build-up of scar tissue or collagen on liver tissues. Lecithin removes the collagen from liver tissue by activating an enzyme which is effective in breaking down collagen [90].

## CONCLUSION

Emulsifiers are one of the most important ingredients used to maintain the quality, safety and integrity of processed foods. The processed foods are complex systems containing interfaces among ingredients, such as fats, protein, starch, water and air. Emulsifiers manage these interfaces, interactions and transitions by allowing the preservation of texture flavour and so on. This ingredient is an innovative solution for leading food manufacturers around the world. It meets the customer's food expectation to craft foods that stay flavorful, fresh and remain safe from the date of production to the date of consumption. The formulations of food emulsions have become an art since it is essential to choose the correct composition and processing conditions. Also, there are many factors involved in the selection of the correct emulsifier and the correct level of usage for food preservation application depending upon the type of food.

## CONSENT FOR PUBLICATION

Not applicable.

## CONFLICT OF INTEREST

The authors declare that there are no conflicts of interest

## ACKNOWLEDGEMENTS

The authors wish to acknowledge the Computational and Bioinformatics facility provided by the Alagappa University Bioinformatics Infrastructure Facility (DBT, Government of India. BT/BI/25/012/2012, BIF) and the instrumentation facilities and grant provided by, DST-FIST (Grant No. SR/FST/LSI-639/2015(C)), UGC-SAP (Grant No. F.5-1/2018/DRS-II(SAP-II)), (DST-PURSE (Grant No. SR/PURSE Phase 2/38 (G)), RUSA 2.0 [F. 24-51/2014-U, Policy (TN Multi-Gen), Dept of Education, Government of India] and the University Science Instrumentation Centre (USIC), Alagappa University.

## REFERENCES

[1]    Hasenhuettl GL, Hartel RW, Eds. Food emulsifiers and their applications. New York: Springer 2008.
[http://dx.doi.org/10.1007/978-0-387-75284-6]

[2]    Friberg S, Larsson K, Sjoblom J, Eds. Food emulsions. USA: CRC Press 2003.
[http://dx.doi.org/10.1201/9780203913222]

[3]    Gudiña EJ, Pereira JF, Costa R, *et al.* Novel bioemulsifier produced by a Paenibacillus strain isolated from crude oil. Microb Cell Fact 2015; 14(1): 14.
[http://dx.doi.org/10.1186/s12934-015-0197-5] [PMID: 25636532]

[4]    Banat IM, Franzetti A, Gandolfi I, *et al.* Microbial biosurfactants production, applications and future potential. Appl Microbiol Biotechnol 2010; 87(2): 427-44.
[http://dx.doi.org/10.1007/s00253-010-2589-0] [PMID: 20424836]

[5]    Franzetti A, Bestetti G, Caredda P, La Colla P, Tamburini E. Surface-active compounds and their role in the access to hydrocarbons in Gordonia strains. FEMS Microbiol Ecol 2008; 63(2): 238-48.
[http://dx.doi.org/10.1111/j.1574-6941.2007.00406.x] [PMID: 18070077]

[6]    Zheng C, He J, Wang Y, Wang M, Huang Z. Hydrocarbon degradation and bioemulsifier production by thermophilic Geobacillus pallidus strains. Bioresour Technol 2011; 102(19): 9155-61.
[http://dx.doi.org/10.1016/j.biortech.2011.06.074] [PMID: 21764302]

[7]    Monteiro AS, Coutinho JO, Júnior AC, Rosa CA, Siqueira EP, Santos VL. Characterization of new biosurfactant produced by Trichosporon montevideense CLOA 72 isolated from dairy industry effluents. J Basic Microbiol 2009; 49(6): 553-63.
[http://dx.doi.org/10.1002/jobm.200900089] [PMID: 19810042]

[8]     Luna-Velasco MA, Esparza-García F, Cañizares-Villanueva RO, Rodríguez-Vázquez R. Production and properties of a bioemulsifier synthesized by phenanthrene-degrading Penicillium sp. Process Biochem 2007; 42(3): 310-4.
        [http://dx.doi.org/10.1016/j.procbio.2006.08.015]

[9]     Perfumo A, Smyth TJP, Marchant R, Banat IM. Production and roles of biosurfactants and bioemulsifiers in accessing hydrophobic substrates.Handbook of hydrocarbon and lipid microbiology. Springer Berlin Heidelberg 2010; pp. 1501-12.
        [http://dx.doi.org/10.1007/978-3-540-77587-4_103]

[10]    Sekhon-Randhawa KK. Biosurfactants produced by genetically manipulated microorganisms: challenges and opportunities. 2014.

[11]    Kaplan N, Zosim Z, Rosenberg E. Reconstitution of emulsifying activity of Acinetobacter calcoaceticus BD4 emulsan by using pure polysaccharide and protein. Appl Environ Microbiol 1987; 53(2): 440-6.
        [http://dx.doi.org/10.1128/AEM.53.2.440-446.1987] [PMID: 3566271]

[12]    Lukondeh T, Ashbolt NJ, Rogers PL. Evaluation of Kluyveromyces marxianus FII 510700 grown on a lactose-based medium as a source of a natural bioemulsifier. J Ind Microbiol Biotechnol 2003; 30(12): 715-20.
        [http://dx.doi.org/10.1007/s10295-003-0105-6] [PMID: 14689315]

[13]    Jagtap S, Yavankar S, Pardesi K, Chopade B. Production of bioemulsifier by Acinetobacter species isolated from healthy human skin Cited: 2010 Available from: http://nopr.niscair.res.in/handle/123456789/6966

[14]    Whitehurst RJ, Ed. Emulsifiers in Food Technology. John Wiley & Sons 2008.

[15]    Flickinger BD, Matsuo N. Nutritional characteristics of DAG oil. Lipids 2003; 38(2): 129-32.
        [http://dx.doi.org/10.1007/s11745-003-1042-8] [PMID: 12733744]

[16]    DeMerlis CC, Howell JC. The use of food additive safety evaluation procedures as a basis for evaluating the safety of new pharmaceutical excipients. Excipient development for Pharmaceutical, Biotechnology, and Drug Delivery systems 2006; 69
        [http://dx.doi.org/10.1201/9781420004137.ch6]

[17]    Gunstone FD, Harwood JL, Dijkstra AJ. The lipid handbook with CD-ROM. USA: CRC press 2007.
        [http://dx.doi.org/10.1201/9781420009675]

[18]    Wang FC, Marangoni AG. Advances in the application of food emulsifier α-gel phases: Saturated monoglycerides, polyglycerol fatty acid esters, and their derivatives. J Colloid Interface Sci 2016; 483: 394-403.
        [http://dx.doi.org/10.1016/j.jcis.2016.08.012] [PMID: 27554171]

[19]    Bastida-Rodríguez J. The food additive polyglycerol polyricinoleate (E-476): structure, applications, and production methods. ISRN Chemical Engineering 2013.

[20]    Norn V, Ed. Emulsifiers in food technology. John Wiley & Sons 2014.

[21]    Food and Drug Administration; Code of federal regulations, 21CFR202. Title 21—Food and drugs. Chapter I—Food and drug administration. Department of Health and Human Services Part 202—Prescription-drug advertisements. . Food and Drug Administration Code of federal regulations . 2005. 21CFR202. Title

[22]    Lamb J, Hentz K, Schmitt D, Tran N, Jonker D, Junker K. A one-year oral toxicity study of sodium stearoyl lactylate (SSL) in rats. Food Chem Toxicol 2010; 48(10): 2663-9.
        [http://dx.doi.org/10.1016/j.fct.2010.06.037] [PMID: 20600527]

[23]    Schaefer EC, Matthews ME. Fatty Acids, C16-18 and C18-Unsaturated, Reaction Products with Lactic Acid and Monosodium Lactate (CAS# 847904-46-5): Ready Biodegradability by the Carbon Dioxide Evolution Test Method, Project No. 645E-101 for Caravan Ingredients. Easton, Maryland: Wildlife

International 2007.

[24]   Bährle-Rapp M, Bährle-Rapp M. Calcium Stearoyl Lactylate. Springer Lexikon Kosmetik und Körperpflege 2007; pp. 83-3.

[25]   Szűts A, Szabó-Révész P. Sucrose esters as natural surfactants in drug delivery systems--a mini-review. Int J Pharm 2012; 433(1-2): 1-9.
[http://dx.doi.org/10.1016/j.ijpharm.2012.04.076] [PMID: 22575672]

[26]   Watanabe T. Sucrose fatty acid esters-past, present and future. Foods and Food Ingredients Journal of Japan 1999; pp. 18-25.

[27]   Long CL, Domingues FJ, Studer V, *et al.* Studies on absorption and metabolism of propylene glycol distearate. Arch Biochem Biophys 1958; 77(2): 428-39.
[http://dx.doi.org/10.1016/0003-9861(58)90090-0] [PMID: 13584006]

[28]   Oke M, Jacob JK, Paliyath G. Effect of soy lecithin in enhancing fruit juice/sauce quality. Food Res Int 2010; 43(1): 232-40.
[http://dx.doi.org/10.1016/j.foodres.2009.09.021]

[29]   Bueschelberger HG. Lecithins. Emulsifiers in Food Technology 2004; pp. 1-39.

[30]   Navon-Venezia S, Zosim Z, Gottlieb A, *et al.* Alasan, a new bioemulsifier from Acinetobacter radioresistens. Appl Environ Microbiol 1995; 61(9): 3240-4.
[http://dx.doi.org/10.1128/AEM.61.9.3240-3244.1995] [PMID: 7574633]

[31]   Becher P, Fishman MM. Emulsions—Theory and Practice. J Electrochem Soc 1959; 106(4): 108C-C.
[http://dx.doi.org/10.1149/1.2427327]

[32]   Dickinson E, Patino JR, Eds. Food emulsions and foams: interfaces, interactions and stability. Cambridge, No 227, Royal Society of Chemistry . 1999.

[33]   Hasenhuettl GL. Emulsifier Trends for the Future.Food Emulsifiers and Their Applications. US: Springer 1997; pp. 281-6.
[http://dx.doi.org/10.1007/978-1-4757-2662-6_11]

[34]   Sezgin AC, Artik N. Determination of saponin content in Turkish tahini halvah by using HPLC. Advance Journal of Food Science and Technology 2010; 2(2): 109-15.

[35]   Guneser O, Zorba M. Effect of emulsifiers on oil separation problem and quality characteristics of Tahin Helva during storage. J Food Sci Technol 2014; 51(6): 1085-93.
[http://dx.doi.org/10.1007/s13197-011-0594-7] [PMID: 24876640]

[36]   Ereifej KI, Rababah TM, Al-Rababah MA. Quality attributes of halva by utilization of proteins, non-hydrogenated palm oil, emulsifiers, gum Arabic, sucrose, and calcium chloride. Int J Food Prop 2005; 8(3): 415-22.
[http://dx.doi.org/10.1080/10942910500267323]

[37]   Aloui F, Maazoun B, Gargouri Y, Miled N. Optimization of oil retention in sesame based halva using emulsifiers and fibers: an industrial assay. J Food Sci Technol 2016; 53(3): 1540-50.
[http://dx.doi.org/10.1007/s13197-015-2116-5] [PMID: 27570279]

[38]   Elleuch M, Besbes S, Roiseux O, *et al.* Date flesh: Chemical composition and characteristics of the dietary fibre. Food Chem 2008; 111(3): 676-82.
[http://dx.doi.org/10.1016/j.foodchem.2008.04.036]

[39]   Sangnark A, Noomhorm A. Effect of particle sizes on functional properties of dietary fibre prepared from sugarcane bagasse. Food Chem 2003; 80(2): 221-9.
[http://dx.doi.org/10.1016/S0308-8146(02)00257-1]

[40]   Arcos JA, Otero C. Enzyme, medium, and reaction engineering to design a low-cost, selective production method for mono-and dioleoylglycerols. J Am Oil Chem Soc 1996; 73(6): 673-82.
[http://dx.doi.org/10.1007/BF02517939]

[41]    Barrault J, Pouilloux Y, Clacens JM, Vanhove C, Bancquart S. Catalysis and fine chemistry. Catal Today 2002; 75(1): 177-81.
[http://dx.doi.org/10.1016/S0920-5861(02)00062-7]

[42]    Zatta P, Alfrey AC. Aluminium Toxicity in Infants' Health and Disease. World Scientific 1997.

[43]    Saiyed SM, Yokel RA. Aluminium content of some foods and food products in the USA, with aluminium food additives. Food Addit Contam 2005; 22(3): 234-44.
[http://dx.doi.org/10.1080/02652030500073584] [PMID: 16019791]

[44]    Ellinger RH. Phosphates as food ingredients. USA: CRC Press 1972.

[45]    Yokel RA, Hicks CL, Florence RL. Aluminum bioavailability from basic sodium aluminum phosphate, an approved food additive emulsifying agent, incorporated in cheese. Food Chem Toxicol 2008; 46(6): 2261-6.
[http://dx.doi.org/10.1016/j.fct.2008.03.004] [PMID: 18436363]

[46]    Ashwini A, Jyotsna R, Indrani D. Effect of hydrocolloids and emulsifiers on the rheological, microstructural and quality characteristics of eggless cake. Food Hydrocoll 2009; 23(3): 700-7.
[http://dx.doi.org/10.1016/j.foodhyd.2008.06.002]

[47]    Kohrs D, Herald TJ, Aramouni FM, Abughoush M. Evaluation of egg replacers in a yellow cake system. Emir J Food Agric 2010; 22(5): 340.
[http://dx.doi.org/10.9755/ejfa.v22i5.4822]

[48]    Yang SC, Baldwin RE. Functional properties of eggs in foods. Egg Science and Technology 1995; p. 4.

[49]    Turabi E, Sumnu G, Sahin S. Rheological properties and quality of rice cakes formulated with different gums and an emulsifier blend. Food Hydrocoll 2008; 22(2): 305-12.
[http://dx.doi.org/10.1016/j.foodhyd.2006.11.016]

[50]    Gomez M, Ronda F, Caballero PA, Blanco CA, Rosell CM. Functionality of different hydrocolloids on the quality and shelf-life of yellow layer cakes. Food Hydrocoll 2007; 21(2): 167-73.
[http://dx.doi.org/10.1016/j.foodhyd.2006.03.012]

[51]    Bailey AE. Industrial oil and fat products. New York: Interscience Publishers 1945.

[52]    O'brien RD. Fats and oils: formulating and processing for applications. USA: CRC press 2008.
[http://dx.doi.org/10.1201/9781420061673]

[53]    Wetterau FP, Olsanski VL, Smullin CF. The determination of sorbitan monostearate in cake mixes and baked cakes. J Am Oil Chem Soc 1964; 41(12): 791-5.
[http://dx.doi.org/10.1007/BF02663958]

[54]    Reilly NR, Green PH. Epidemiology and clinical presentations of celiac disease. 2012.
[http://dx.doi.org/10.1007/s00281-012-0311-2]

[55]    Gallagher E, Gormley TR, Arendt EK. Recent advances in the formulation of gluten-free cereal-based products. Trends Food Sci Technol 2004; 15(3): 143-52.
[http://dx.doi.org/10.1016/j.tifs.2003.09.012]

[56]    Sarabhai S, Indrani D, Vijaykrishnaraj M, Milind , Arun Kumar V, Prabhasankar P. Effect of protein concentrates, emulsifiers on textural and sensory characteristics of gluten free cookies and its immunochemical validation. J Food Sci Technol 2015; 52(6): 3763-72.
[PMID: 26028761]

[57]    Marcoa C, Rosell CM. Effect of different protein isolates and transglutaminase on rice flour properties. J Food Eng 2008; 84(1): 132-9.
[http://dx.doi.org/10.1016/j.jfoodeng.2007.05.003]

[58]    Juliano BO. Grain quality problems in Asia.Aciar Proceedings. 1996; pp. 15-22.

[59]    Kaur L, Singh N, Kaur K, Singh B. Effect of mustard oil and process variables on extrusion behaviour

of rice grits. J Food Sci Technol 2000; 37(6): 656-60.

[60]   Smith DA, Rao RM, Liuzzo JA, Champagne E. Chemical Treatment and Process Modification for Producing Improved Quick-Cooking Rice. J Food Sci 1985; 50(4): 926-31.
[http://dx.doi.org/10.1111/j.1365-2621.1985.tb12981.x]

[61]   Wang JP, An HZ, Jin ZY, Xie ZJ, Zhuang HN, Kim JM. Emulsifiers and thickeners on extrusion-cooked instant rice product. J Food Sci Technol 2013; 50(4): 655-66.
[http://dx.doi.org/10.1007/s13197-011-0400-6] [PMID: 24425967]

[62]   Jukes DJ. Food Legislation of the UK: A concise guide. Elsevier 2013.

[63]   Holdt SL, Kraan S. Bioactive compounds in seaweed: functional food applications and legislation. J Appl Phycol 2011; 23(3): 543-97.
[http://dx.doi.org/10.1007/s10811-010-9632-5]

[64]   Marangoni AG, Rousseau D. Engineering triacylglycerols: the role of interesterification. Trends Food Sci Technol 1995; 6(10): 329-35.
[http://dx.doi.org/10.1016/S0924-2244(00)89167-0]

[65]   Nash NH, Brickman LM. Food emulsifiers—science and art. J Am Oil Chem Soc 1972; 49(8): 457-61.
[http://dx.doi.org/10.1007/BF02582479]

[66]   Orten JM, Dajani RM. A study of the effects of certain food emulsifiers in hamsters. J Food Sci 1957; 22(6): 529-41.
[http://dx.doi.org/10.1111/j.1365-2621.1957.tb17513.x]

[67]   Ferber E. Nutritional Conditions in Yugoslavia and their Reflection on Health.World Review of Nutrition and Dietetics. Switzerland: Karger Publishers 1973; Vol. 18: pp. 263-74.

[68]   Younes M, Aggett P, Aguilar F, *et al.* Re-evaluation of mono-and di-glycerides of fatty acids (E 471) as food additives. EFSA J 2017a; 15(11)

[69]   Babayan VK. Modification of food to control fat intake. J Am Oil Chem Soc 1974; 51(6): 260-4.
[http://dx.doi.org/10.1007/BF02642632] [PMID: 4853240]

[70]   King WR, Michael WR, Coots RH. Subacute oral toxicity of polyglycerol ester. Toxicol Appl Pharmacol 1971; 20(3): 327-33.
[http://dx.doi.org/10.1016/0041-008X(71)90276-6] [PMID: 5132776]

[71]   Younes M, Aggett P, Aguilar F, *et al.* Re-evaluation of polyglycerol esters of fatty acids (E 475) as a food additive. EFSA J 2017b; 15(12)

[72]   Bevan C, Tyler TR, Gardiner TH, Kapp RW Jr, Andrews L, Beyer BK. Two-generation reproduction toxicity study with isopropanol in rats. J Appl Toxicol 1995; 15(2): 117-23.
[http://dx.doi.org/10.1002/jat.2550150210] [PMID: 7782556]

[73]   Joint FAO/WHO Expert Committee on Food Additives. Meeting, & World Health Organization Evaluation of Certain Food Additives: Seventy-first Report of the Joint FAO/WHO Expert Committee on Food Additives. World Health Organization 2010; Vol. 71.

[74]   Benninga H. C.J. Patterson Finds a New Use for Lactic Acid (The Story of Stearoyl Lactylates, Conditioners of Bread) 1990.

[75]   Joint FAO. WHO Expert Committee on Food Additives, & World Health Organization Toxicological evaluation of certain food additives with a review of general principles and of specifications: seventeenth report of the Joint FA. World Health Organization 1974.

[76]   Lamb J, Hentz K, Schmitt D, Tran N, Jonker D, Junker K. A one-year oral toxicity study of sodium stearoyl lactylate (SSL) in rats. Food Chem Toxicol 2010; 48(10): 2663-9.
[http://dx.doi.org/10.1016/j.fct.2010.06.037] [PMID: 20600527]

[77]   Chesterman H, Andrew JE, Heywood R. Celynol MSPO 11 Preliminary dietary toxicity study in beagle dogs Unpublished report no 2307 from Huntingdon research centre submitted to WHO by

Rhône poulenc 1980.

[78]   Chesterman H, Heywood R, Allen TR, Street AE, Read R, Gapinath C. Sucrose ester of mixed stearic and palmitic acid dietary study in beagle dogs. Unpublished report from Huntingdon research centre submitted to Ryoto company Ltd 1979.

[79]   Lamb J, Hentz K, Schmitt D, Tran N, Jonker D, Junker K. A one-year oral toxicity study of sodium stearoyl lactylate (SSL) in rats. Food Chem Toxicol 2010; 48(10): 2663-9.
       [http://dx.doi.org/10.1016/j.fct.2010.06.037] [PMID: 20600527]

[80]   Chengelis CP, Kirkpatrick JB, Marit GB, Morita O, Tamaki Y, Suzuki H. A chronic dietary toxicity study of DAG (diacylglycerol) in Beagle dogs. Food Chem Toxicol 2006; 44(1): 81-97.
       [http://dx.doi.org/10.1016/j.fct.2005.06.005] [PMID: 16084638]

[81]   Lerner A, Matthias T. Changes in intestinal tight junction permeability associated with industrial food additives explain the rising incidence of autoimmune disease. Autoimmun Rev 2015; 14(6): 479-89.
       [http://dx.doi.org/10.1016/j.autrev.2015.01.009] [PMID: 25676324]

[82]   Long CL, Zeitlin BR, Thiessen R Jr. An investigation of the *in vivo* hydrolysis and absorption of propylene glycol distearate. Arch Biochem Biophys 1958; 77(2): 440-53.
       [http://dx.doi.org/10.1016/0003-9861(58)90091-2] [PMID: 13584007]

[83]   Rigler MW, Patton JS. The production of liquid crystalline product phases by pancreatic lipase in the absence of bile salts. A freeze-fracture study. Biochim Biophys Acta 1983; 751(3): 444-54.
       [http://dx.doi.org/10.1016/0005-2760(83)90305-3] [PMID: 6849954]

[84]   Adams CA. Nutricines: food components in health and nutrition. Nottingham University Press 1999.

[85]   Dobson KS, Williams KD, Boriack CJ. The preparation of polyglycerol esters suitable as low-caloric fat substitutes. J Am Oil Chem Soc 1993; 70(11): 1089-92.
       [http://dx.doi.org/10.1007/BF02632147]

[86]   Yin LJ, Kobayashi I, Nakajima M. Effect of polyglycerol esters of fatty acids on the physicochemical properties and stability of β-carotene emulsions during digestion in simulated gastric fluid. Food Biophys 2008; 3(2): 213-8.
       [http://dx.doi.org/10.1007/s11483-008-9077-4]

[87]   Wood JL, Allison RG. Effects of consumption of choline and lecithin on neurological and cardiovascular systems. Fed Proc 1982; 41(14): 3015-21.
       [PMID: 6754453]

[88]   Canty DJ, Zeisel SH. Lecithin and choline in human health and disease. Nutr Rev 1994; 52(10): 327-39.
       [http://dx.doi.org/10.1111/j.1753-4887.1994.tb01357.x] [PMID: 7816350]

[89]   Knuiman JT, Beynen AC, Katan MB. Lecithin intake and serum cholesterol. Am J Clin Nutr 1989; 49(2): 266-8.
       [http://dx.doi.org/10.1093/ajcn/49.2.266] [PMID: 2916447]

[90]   Lieber CS, DeCarli LM, Mak KM, Kim CI, Leo MA. Attenuation of alcohol-induced hepatic fibrosis by polyunsaturated lecithin. Hepatology 1990; 12(6): 1390-8.
       [http://dx.doi.org/10.1002/hep.1840120621] [PMID: 2258155]

[91]   Regulation (EU) No 1129/2011 of 11 November 2011 amending Annex II to Regulation (EC) No 1333/2008 of the European Parliament and of the Council by establishing a Union list of food additives. Off J Eur Union L 2011; 295(4): 12-.

# CHAPTER 12

# Stabilizers (Including pH Control Agents and Phosphates)

**Tarun Belwal[1,*], Hari Prasad Devkota[2,3], Ankur Kumar Goel[4] and Indra D. Bhatt[1,*]**

[1] *G.B. Pant National Institute of Himalayan Environment and Sustainable Development, Kosi-Katarmal, Almora, Uttarakhand, India*

[2] *School of Pharmacy, Kumamoto University, 5-1 Oe-honmachi, Chuo ku, Kumamoto 862-0973, Japan*

[3] *Program for Leading Graduate Schools, Health life science: Interdisciplinary and Glocal Oriented (HIGO) Program, Kumamoto University, Kumamoto, Japan*

[4] *Jubilant Generics Limited, Sikandarpur Bhainswal, Bhagwanpur, Roorkee, Uttarakhand, India*

**Abstract:** The continuous availability of food, as a very basic requirement of life, has always been a difficult aspect due to food contamination and decomposition. It is a difficult task for food scientists to make food products available in good condition after harvest and/or processing, storage and transportation to other places from their place of origin. The use of food additives allows food products to maintain their quality during storage as well as improve shelf-life and maintain their palatability and nutritional quality. The role of stabilizers as food additives is becoming crucial in controlling the pH of the product as well as stabilizing the product texture and its structure. These stabilizers are becoming more popular and widely used in various food products and are chosen based on different criteria. Their origin, either natural or synthetic, is one of the most important criteria regarding consumer acceptability. Various physiological and toxicological profiles of these stabilizers have also been studied. This chapter describes the general aspects of food stabilizers and their application in various food products. Further research is necessary to widen their applications and consumer acceptability as well as to determine possible toxicological effects.

**Keywords:** Food additives, pH control agents, Safety, Stabilizers.

## INTRODUCTION

Food, as a regular consumable item, needs to be produced and sold in a more

---

\* **Corresponding author Tarun Belwal and Indra D. Bhatt:** G.B. Pant National Institute of Himalayan Environment and Sustainable Development, Kosi-Katarmal, Almora, Uttarakhand, India; E mail: tarungbpihed@gmail.com; id_bhatt@yahoo.com

**Seyed Mohammad Nabavi *et al.* (Eds.)**

structured way. Many food items cannot be made readily available to consumers in fresh form, thus prior processing is required to make them durable for a certain period of time. The food products, in some cases, require a long distance of transport with changing climatic conditions and thus require modification by adding additives. Food processing not only requires technical and scientific inputs regarding the raw materials but also need prior knowledge of the additives that can be best suited to the product quality. Various additives, such as anti-caking agents, acidity regulators, bulking agents, colouring agents, preservatives, stabilizers,and sweeteners, among others, have been used in food product formulations. Among these, stabilizers are required to stabilize the texture or structure of the formulation. Similar to stabilizers, acidifying agents, also known as pH control agents, are crucial for product quality. This book chapter will elaborate the commonly used stabilizers and acidifying agents with their origin, uses and food applications, legislative and toxicological data for a better understanding of their use in various food products.

## STABILIZERS AND ACIDIFYING AGENTS

The role of stabilizers is crucial to maintain the proper texture of the product [1]. For instance, if the food product lacks stabilizers, after a certain period of time, it will lead to the separation of oil and water in the case of emulsions [2]. The lack of stabilizers in frozen food leads to the formation of ice crystals [3], and in the case of products such as jams, jelly, ketchup, it leads to the setting of the ingredients [4]. Therefore, to prevent all these problems, the role of stabilizers is important. The commonly used stabilizers are alginates, agar, carrageenan, guar gums, tragacanth, tara gum, *etc*. The list of commonly used stabilizers, along with their origin, uses and food applications, is given in Table **1**. Most of them are of natural origin. Their role in food products is well defined and depends upon the need as well as the type of food products, and some of them have also been tested regarding their safety level. Nowadays, the market of these stabilizers is growing faster; especially, the demand for safer and compatible stabilizers is increasing. An analysis predicted the market of global food stabilizers to grow at a compound annual growth rate (CAGR) of 4.14% during the period 2016-2020 [5].

Table 1. List of commonly used stabilizers, including name, origin, uses and food applications [6 - 8].

| S.No. | Name (E No.) | Origin | Used as | Food Applications |
|---|---|---|---|---|
| 1 | Alginic acid (E 400) | Natural, derived from seaweed | Gelling agent, stabilizer | Used in custard mix, flavoured mix, cream and yogurt |

*(Table 1) cont.....*

| S.No. | Name (E No.) | Origin | Used as | Food Applications |
|-------|--------------|--------|---------|-------------------|
| 2 | Sodium alginate (E 401) | Natural polysaccharide product extracted from the cell wall of brown seaweed | Gelling agent, stabilizer | Prevent ice crystal formation, maintaining a smooth texture and discouraging product melt, thickening agent |
| 3 | Propylene glycol alginate (E405) | Extracted from natural algae | Thickener, texture stabilizer, emulsifier, swelling, acid resistance, gelling agents | Fruit juice, salad dressing, dairy products, lactic acid beverages, beer, and instant food |
| 4 | Agar (E 406) | Derived from red seaweed | Thickener, gelling agent, coagulant, suspending agents, emulsifiers, preservatives, stabilizers | Drinks, jelly, ice cream, cakes, candy, jellies canned food, meat products, |
| 5 | Carrageenan (E407) | Derived from red seaweed | Binder, thickening agent and stabilizer | Ice cream and frozen products, Milk-based beverages, Ready-to-eat dairy desserts, jellies |
| 6 | Locust bean gum/Carobgum (E410) | Derived from locust bean tree (*Ceratonia siliqua*) | Texturizer, gelling agent | Ice cream and frozen products, fruit juice, caffeine-free chocolate substitute |
| 7 | Guar gum (E412) | From seeds of *Cyamopsis tetragonoloba* | Thickening agent, texturing and binding agent | Beverages, candies, ice-creams, cheese products, puddings, salad dressings, jams, mayonnaise, sauce, ketchup, jellies, fruit spreads |
| 8 | Tragacanth (E413) | Resin from the tree *Astracantha gummifera* | Thickening agent, suspending agent, emulsifier | Beverages, soup and cake mixes |
| 9 | Acacia gum (E414) | Derived from the sap of *Acacia senegal* | stabilizing, suspending and emulsifying agent | Beverage, fruit-flavored water, milk-based beverages, smoothies, soft-alcoholic drinks, light-coloured or dark aromatic emulsions |
| 10 | Xanthan gum (E415) | Derived from the fermentation of corn sugar with a bacterium | Thickening agent, stabilizer | Bakery products, beverages, ice cream, ice milk, sherbet, milkshakes and water ices, salad dressings, frozen fish, buttermilk, frozen egg products, canned or bottled (pasteurized) fruit juice |

*(Table 1) cont.....*

| S.No. | Name (E No.) | Origin | Used as | Food Applications |
|---|---|---|---|---|
| 11 | Karaya gum (E416) | Derived from tree *Sterculia urens* | Thickening agent, emulsifying agent, stabilizer | Beverages, ice cream, custard and sweets |
| 12 | Tara gum (E417) | Derived from *Caesalpinia spinosa* | Thickening agent, stabilizer | Convenience foods, dairy products |
| 13 | Sorbitol (E420) | Derived from glucose | Moisturizer and stabilizer | Confectionery, bakery foods, frozen dessert, biscuit, cake, sugar-coat and chocolate |
| 14 | Pectin (E440) | Produced from citrus peels, apple | Gelling, thickening and stabilizing agent | Jams and fruit jellies, Fruit preparations for dairy applications, Acidified milk and protein drinks, yoghurts (thickening) |
| 15 | Gelatin (E441) | Obtained from animal connective tissue (collagen) | Gelling agent | Mostly gummy candy, as well as other products such as marshmallows, gelatin desserts, and some ice creams, dips, and yogurts |
| 16 | Microcrystalline cellulose (MCC) (E460i) | Cellulose derivative formed by physically interacting crystalline cellulose with colloids, particularly CMC | Gelling agent | Icecream |
| 17 | Carboxymethyl cellulose (CMC) (cellulose gum) (E466) | Extracted from the plant's cell walls especially from the wood pulp and cotton seeds, also the addition of carboxymethyl group to cellulose | Gelling agent, thickener | Icecream, dairy beverages, bakery products, desserts and toppings, sauces, soups, fried foods, candies, chewing gum |

Acidifying agents, as pH stabilizers, are crucial for product quality. They are of natural as well as synthetic origin. Commonly known acidifying agents are malic acid, tartaric acid, fumaric acid, adipic acid and their sodium, potassium, calcium salts, including phosphates. Their role in maintaining the proper pH of food products is crucial as they prevent the growth of microorganisms, development of unpleasant odour and taste (organoleptic properties), and changes in physicochemical characteristics of food ingredients and products. The concentration of these acidifying agents in the food products must be in a desirable level, as a higher or lower concentration will not only affect the product quality but also cause serious complications to health. The list of commonly used acidifying agents along with their origin, uses and food applications is given in

Table **2.**

**Table 2. List of commonly used acidity regulators, including their origin, uses and food applications.**

| S.No. | Name (E No.) | Origin | Used as | Food Applications |
|---|---|---|---|---|
| 1 | Ammonium lactate (E328) | Produced by the fermentation of lactose, carbohydrate and molasses | Preservative, acidity regulator and anti-microbial | Beverages |
| 2 | Adipic acid (E355) | Chemically synthesized | Flavouring, gelling agent, acidity regulator | Beverages |
| 3 | Calcium phosphate (E341) | Produced from phosphoric acid | Acidity regulator | Bakery products |
| 4 | Potassium carbonate (E510) | Produced from potassium chloride | Acidity regulator, alkali and rising agent | Noodles |
| 5 | Sodium fumarate (E365) | Produced from fumaric acid | Acidity regulator | Wine, cold drink, sweet products, canned fruit, jam, jelly, confectionary and bakery products |
| 6 | Malic acid (E296) | Chemically synthesized | Acidity regulator, flavouring agent, colour stabilizer | Juices, jams, jelly and frozen vegetables |
| 7 | Tartaric acid (E334) | Produced by the waste products of the wine industry (grape skins) | Acidity regulator and taste enhancer | Confectionary, soft drinks, wine, candies and jams |
| 8 | Sodium carbonate (E500(i)) | Produced from sea water/salt | Acidity regulator, alkali and rising agent | Beverages |
| 9 | Acetic acid (E206) | Bacterial fermentation and chemical synthesis | Antimicrobial, acidity regulator and aroma component | Fish products, butter, processed cheese and cooking oil |
| 10 | Fumaric acid (E297) | Fermentation product of sugar/chemical synthesis | Acidity regulator and structure stabilizer | Beverages |
| 11 | Sodium acetate (E262) | Fermentation of sugar, molasses/chemical synthesis | Acidity regulator, preservative | Beverages |
| 12 | Potassium phosphate (E340) | Produced from phosphoric acid | Acidity regulator and chelating agent | different food products include sauce and dessert mixes, jelly *products*, cooked and other cured meats, milk and cream products |
| 13 | Propionic acid (E280) | Chemically synthesized | Preservative and acidity regulator | Bakery products, meat products |

*(Table 2) cont.....*

| S.No. | Name (E No.) | Origin | Used as | Food Applications |
|-------|--------------|--------|---------|-------------------|
| 14 | Potassium hydroxide (E525) | Produce from natural salt potassium chloride | Acidity regulator | Bakery products, cocoa products and black olives |
| 15 | Magnesium carbonate (E504) | Produced from magnesium hydroxide | Acidity regulator, alkali and anti-caking agent | Beverages, bakery products |
| 16 | Sodium adipate (E356) | The sodium salt of adipic acid | Acidity regulator | different food products |
| 17 | Sodium lactate (E325) | Fermentation product of starch and molasses | Preservative, acidity regulator | Cheese, confectionary, ice-cream, fruit jelly, soups and canned fruits |
| 18 | Sodium ascorbate (E301) | Fermentation product of glucose and chemical oxidation | Antioxidant, acidity regulator | Different food products |
| 19 | Succinic acid (E363) | Synthesis from acetic acid | Acidity regulator and flavor enhancer | Confectionary and bakery products |
| 20 | Phosphoric acid (E338) | Chemically synthesized | Acidity regulator, flavoring agent | Soft drinks (soda and cola), jams |
| 21 | Sodium citrate (E331) | Fermentation of molasses | Antioxidant, acidity regulator, aroma compounds and preservatives | Fruits and fruit products |
| 22 | Tripotassium citrate (E332 ii) | Chemically synthesized | Acidity regulator, chelating agent, antioxidant, flavoring agent | Bakery products, cocoa products, coffee creamer and black olives |

## LEGISLATION RELATED TO FOOD ADDITIVES

As food additives, including stabilizers and acidifying agents, are consumed on a daily basis, their impact on human health must be closely monitored. Thus, food regulatory bodies in different countries have regulations regarding food additives. In the United States of America, food additives must get a premarket approval from the Food and Drug Administration [9] unless the use of the substance is generally recognized as safe (GRAS). In the European Union (EU) countries, food additives are regulated by Regulation EU no.1333/2008 [7]. In Japan, food additives are regulated by the Ministry of Health, Labour and Welfare under the Food Sanitation Act [10].

## TOXICOLOGICAL STUDIES

Stabilizers are known to be an important part of food additives. A number of applications of these stabilizers in different food items have been discussed above. Besides the applications of these stabilizers in different food items, studies have also been conducted on the toxicological profile of these additives; some of them are discussed below.

Pectin digestion has been tested for toxicological effects in rats [11]. Pectin was given in different doses to both male and female rats. Body weight was found to be increased in male rats by 5% as compared to the control. Also, a significant increase in blood urea nitrogen (BUN) and creatinine (CRN) was found in male rats, while the liver weight increased in females. No cell damage and/or death was recorded in both the sexes [11]. In another chronic toxicity study on pectin, a dose up to 5000 mg/kg/day showed no adverse effect. Also, a dose of 36g/day for 6 weeks in humans showed no adverse effects [12]. Pectin was administered at 0, 5, 10 and 15% to 10 male and 10 female rats for 90 days. The growth of the rats slightly decreased at a diet with 15% pectin, with a decrease in total serum protein and albumin. Other studies on blood chemistry and haematological features showed no side effects [13].

Carrageenan was also tested for its toxicity in rats for 3 months. It was found that by increasing the dose up to 50 times of the accepted doses, carrageenan showed no adverse effects [14]. A study was conducted on male albino rats fed with 0, 5, 10 or 20% of carrageenan for 10 weeks [15] that reported a significant rate of death at a higher dose. In another study, male and female rats were fed with carrageenan at 2.5, 10, 15 or 20% concentration for 23 to 143 days [16]. The rats were found to have a reduced growth rate at a higher carrageenan dose. After 20 days, 2 rats were found to have ulcer lesions in the caecum, while 6 had lesions after 30 days of treatment. In a similar study, 5% of carrageenan was given to guinea pigs for 56 days who developed pinpoint caecal and colonic ulceration [17]. Similar reports are available elsewhere [18]

An acute toxicological study showed that tragacanth gum was found safe; however, a diet containing 2% of tragacanth gum resulted in a significant reduction in growth in chickens. The topical application of tragacanth gum induced irritation to rabbits. Also, they found that no significant toxic and teratogenic effect when tragacanth was orally given to pregnant mice. Tragacanth was found to be a powerful allergen [19]. When tragacanth was administered *via* an intraperitoneal injection of 1% aqueous tragacanth (1ml) to mice (11 to 15 days of gestation), the death of all the foetuses of mice was recorded [20]. In another study, pregnant mice, hamsters, rats and rabbits were administered a tragacanth dose of 700, 900 and 1200 mg/kg [21]. No evidence of maternal toxicity after oral administration up to 1200 mg/kg tragacanth was recorded in hamsters and mice; however, significant mortality rates were observed in rats at a dose of 1200 mg/kg and in rabbits at a dose of 700 mg/kg, which was due to the haemorrhage in the mucosa of small intestine.

In another study, guar gum was given in diet (6% of diet) to male rats for 91 days. No significant change in weight gain was observed [22]. In another study, weight gain was observed when 15 rats were fed a diet containing 0.5% guar gum for 21 days [23]. Guar gum in the diet (0,1,2 or 5%) was administered to 10 female and male rats. At the end of the $90^{th}$ day, no significant changes in behaviour were found, however, growth in male rats and food efficiency were slightly reduced at a 5% diet. Also, haematological, urine analysis and blood enzyme activity showed no changes. However, blood urea was slightly increased in male rats at a higher dose [13]. In another study, 20 chickens were given 2% of guar gum in the diet for 21 days, which showed lower growth. The pancreatic weight also increased [24]. A mixture of guar gum and carob bean gum was administered to five male and five female dogs at different concentrations (0-10%) for 30 weeks. Hypermotility and bulky faeces were observed at a higher dose with reduced digestion. No other side effect was noticed [25]. In the case of rats (15 male and 15 female) administered 0 to 5% of guar gum flour in diet, only 7 male and 7 female survived which was further observed for 24 months. Out of these, one rat died after 12, 18, 19 and 22 months and no further abnormality was recorded [26]. A trial conducted on humans showed no side effects [27].

Gelatin was administered by vein for 2 to 3 days (1 to 3g/kg/day) to dogs and was found to produce no side effects. However, when the time increased to 1 to 2 weeks, the plasma protein and haemoglobin production was disturbed and interfered with the utilization of amino acids and food proteins [28].

Guar gum, when administered to animals such as mice, rats and hamsters, did not show any toxicological activity [29]. In another experiment, guar gum in cocoa butter at 30% administered to rats for 48 h, showed no adverse effect [26]. However, 27% guar gum administered to rats caused death due to intestinal blockage [30]. (Anonymous, 1964).

Rats (10 male and 10 female) administered 0-15% of pectin for 90 days showed a slight decrease in growth at higher pectin levels. Also, total serum protein and albumin level was reduced. A slight degree of hyperkeratosis of the stomach was seen in some male rats at 10 and 15% pectin level [31]. In a longer period of toxicological study, pectin was fed in the diet (10%) to 20 male Wister rats for two years. Mortality was not found to be significantly different as compared to control. However, body weight was found to be significantly lower in pectin treated rats. Other examinations such as blood chemistry, histology of heart, kidney, liver, lungs, spleen and testes were found to be unaffected [32, 33].

Locust bean gum was tested for teratogenicity in rats, mice, hamsters and rabbits and showed no teratogenicity at 280 mg/kg and 1300 mg/kg doses. However, at a 1300 mg/kg dose, some of the dams died while in rabbits, most of the pregnant dams died at a 910 mg/kg dose [34].

Tara gum was tested for toxicity in a group of 10 male and 10 female rats [14]. A dose of 0, 1, 2 or 5% of tara gum in the diet was given for 90 days. The body weight of male rats was found to be lower at 2% tara gum, while blood urea concentration increased at 5%. Also, an increase in the weight of thyroid at 2 and 5% and in the kidney at 5% concentration of tara gum was recorded in males. In a similar study, a group of 3 male and 3 female dogs were given a dose of tara gum at 0, 1 or 5% concentration in the diet for 90 days [365]. No significant change in behaviour, mortality, haematology, urine analysis and clinical chemistry was found. A long term animal testing (50 male and 50 female rats) was conducted for toxicity against tara gum [36]. A dose of 5% for 2 years was given in the diet. The results revealed a significant decrease in body weight in both male and female rats. A decrease in haematocrit and leukocyte count in male rats at 99 weeks and a decrease in monocyte count in female rats at 12 months and reticulocytes in female rats at 18 months were recorded. A significant increase in haemoglobin concentration in female rats at 99 weeks was recorded. The enzyme level was also tested in rats and it was found that SGPT activity in males at 12 months, fasting serum glucose and BUN at 12 months in female rats and SGOT activity in females at three months increased significantly.

Gum Arabic was tested in 50 male and 50 female mice at a dose of 0, 25000 or 50000ppm for 103 weeks [37]. The mean daily consumption of food decreased in both the sexes. Hepatocellular adenoma of the liver was recorded in female mice at a higher dose; however male mice did not show any tumour growth in the liver.

In a study, 12 food grade gums (sodium and calcium carrageenan, tragacanth, ghatti, locust bean, Arabic, guar, karaya, propylene glycol, alginate, furcellaran, agar agar and sodium carboxymethyl cellulose) were provided to 5 groups of 10 animals (5 male and 5 female). Rabbits were found to be the most sensitive to these gums, while rats and mice were the least sensitive [38].

Chickens (7 per group) were tested for toxicity against tragacanth. A soybean diet containing 2% tragacanth was provided for 24 days. Tragacanth was found to decrease the body weight with reduced digestibility [39].

When karaya gum was administered to pregnant mice at a dose of 170 mg/kg and 800 mg/kg for 10 days, a significant number of maternal deaths were recorded at a higher dose [40, 41].

Sodium alginate was also tested for its toxicity in an animal model. 4 male and 4 female rats were administered 10% sodium alginate for 12 days [42]. In these rats, faecal lipids increased 5 times, and faecal sterols also increased. In a similar study, 5-7 rats were given 5% sodium alginate for 2 to 4 weeks [43]. In these rats, pancreatic bile secretion was elevated.

## CONCLUSION AND FUTURE PERSPECTIVES

Food stabilizers and acidifying agents are one of the most widely used food additives in various food products, including dairy products, beverages, breads, among others. With the advancement in food technology, the increase in the consumption of packaged foods and convenient lifestyles, the use of food additives will grow more in the future. However, their safety and efficacy in human health must be closely monitored. There is also a high demand for natural agents as compared to synthetic ones for their safety.

## CONSENT FOR PUBLICATION

Not applicable.

## CONFLICT OF INTEREST

The authors declare no conflict of interest.

## ACKNOWLEDGEMENTS

Declared none.

## REFERENCES

[1]     Lal SN, O'Connor CJ, Eyres L. Application of emulsifiers/stabilizers in dairy products of high rheology. Adv Colloid Interface Sci 2006; 123-126: 433-7.
        [http://dx.doi.org/10.1016/j.cis.2006.05.009] [PMID: 16806031]

[2]     Dickinson E. Hydrocolloids as emulsifiers and emulsion stabilizers. Food Hydrocoll 2009; 23(6): 1473-82.
        [http://dx.doi.org/10.1016/j.foodhyd.2008.08.005]

[3]     Petzold G, Aguilera JM. Ice morphology: fundamentals and technological applications in foods. Food Biophys 2009; 4(4): 378-96.
        [http://dx.doi.org/10.1007/s11483-009-9136-5]

[4]     Sila DN, Van Buggenhout S, Duvetter T, *et al.* Pectins in processed fruits and vegetables: Part II—Structure–function relationships. Compr Rev Food Sci Food Saf 2009; 8(2): 86-104.

[http://dx.doi.org/10.1111/j.1541-4337.2009.00071.x]

[5]  Research and Markets. 2018.Global Food Stabilizers Market Available from: https://www.research andmarkets.com/research/2179ls/global_food

[6]  FAO. Joint FAO/WHO Expert Committee on Food Additives Combined Compendium of Food Additive Specifications: Analytical methods, test procedures and laboratory solutions used by and referenced in food additive specifications 2005.

[7]  Sensible Bites: little bites of digestible nutrition information Available from http://www.sensi blebite.com/

[8]  Regulation EC. No 1333/2008 of the European Parliament and of the Council of 16 December 2008 on food additives (L354). Off. Journal of European Union 2008; 51: 16-33.

[9]  U.S. Food and Drug Administration. 2018.Determining the Regulatory Status of a Food Ingredient https://www.fda.gov/Food/IngredientsPackagingLabeling/FoodAdditivesIngredients/ucm228269.htm

[10]  Japan's Specifications and Standards for Food Additives. 8th ed., Japan: The Ministry of Health, Labour and Welfare 2009.

[11]  Takagi H, Yasuhara K, Mitsumori K, Onodera H, Takegawa K, Takahashi M. A 13-week subacute oral toxicity study of pectin digests in rats Bull Nat Inst Health Sci 1997; 115: 119-24.

[12]  Mortensen A, Aguilar A, Crebelli R, *et al.* [12] EFSA ANS Panel (EFSA Panel on Food Additives and Nutrient Sources added to Food) Scientific Opinion on the re-evaluation of pectin (E 440i) and amidated pectin (E 440ii) as food additives EFSA J 2017; 15(7): 4866-62.

[13]  Til HP, Spanjers MT, de Groot AP. Sub-chronic toxicity study with locust bean gum in rats. Unpublished report from Centraal Instituutvoor Voedingsonderzoek TNO submitted to the World Health Organization by Hercules BV and Institut Européen des Industries de la Gomme de Caroube 1974.

[14]  Kintanar QL, Lim-Sylianc CY, Gutierrez OG, *et al.* Toxicological studies on Philippine natural grade carrageenan. National Academy of Science and Technology 1997; 19: 183-208.

[15]  Nilson HW, Schaller JW. Nutritive value of agar and Irish moss. J Food Sci 1941; 6: 461-9.
[http://dx.doi.org/10.1111/j.1365-2621.1941.tb16304.x]

[16]  Hawkins WW, Yaphe W. Carrageenan as a dietary constituent for the rat: Faecal excretion, nitrogen absorption, and growth. Can J Biochem 1965; 43(4): 479-84.
[http://dx.doi.org/10.1139/o65-056] [PMID: 14325985]

[17]  Grasso P, Sharratt M, Carpanini FMB, Gangolli SD. Studies on carrageenan and large-bowel ulceration in mammals. Food Cosmet Toxicol 1973; 11(4): 555-64.
[http://dx.doi.org/10.1016/S0015-6264(73)80326-8] [PMID: 4202364]

[18]  Sharratt M, Grasso P, Carpanini F, Gangolli SD. Carrageenan ulceration as a model for human ulcerative colitis. Lancet 1971; 1(7691): 192-3.
[http://dx.doi.org/10.1016/S0140-6736(71)91971-4] [PMID: 4102221]

[19]  Gelfand HH. The allergenicity of vegetable gums, a case of asthma due to tragacanth. J Allergy 1943; 14(3): 203.
[http://dx.doi.org/10.1016/S0021-8707(43)90640-9]

[20]  Frohberg H, Oettel H, Zeller H. [Mechanism of the fetotoxic effect of tragacanth]. Arch Toxikol 1969; 25(3): 268-95.
[http://dx.doi.org/10.1007/BF00577782] [PMID: 5394007]

[21]  FDRL (Food and Drug Research Laboratories). Teratologic evaluation of FDA 71-17 in mice, hamsters and rats Contract No FDA 71-260 NTIS Report PB 221789 1972.

[22]  Booth AN, Hendrickson AP, Deeds F. Physiologic effects of three microbial polysaccharides on rats. Toxicol Appl Pharmacol 1963; 5(4): 478-84.

[http://dx.doi.org/10.1016/0041-008X(63)90019-X] [PMID: 14013824]

[23]    Keane KW, Smutko CJ, Krieger CH, Denton AE. The addition of water to purified diets and its effect upon growth and protein efficiency ratio in the rat. J Nutr 1962; 77: 18-22.
[http://dx.doi.org/10.1093/jn/77.1.18] [PMID: 14454722]

[24]    Kratzer FH, Rajaguru RW, Vohra P. The effect of polysaccharides on energy utilization, nitrogen retention and fat absorption in chickens. Poult Sci 1967; 46(6): 1489-93.
[http://dx.doi.org/10.3382/ps.0461489] [PMID: 6081746]

[25]    Cox GE, Baily DE, Morgareidge K. Subacute feeding in dogs with a pre-cooked gum blend. Unpublished report from the Food and Drugs Latoratories, Inc, submitted to the World Health Organization by Hercules BV In: Carob (locust) bean gum. WHO Food Additives Series. 1974; 16

[26]    Krantz JC Jr, Carr CJ, Farson DB. Guar polysaccharide as a precursor of glycogen. J Am Diet Assoc 1948; 24(3): 212.
[PMID: 18905027]

[27]    Krantz JC. Unpublished report from General Mills, Inc. submitted to the World Health Organization, cited in JECFA 1975b; 1947

[28]    Robscheit-Robbins FS, Miller LL, Whipple GH. Gelatin—Its Usefulness and Toxicity. J Exp Med 1944; 80(2): 145-64.
[http://dx.doi.org/10.1084/jem.80.2.145] [PMID: 19871403]

[29]    Teratologic evaluation of FDA 71-16 (guar gum) in mice, rats, hamsters and rabbits. Unpublished report from the Food and Drug Research Labs, Inc submitted to the World Health Organization by the Food and Drug Administration 1972.

[30]    Evaluation of Jaguar A-20 and Karaya gum. Assay report No. 3110860 and 3110861. Unpublished report from the Wisconsin Alumni Research Foundation submitted to the World Health Organization 1964.

[31]    Til HP, Seinen W, De Groot AP. Sub-chronic (90-day) toxicity study with two samples of pectin (Melange A2 and C2) in rats Unpublished CIVO Report No 3843 studied August 1972, Submitted to the World Health Organization by the Inst Eur DesInd de la Pectine 1972.

[32]    Palmer GH, Jones TR. Two-year pectin feeding study. Unpublished report from Sunkist Growers, Inc submitted to the World Health Organization by Sunkist Growers, Inc 1974.

[33]    Abdul Haq, Palmer GH. Two-year pectin feeding study: histopathological studies Unpublished report from Sunkist Growers, Inc submitted to the World Health Organization by Sunkist Growers, Inc 1974.

[34]    Morgareidge K. Teratological evaluation of FDA-71-14 (locustbean gum). Unpublished report from the Food & Drug Research Laboratories, Inc, submitted to the World Health Organization by Hercules BV 1972.

[35]    Oshita G, Burtner BR, Kennedy GL, Kinoshita FK, Keplinger ML. 90 day subchronic oral toxicity study with tara gum in beagle dogs. Unpublished report from Industrial Bio-Test Laboratories, Inc, Northbrook, IL, USA Submitted to WHO by Hercules Incorporated 1975.

[36]    Carlson WA, Domanski J. Two-year chronic oral toxicitystudy with tara gum in albino rats. Unpublished data IndustrialBio-Test, Northbrook, Illinois, United States of America 1980.

[37]    National Toxicology Program. Carcinogenesis bioassay of gumarabic. Unpublished National Toxicology Program, Research Triangle Park, North Carolina, 1980; 134. Submitted to the World Health Organization by the US Food and Drug Administration

[38]    Bailey D, Morgareidge K. Comparative acute oral toxicity of 12 food grade gums in mouse, rat, hamster, and rabbit. Fd Drug Res Lab Papers 1976; (124):

[39]    Vohra P, Shariff G, Kratzer FH. Growth inhibitory effect of some gums and pectin for Tribolium castaneum larvae, chickens and Japanese quail. Nutr Rep Int 1979. [Nutritional evaluation of dietary fiber].

[40]    US FDA. Teratogenic evaluation of gum karaya. NTIS ReportPB-221-789 1972.

[41]    US FDA. Teratological evaluation of gum karaya. NTIS ReportPB-223-818AS 1973.

[42]    Mokady S. Effect of dietary pectin and algin on blood cholesterol level in growing rats fed a cholesterol-free diet. Nutr Metab 1973; 15(4): 290-4.
[http://dx.doi.org/10.1159/000175452] [PMID: 4748994]

[43]    Ikegami S, Tsuchihashi F, Harada H, Tsuchihashi N, Nishide E, Innami S. Effect of viscous indigestible polysaccharides on pancreatic-biliary secretion and digestive organs in rats. J Nutr 1990; 120(4): 353-60.
[http://dx.doi.org/10.1093/jn/120.4.353] [PMID: 2158535]

**CHAPTER 13**

# Indirect Additives

**Mariana A. Andrade[1], Regiane Ribeiro-Santos[2], Seyed M. Nabavi[3] and Ana Sanches-Silva[4,5,*]**

[1] *Department of Food and Nutrition, National Institute of Health Dr Ricardo Jorge, I.P., Lisbon, Portugal*

[2] *Federal Institute of Education, Science and Techology of Pernambuco, IFPE campus, Vitória de Santo Antão, PE, Brazil*

[3] *Applied Biotechnology Research Center, Baqiyatallah University of Medical Sciences, Tehran 1435916471, Iran*

[4] *National Institute for Agricultural and Veterinary Research (INIAV), Vairão, Vila do Conde, Portugal*

[5] *Center for Study in Animal Science (CECA), ICETA, University of Oporto, Oporto, Portugal*

**Abstract:** Indirect food additives are the additives that are not intended to be added directly to foods but are added to food contact articles namely, food packaging. In this chapter, the main indirect additives are reviewed, as well as, the legal aspects and regulatory control applied to these kinds of substances in the USA and the European Union. The migration of some of these compounds to foods is undesired and, in some cases, may represent a threat to human health. This chapter also highlights some specific groups of indirect additives including monomers, plasticizers, antioxidants and antimicrobials, catalysts, initiators, curing and cross-linking agents, stabilizers, and solvents. Future trends in the use of indirect additives are also discussed in this chapter. Innovative technologies in the food packaging industry are emerging every day, so the regulations and the regulatory agencies must be updated.

**Keywords:** Antimicrobials, Antioxidants, Catalysts, Cross-linking agents, Curing agents, Initiators, Indirect additives, Monomers, Plasticizers, Stabilizers.

## INTRODUCTION

Food contact materials and articles (FCM) comprise a wide variety of materials, including plastic, paper, wood, metals, lacquers, adhesives and printing inks. They can be used as a single material or in combination. (*e.g.*, multilayer multi-mater-

* **Corresponding author Mariana A. Andrade:** National Institute for Agricultural and Veterinary Research (INIAV), Vairão, Vila do Conde, Portugal and Center for Study in Animal Science (CECA), ICETA, University of Oporto, Oporto, Portugal

**Seyed Mohammad Nabavi *et al*. (Eds.)**

ials). A broad number of substances can be used in the manufacture of these materials and they can represent a potential source of food contamination during manufacturing, packaging, preparation, and storage. FCM should comply with legislation and the food industry should implement strict control in order to avoid the violation of the legislation.

The substances used in food-contact articles are also recognized as "indirect additives". Although they can come into contact with food (as part of the processing equipment or the packaging), they are not intended to be added directly to food. The U.S. Food and Drug Administration (FDA) Center for Food Safety and Applied Nutrition (CFSAN) under an ongoing program known as the Priority-based Assessment of Food Additives (PAFA) has a database with administrative and chemical information on over 3000 substances in Title 21 of the U.S. Code of Federal Regulations (21CFR) [1]. Parts 175 to 178 of 21CFR deal with indirect additives, including adhesives and components of coatings (Part 175), paper and paperboard components (Part 176), polymers (Part 177) and adjuvants and production aids (Part 178) [1 - 5]. Additional "indirect" additives can be found in separate inventories when they are effective as part of the food contact substance notification program or that are exempted from regulation as food additives in accordance with 21 CFR 170.39 "Threshold of Regulation (TOR) exemptions for substances used in food-contact articles."

The FDA has a list of approved indirect food additives (continually updated), which includes the identity, intended use, and conditions of use of each authorized substance [1].

In the European Union, there are several binding rules concerning FCM in order to ensure their safety, to facilitate the effective functioning of the internal market and to protect the human health and the Consumer's interest. FCMs should be inert so that their components do not affect consumer health or influence food quality.

EU legislation on FCM includes regulations of general scope, *i.e.*, applied to all types of FCMs and regulations applied only to specific materials or compounds. In the absence of specific rules at the EU level, community legislation can be complemented by the national legislation of the Member States [6]. The safety of FCMs is assessed by the European Food Safety Authority (EFSA). The safety of these materials is tested by the companies placing them in the market and by the competent authorities of the Member States during official controls. The scientific knowledge and technical competence of the methods for testing the safety of FCM are guaranteed by the European Reference Laboratory for Food Contact Materials (EURL-FCM).

Regulation (EC) No 1935/2004 provides for harmonization in the EU with regard to FCM, laying down the general safety principles for these materials. According to Article n° 3 of this regulation, FCM should not transfer chemical substances to foods that might raise food safety concerns, alter food composition, taste and aroma in an unacceptable manner. Due to the possibility of migration of chemicals to food, FCM must be evaluated. This regulation provides special rules for active and intelligent materials (which are not inert by virtue of their concept); the adoption of additional measures at EU level for specific materials; the procedure for conducting tests to assess the safety of FCM; labeling rules indicating which materials are likely to come into contact with food and compliance and traceability documentation. This regulation applies to FCM, including active and intelligent FCM, which in their finished state are: intended to be brought into contact with food, or already brought into contact with food and are intended for that purpose, or can reasonably be expected to be brought into contact with food or to transfer their constituents to food under normal or foreseeable conditions of use. However, the regulation does not apply to FCM which are supplied as antiques, covering or coating materials, such as the materials covering cheese rinds, prepared meat products or fruits, and which form part of the food and may be consumed together with this food nor to fixed public or private water supply equipment.

Regulation (EC) No 2023/2006 (2006) is also transversal to all FCM and concerns good manufacturing practices. According to this regulation: (i) the facilities in which the FCM are manufactured must be appropriate to the purpose and staff should be sensitized to the critical stages of production; quality assurance must be documented and quality control systems must be in place and the raw materials (starting materials) must be suitable for the manufacturing process for safety purposes and the final articles must be inert. Good manufacturing practices must be applied throughout the entire process, although the production of the starting substances is covered by other legislation [7].

## MIGRATION

The evaluation of migration (mass transference of compounds from FCM to foods) is driven by regulation and demands that evaluate all known intentionally added substances (IAS) as well as "unknown" non-intentionally added substances (NIAS). Factors affecting migration include the temperature of contact (higher temperatures increase migration); food type (fatty and acidic foods have an influence on migration); and packaging size (ratio of packaging surface to foodstuff volume).

Although Regulation (EC) No 1935/2004 indicates that specific measures should be established for 17 groups of materials, there are only specific measures to: active and intelligent materials (Regulation EC No 450/2009), ceramic materials (Directive No 84/500/EEC), regenerated cellulose film (Directive No 2007/42/CE), plastics (Regulation EU No 10/2011) and recycled plastic materials (Regulation EC No 282/2008) [6, 8 - 12]. There are also specific rules on certain starting substances used in the production of FCM.

Regulation (EU) No 10/2011 lays down specific rules for the safe use of plastic materials and articles. It repeals Commission Directive 2002/72/EC (2002), which applies to materials and articles consisting exclusively of plastics and plastic liner seals. This regulation is more comprehensive as it applies to (i) materials and articles and parts thereof consisting exclusively of plastics; (ii) materials and articles with multiple layers of plastic (multilayer) bound together by adhesives or other means; (iii) Prior materials and articles (items i and ii) printed and/or covered by a coating; (iv) plastic layers or plastic coatings, forming gaskets in caps and closures, that together with those caps and closures compose a set of two or more layers of different types of materials; (v) plastic layers in multi-material multi-layer materials and articles [11, 13].

This Regulation lays down rules on the composition of plastic FCM and establishes a positive list which includes all substances that are permitted for use in the manufacture of plastic FCM. The Regulation also specifies restrictions on the use of these substances and lays down rules for determining the conformity of plastic materials and articles. This positive list includes monomers and other starting substances; additives other than colorants; polymer production aids, excluding solvents; and macromolecules obtained from microbial fermentation [11].

Moreover, this Regulation establishes two migration limits, the Overall Migration Limit (OML) and the Specific Migration Limit (SML). OML is the maximum permitted amount of non-volatile substances released from a material or article into food simulants (test medium representing the food, its behavior replicates the migration from the plastic FCM). OML is 10 mg/dm$^2$ plastic surface area [11].

On the other hand, SML is the maximum permitted amount of a given substance released from a material or article into food or food simulants. The Total Specific Migration Limit (SML (T)) is the maximum permitted sum of particular substances released in food or food simulants expressed as a total of the moiety of the substances indicated. Not all substances included in the EU positive list contain SML or SML(T). Regulation (EU) No 10/2011 also sets out the food simulants that can be used. Table **1** lists the authorized simulants and the types of food they represent.

**Table 1. Authorized Food simulants according to Regulation (EU) No 10/2011.**

| | Simulants | Foods they represent |
|---|---|---|
| A | Ethanol 10% (v/v) | Foods that have a hydrophilic character |
| B | Acetic acid 3% (w/v) | Foods which have a pH below 4.5 |
| C | Ethanol 20% (v/v) | Alcoholic foods with an alcohol content of up to 20% and those foods which contain a relevant amount of organic ingredients that render the food more lipophilic |
| D1 | Ethanol 50% (v/v) | Foods that have a lipophilic character and for alcoholic foods with an alcohol content of above 20% and for oil in water emulsions |
| D2 | Vegetable oil | Foods that have a lipophilic character and foods which contain free fats at the surface |
| E | Poly(2,6-diphenyl-p-phenylene oxide), particle size 60-80 mesh, pore size 200 nm | Dry foods |

Regulation (EU) No 10/2011 also indicates which simulants represent the food by category of food. The regulation also provides the time and temperature conditions of the migration tests.

Additives which are also authorized as food additives by Regulation (EC) No 1333/2008 or as flavorings by Regulation (EC) No 1334/2008 should not migrate to food in quantities which have a technical effect on the final food and should not [14, 15]:

i. exceed the restrictions laid down in these Regulations or in Annex I of Regulation (EU) No 10/2011 for foods for which they are authorized as food additives or flavoring substances; or

ii. exceed the restrictions laid down in Annex I of this Regulation in foods for which they are not authorized as food additives or flavouring substances.

According to Regulation (EU) No 10/2011, it is also possible to use recognized diffusion models based on scientific evidence to predict migration. These diffusion models are designed to overestimate the actual migration [16, 17].

Regulation (EU) No 10/2011 is being continually updated. Up-to-now there are nine amendments, most of them dealing with the positive list of substances. Based on EFSA scientific reports [18 - 22], the use of some nanoforms (*e.g.* (butadiene, ethyl acrylate, methyl methacrylate, styrene) copolymer; zinc oxide, nanoparticles, uncoated and coated with [3-(methacryloxy)propyl] trimethoxysilane; (methacrylic acid, ethyl acrylate, n-butyl acrylate, methyl methacrylate and butadiene) copolymer; montmorillonite clay modified by dimethyldialkyl(C16-C18)ammonium chloride; zinc oxide, nanoparticles) is permitted according to Regulation (EU) No 10/2011 and its amendments Commission Regulation (EU) No 1282/2011 [23]; Commission Regulation (EU) No 1183/2012 [24]; Commission Regulation (EU) No 202/2014 [25]; Commission Regulation (EU) No 865/2014 [26]; Commission Regulation (EU) No 2015/174 [27]; Commission Regulation (EU) No 2016/1416 [28]; Commission regulation (EU) No 2017/752 [29]; Commission Regulation (EU) No 2018/79 [30].

## MONOMERS

According to the EU Regulation n° 10/2011, a monomer is *"a substance undergoing any type of polymerisation process to manufacture polymers; or a natural or synthetic macromolecular substance used in the manufacture of modified macromolecules; or a substance used to modify existing natural or synthetic macromolecules"* [11]. The positive list of substances included in EU Regulation n° 10/2011, has a column which indicates if the substances can be used as monomers or other initiator substances or as macromolecules obtained by microbial fermentation. Due to the vast number of substances that can be used as monomers, this chapter will only focus on two of them: bisphenol A and glycerol.

Bisphenol A (BPA - 2,2-bis(4-hydroxyphenyl)propane) is a monomer used in food packaging. It is considered an endocrine-disrupting chemical, which has been associated with altered reproductive function in humans, breast cancer, abnormal growth, alterations in immune function and neurodevelopmental delays in children [31]. On the European Regulation, BPA (substance number 151) is authorized to be used as a monomer in plastic packages with a Specific Migration Limit (SML) of 0.05 mg of the substance/kg of food [32]. This monomer is widely used in the manufacturing of epoxy resins and polycarbonate and can be found in most plastic packages such as baby bottles, plastic food containers, coatings of metal cans, medical devices, dental composites and sealants, kitchen utensils and others [33, 34]. BPA, being an endocrine-disrupting chemical, can be a danger to human health, and so the migration of the BPA from containers to foods must be minimal or non-existing. When used in the plastic applications, its chemical structure is submitted to the polymerisation process, which is not always complete, producing residuals monomers of BPA. Not so often, BPA residual monomers can also be derived from the polymer's degradation during the production process or when the package is submitted to high-temperatures or aggressive detergents [35]. Due to these health concerns, the European Commission forbids the use of BPA in the manufacture of polycarbonate infant feeding bottles and drinking cups or bottles intended for infants and young children [32]. Due to the growing concerns about this monomer, the industry tried to substitute this component with other bisphenols (Fig. **1**). Some examples are bisphenol S (4,4'-sulfonyldiphenol, BPS), bisphenol F (4,4'-dihydroxydiphenylmethane, BPF), bisphenol B (2,2-bis(4-hydroxyphenyl)butane, BPB), bisphenol E (1,1-Bis(4-hydroxyphenyl)ethane, BPE), bisphenol AF (4,4'-(hexafluoroisopropylidene)diphenol, BPAF), bisphenol AD (ethylidenebisphenol, BPAD), tetrabromobisphenol A (2,2-bis-(3,5-dibromo-4-hydroxyphenyl)propane, TBBPA), tetramethylbisphenol A (2,2-bis-(3,5-dimeth-l-4-hydroxyphenyl)propane, TMBPA) and 3,3'-dimethylbisphenol A [33, 36].

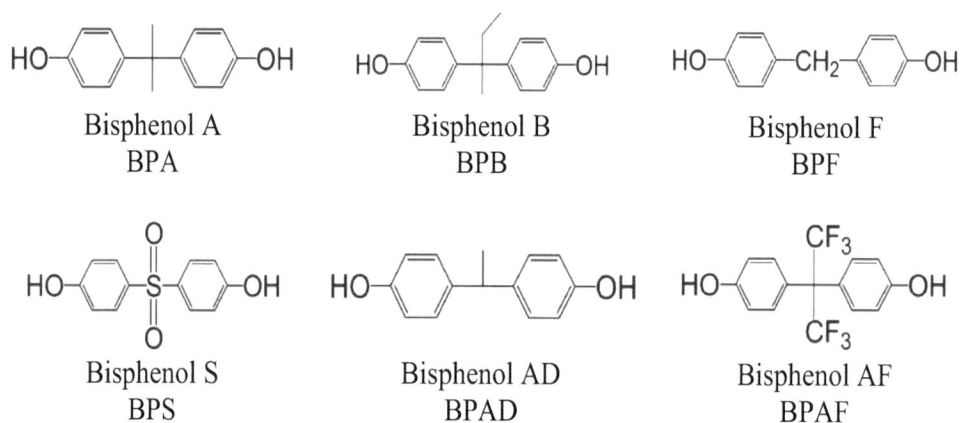

Fig. (1). Chemical structures of BPA, BPB, BPF, BPS, BPAD and BPAF [36].

Regarding their effect in human health, Kitamura *et al.* (2005) reported that BPA and other bisphenols exhibit estrogenic activity in the human breast cancer cell line MCF-7, being the Tetrachlorobisphenol A (2,2-bis-(3,5-dichlo-o-4-hydroxyphenyl)propane), the one with the highest activity, followed by BPB and BPA. Antiestrogenic activity against 17β-estradiol, an important female hormone involved in the estrous and menstrual female reproductive cycle's regulation, was observed in TMBPA and TBBPA. In this study, TCBPA (Tetrachlorobisphenol A (2,2-bis-(3,5-dichloro-4-hydroxyphenyl)propane), TBBPA and BPA presented positive responses in *in vivo* uterotrophic assay in mice [36]. Brede and others (2003) carried out another study to determine the possible migration of BPA from polycarbonate (PC) baby bottles submitted to several washing processes. The authors found that after the first wash, the new bottles exhibited migration levels below 1 µg/L, while the bottles washed in the dishwasher and submitted to brushing and boiling exhibited migration values between 2.5 and 17 µg/L [37]. Howdeshell *et al.* (2003) tested new and used animal cages for a possible BPA migration at room temperature. The authors found that the migration of BPA from the PC cages to water was much higher in the old and used PC cages than in the new ones [38].

Glycerol, substance number 103 with the EEC packaging material reference number 18100 and 55920, is categorized by the European Commission as an additive and also as a monomer [11]. The Food and Drug Administration considers glycerol as a plasticizer [39]. Glycerol can be naturally found in oils and fats and is also an important intermediate in the metabolism of organisms. It can be produced as a by-product of the biodiesel and, due to its chemical and physical characteristics, it is widely applied in food, cosmetic and pharmaceutical industries [40, 41]. Glycerol is normally used in edible coatings in order to improve their flexibility and to overcome the coating's brightness [42]. This monomer and plasticizer are considered safe and also present antibacterial and antiviral properties [43].

## PLASTICIZERS

The vast majority of food packaging is made from plastic since it presents several advantages. The flexibility of the plastic allows a vast number of shapes and forms that best adapt to the food intended to be packaged. Other advantages are the lightweight, low price and great resistance of the plastic: a plastic package can be heated or frozen, printed and sealed in the same production line. Still, this amazing matrix presents light, gases and vapors permeability and the final product presents low molecular weight molecules. These molecules present a major concern because, depending on what the packages hold or the treatment that is submitted (temperature variations, light, aggressive detergents, *etc.*) by the consumers, they can migrate to foods representing a health concern [44].

Plasticizers are substances that are used to increase the plasticity of a certain material. In this chapter, some examples have been focused. Phthalates, or phthalic acid (PA) diesters, are a category of plasticizers, widely used, not only in the food packaging industry but also in cosmetic, pharmaceutical, *etc*. In fact, phthalates are so important in the modern world that the global market for phthalic anhydride ($C_8H_4O_3$ – principal constituent of phthalates) is set to reach the 10 billion USD mark by 2020, because of the increasing plastic demand [45]. The most used phthalates in the world are diisononyl phthalate (bis(7-methyloctyl)benzene-1,2-dicarboxylate, DINP) and diethylhexyl phthalate (bis(2-ethylhexyl) phthalate, DEHP), being the DEHP used in food packaging and listed as "*warranting immediate attention*" by the Environmental Protection Agency (EPA) [45].

Substance number 283 is phthalic acid, bis(2-ethylhexyl) ester (EEC number 74640), with the SML of 1.5 mg/kg, only authorized to be used as *"plasticizer in repeated use materials and articles contacting non-fatty foods"* and as *"technical support agent in concentrations up to 0,1% in the final product"* [11]. This compound is one of the phthalic acid esters (PAEs) which are physically and not chemically bound to a polymeric matrix. This fact makes their migration into the substance of contact easier once in the presence of some factors, such as temperature variations, UV radiation, among others described above [45, 46].

Epoxidized soybean oil (ESBO) is listed as the substance number 532 (EEC number 88640) authorized to be used as additive or polymer production aid. The SML is 60 mg/kg or 30 mg/kg bwt. *"in the case of PVC gaskets used to seal glass jars containing infant formulae and follow-on formulae as defined by Directive 2006/141/EC or processed cereal-based foods and baby foods for infants and young children as defined by Directive 2006/125/EC"* [11]. The ESBO, besides being used as a plasticizer, can be used as a lubricant, a cross-linking agent and a stabilizer [47]. This plasticizer is a biomass-derived resource with the potential of increasing the thermal stability and flexibility of PVC films [48] and also showed good thermal stability and non-flammability and reduced water and oxygen vapor permeabilities of ethyl cellulose films [49].

## ANTIOXIDANTS AND ANTIMICROBIALS

According to the European Commission, a food additive is *"any substance not normally consumed as a food in itself and not normally used as a characteristic ingredient of food, whether or not it has nutritive value, the intentional addition of which to food for a technological purpose in the manufacture, preparation, processing, treatment, packaging, transport or storage of such food results, or may be reasonably expected to result, in it or its by-products becoming directly or indirectly a component of such foods"* [14].

The Regulation N° 1333/2008 distributes the additives for 26 functional groups depending on their action on foods. The antimicrobial agents are placed in the group of "Preservatives". This group, from E200 to E399, contains the food additives that prolong food's shelf-life by protecting them against microorganisms [14, 50].

Benzoic acid and their derivatives (E210-219, E928, and E1519) are widely used food additives with antimicrobial activity. Benzoic acid (E210) is produced by the oxidation of toluene and is present naturally in plants, as an intermediate in the formation of other compounds, and in some animals [50 - 53]. The main benzoic acid salts are sodium benzoate (E211), potassium benzoate and calcium benzoate, besides being used as antimicrobial agents, are commonly used as plasticizers in the manufacturing of plastic of food packaging material [50, 52]. Sodium benzoate is mainly applied in soft drinks, fruit juices, sauces, pickles, edible coatings, seafood products, toothpaste, lotions, creams and some pharmaceutical products [50, 53 - 55].

The use of benzoic acid and its derivatives as food additives is controversial due to the findings of their toxicity. Yadav *et al.* (2016) reported cytotoxicity when applied sodium benzoate to splenocytes at 2500 µg/ml. Noorafshan *et al.* (2014) investigated anxiety and motor impairment in rats treated with sodium benzoate. The authors found that the motor skills of the rats treated with sodium benzoate in the maze were impaired when compared to the control group (without sodium benzoate). These rats also showed higher levels of anxiety than the control group [56]. Other studies found an association with the consumption of sodium benzoate and hyperactivity in children. McCann *et al.* (2007) tested the effect of food colorants and sodium benzoate on 3-years-old and 8/9-years-old children. The authors found adverse effects of the tested food additives on the hyperactive behaviour of the tested children [57]. The effect of sodium benzoate was tested on micronucleus induction and chromosome break in *in vitro* tests at the concentration of 0.5, 1.0, 1.5 and 2.0 mg/ml. The authors concluded that this food additive may have negative effects on human DNA [58].

Nitrates and nitrites (E240-E259) are other groups of antimicrobials mainly used in the meat industry for curing purposes. In the human organism, high concentrations of nitrates can bind to hemoglobin ($Fe^{2+}$) cells, turning them into methemoglobin ($Fe^{3+}$) cells, which are unable to carry oxygen, eventually causing cyanosis, a condition that turns the skin blue [59, 60]. The intake of nitrates and nitrites is also associated with the carcinogenesis promotion [61 - 63]. For these reasons, in Europe, the application of nitrates is only allowed in specific slow curing meats [50]. Regarding nitrites, naturally present in some non-treated fruits and vegetables (spinach, beet, amaranth, *etc.*), they are the only food additive that can prevent the formation of the botulinum toxin from *Clostridium botulinum*. In addition, they are used for the formation of color and inhibit the lipid oxidation of cured meats [50, 64]. Despite these advantages, nitrites lead to the formation of nitrosamines, which are carcinogenic molecules formed in very specific conditions, such as the acidity of the human stomach [50, 64 - 66].

As can be observed, the advantages and disadvantages of the direct application of food additives into foods are not clear. On one side, these additives are low-priced, easy to apply, help to prevent fatal foodborne diseases and can extend food's shelf-life, preventing food spoilage. Although, on the other side, these additives can also be a threat to human health since their effects on long-term exposure are yet to be proven safe. One possible resolution for this problem is the application of active and intelligent food packaging. These types of packaging present advantages when compared to conventional or traditional packages. The intelligent packaging gives the consumer information about one condition of the packaged food, for instance, it indicates if there are leaks in vacuum packaging or informs about the history of temperatures to which the food was submitted. On the contrary, the active packaging interferes directly with the packaged foods, absorbing/emitting substances from/to foods [67, 68].

Packaging with antimicrobial and antioxidant capacity is being developed and tested by several research groups. One of the polymeric matrices with high potential to be applied in active packages is polylactic acid (PLA). This polymer is thermoplastic, biodegradable, biocompatible and has high-strength, high-modulus and good processability [69]. This biodegradable polymer can be obtained from corn starch, sugar cane, tapioca roots and other renewable sources [70]. Rhim *et al.* (2009) tested the tensile, water vapor barrier and antimicrobial properties of a PLA active film incorporated with nanoclay composites. The authors concluded that the PLA with nanoclay composites is less transparent and thicker than the PLA films. The nanoclay composites also had some influence on the water vapour permeability, on the used nanoclay. Regarding the antimicrobial activity, only the PLA with Cloisite 30B presented bacteriostatic activity against *Listeria monocytogenes* [69]. Vilarinho *et al.* (2017) tested the effect of a PLA incorporated with montmorillonite clay on retarding the lipid oxidation of salami slices during several storage periods. The authors found that the montmorillonite clay can inhibit the lipid oxidation of the salami slices for at least 30-days due to their enhanced barrier properties [70]. Jammshidian *et al.* (2011) tested the release to food simulants of natural (ascorbyl palmitate and α-tocopherol) and synthetic (butylated hydroxytoluene, butylated hydroxyanisole, propyl gallate and tert-butylhydroquinone) antioxidants from a PLA film. Only the ascorbyl palmitate presented problems in the film making process, having been completely degraded. The authors considered PLA a good carrier for antioxidants aimed to be released into foods in order to avoid oxidation reactions [71].

Ribeiro-Santos *et al.* (2017) tested the antimicrobial and antioxidant properties of a whey protein film incorporated with a blend of essential oils. The developed active film was able to inhibit *Escherichia coli*, *Staphylococcus aureus* and *Penicillium* sp. using just 5% of the blend in the whey protein film. The antioxidant properties of the films, performed in a fatty food simulant at different temperatures, were higher in all the active films, with 1, 2, 2.7 and 5% of the essential oils blend, when compared with the control active film, showing that the incorporation of essential oils in active food packaging is a possible and viable way to inhibit lipid oxidation and some pathogenic microorganisms [72].

Wen *et al.* (2016) developed a polyvinyl alcohol film with encapsulated cinnamon essential oil containing β-cyclodextrin, through electrospinning technique. The authors encapsulated the cinnamon oil in order to minimize its strong flavor, maintaining its powerful antimicrobial properties. The active film presented good antimicrobial activity against *E. coli* and *S. aureus* and proved to be effective in prolonging shelf-life in strawberries [73].

In another study, Suppakul *et al.* (2008) tested a low-density polyethylene (LDPE) based film with antimicrobial properties. The authors developed two active films applying the extrusion film-blowing technique and incorporated linalool and methylchavicol. The films presented antimicrobial activity against *E. coli* and *Listeria innocua* [74].

## CATALYSTS, INITIATORS, CURING AND CROSS-LINKING AGENTS

Catalysts, initiators, curing and cross-linking agents are the compounds that are more prone to migration from different FCMs to food [75]. Crosslinking is defined as a stabilization process in polymer chemistry, which leads to a multidimensional extension of the polymeric chain resulting in a strong and flexible network structure. Both natural polymers or synthetic polymers can be crosslinked [76]. Crosslink agents or cross-linkers are monomers that link different polymer chains together. They link by covalent or noncovalent bonds, one polymer chain to the other [77]. Adding crosslinks between polymer chains affects the physical properties of the polymer depending upon the degree of cross-linking and presence and absence of crystallinity. Crosslinking results in elasticity, decrease in the viscosity (the resistance to flow), insolubility of the polymer, increase strength, improving mechanical and barrier properties, as well as enhancing water resistance, makes the structure more resistant to heat and light, improves dimensional stability, and chemical and solvent resistance, and may also retard the biodegradation of biopolymeric materials [77 - 79]. Several crosslinking agents are known, being the most commonly used the phosphorous oxychloride (POCl$_3$), sodium trimetaphosphate (STMP), epichlorohydrin (EPI), formaldehyde and carboxylic acids such as citric acid and malic acid, which are preferred as crosslinking agents to crosslink proteins and cellulose because of their relatively low cost, low toxicity, and high ability to improve the desired properties [80, 81]. Packaging polymers may be synthesized by chemical, physical or enzymatic crosslinking (Table **1**). Though, the use of crosslinking agents is avoided in physical crosslinking [82]. Moreover, crosslinkers intended for use in FCMs must present low toxicity.

Regarding initiators, an initiator is a chemical compound that helps trigger (start) a chemical reaction such as free radical polymerization. This reaction is the most common and useful reaction for making polymers, including polystyrene, poly(methyl methacrylate), poly(vinyl acetate) and branched polyethylene, and the whole process starts with an initiator [83]. A large number of free radical initiators are available, they may be classified into thermal initiators and photoinitiators, according to the fact that they form radicals by exposure to heat or under influence of light, respectively [84]. Organic peroxides like a molecule of benzoyl peroxide, or azo compounds like 2,2′-azo- bis-isobutyrylnitrile (AIBN) are widely used as initiators, for many polymerization reactions, because they easily decompose to form free radicals to start the reaction, forming a three-dimensional network. Peroxides and azo compounds dissociate photolytically as well as thermally [84]. The initiating free radical adds (nonradical) monomer units, thereby growing the polymer chain. Initiators are not true catalysts, as they become an integral part of the end product, unlike catalysts [85]. Catalysts are compounds that increase the rate of chemical reactions without themselves being used or incorporated into the finished products. They are used to aid in the polymer formation reaction, helping the monomers join and /or cross-link [75, 83]. Heterogeneous catalysts are mainly metals and metal oxides, while homogeneous catalysts are cations of certain metals or complexes of metal atoms with an organic molecule (ligands) [83]. The most common catalyst used for polymer synthesis is antimony trioxide but gallium, germanium, manganese, cobalt, magnesium, zinc and salts of titanium are also used [86]. In particular, residual organic parts of the organo-metal compounds will remain as breakdown products in the plastic after completion of polymer synthesis and elimination of catalysts [83]. Some catalysts are called initiators and are used to polymerize and crosslink thermoplastics such as polyvinyl chloride (PVC), polystyrene (PS), low-density polyethylene (LDPE), ethylene-vinyl acetate (EVA) and high-density polyethylene (HDPE) [85]. Curing agents are a group of chemicals that cause cross-linking. These chemicals cause the ends of the monomers to join, forming long polymer chains and cross-linkages. They are added to cause polymerization, resulting in a hardened product [85]. Curing of polymers is a process by which liquid reactive polymers of low molecular weight (oligomers) are irreversibly converted into solid, insoluble, and infusible three-dimensional polymers. The term "curing" may apply to the earlier stages of polymerization wherein fluids increase in viscosity prior to gelation and hardening, it is generally used in the processing of plastics, varnishes, adhesives, and sealing compounds. Curing of polymers may involve polycondensation (for example, the curing of phenol-formaldehyde resins) or polymerization (curing of polyester resins). Curing agents may be some type of catalysts (*i.e.*, crosslinkers) or initiators [85]. Organic peroxides are important curing agents. Unsaturated polyester, vinylester and acrylic resins are cured by free radicals, which are formed when organic peroxides decompose [87].

## STABILIZERS

Stabilizers are used to prevent deterioration of mechanical properties of polymeric materials when they are heated, or exposed to ultraviolet radiation. Stabilizers may migrate from different FCM to food [75]. Stabilizers are a necessary additive to unplasticized packaging. Common stabilizers include, carbon black, lead, cadmium, barium, calcium or zinc with epoxides, and salts of tin [88]. Heat stabilizers are abundantly used additives in plastics. They are added to plastics to prevent thermal degradation. Materials such as PVC, PVDC (polyvinylidene chloride), vinyl chloride copolymers (vinyl chloride/vinyl acetate), and polystyrene require the addition of heat stabilizers to retain functionality.

**Table 1. The most commonly used crosslinker agents for specific food contact materials.**

| Packaging | Cross-linking agent | References |
|---|---|---|
| Polysaccharides and proteins films | Aldehydes (formaldehyde and glutaraldehyde) | [79, 97] |
| Proteins films | Phenolic compounds (tannic acid, ferulic acid and gallic acid) | [79, 98] |
| Collagen films | Alginic acid | [79] |
| Polysaccharide films | Carboxylic acid (Citric acid) | [79] |
| PVA film | Boric acid | [99] |
| Proteín | Enzymes transglutaminase | [100] |
| Hydrogel from Protein and gelatin | Glyoxal | [77] |
| Proteins films | Oxidized polysaccharides | [79] |
| Proteins films | Genipin | [101] |
| Wheat Gliadins | Cinnamaldehyde | [102] |
| Polysaccharides and proteins films | Proanthocyanidin | [103] |
| Gelatin | glutaraldehyde (GTA), N-hydroxysuccinimide (NHS), Bis(succinimidyl) nona(ethylene glycol) (BS(PEG)$_9$) and ferulic acid | [104] |
| Whey protein | Formaldehyde and calcium chloride | [105] |
| Sodium alginate film | Calcium ions | [106, 107] |

Poly (vinyl alcohol).

Generally, epoxidized seed and vegetable oils such as ESBO are widely used in a range of food contact plastics heat stabilizers [89]. While light stabilizers protect plastics from degradation due to light and weather exposure. Chimassorb 81 and Tinuvin 770 are examples of UV stabilizes [88].

## SOLVENTS AND OTHER ADDITIVES

During the process of manufacturing, shipping or storage, FCMs might leach residual solvents found in the adhesives, dyes, printing inks or finishes and in other processes involved in manufacturing food packaging materials into the packaged food [90]. These residual solvents include ethanol, isopropanol, isooctane, ethylacetate, cyclohexane, tributyrin, tricaprylin, toluene, methanol, ethanol, methyl ethyl ketone (MEK), isopropyl alcohol (IPA) and acetone [91]. Seo and Shin (2010) reported the results of residual solvents (methanol, ethanol, ethyl acetate, MEK, isopropyl alcohol, acetone and toluene) in 94 food packaging materials. In samples for natural seasoning products consisting of polyethylene (PE), ethanol and isopropyl alcohol were not detected, while in nylon-polyethylene (Ny /PE) the solvents ethanol, IPA, MEK and toluene were not detected. The packaging materials for processed meat products consisted of layers of nylon-ethylene vinylalcohol (NY/EVOH), polypropylene (PP), polyethylene terephthalate (PET), oriented nylon - linear low-density polyethylene (ONY-LLDPE), ethyl acetate was the residual solvent found in all packaging except in PP, in which acetone was found. Packaging materials for food ingredients consisted of layers of NY-LLDPE, ethyl acetate followed MEK found in most of the samples. Ethanol and isopropyl alcohol residual solvents were not found. In packaging materials for synthetic seasoning products produced with an oriented polypropylene-polyethylene (OPP-PE) film, ethyl acetate and IPA were detected. The samples for bakery products were made up of 5 packaging materials, which consisted of layers of carton, oriented polypropylene- oriented polypropylene (OPP-OPP), polyethylene-oriented polypropylene (PE-OPP), corrugated cardboard, and low-density polyethylene (LDPE). MEK and acetone residual solvents were detected in one carton sample. Four samples for bakery ingredients were produced with packaging materials consisting of NY-LLDPE and residual ethanol was detected in two samples. There are various other additives that provide additional properties such as degradation additives that are used to encourage a polymeric material to break down. There are also nucleating/clarifying agents that can be used to increase stiffness, hardness, impact properties, tensile strength, and to control the size and distribution of pores in polymers. Lubricants are also used to get better mixing, extrusion, and calendaring behavior of materials. An internal lubricant is a type of additive that acts by modifying material viscosity [92]. Fatty acid amides, fatty acid esters, metallic stearates and waxes are used as slip additives in plastics as polyolefins, polystyrene and polyvinyl chloride, where they gradually bloom to the surface to act as a lubricant, thus preventing films from sticking together, reducing the coefficient of friction of the surface of a polymer [88, 89]. There are still antifogging agents such as poly(oxyethylene) sorbitan monooleate, which are effectively used in films where condensation of water vapor as small droplets on the inside surface of the plastic film are undesirable [93]. The photoinitiators (PIs) are used as catalyzers for inks and lacquers that are cured with ultraviolet (UV) light. They are components used in the printing of food packaging [94 - 96]. Coupling agents promote chemical links among molecules, they can encourage materials that are normally incompatible to bond together [92].

## CONCLUSION AND FUTURE PERSPECTIVES

The packaging is an utmost component of the food chain. This chapter addressed the main indirect additives, namely monomers, plasticizers, antioxidants and antimicrobials, catalysts, initiators, curing and cross-linking agents, stabilizers and solvents. These indirect additives are used in the manufacture of FCM (IAS or NIAS) and their migration into food has to be monitored due to potentially be responsible for the change in the composition and organoleptic characteristics of the food that might lead to the rejection of goods by the consumers. Moreover, migration can also result in human health concerns as regard to potentially toxic compounds. Therefore, more investigation and further developments are required in this area until it is possible to effectively control the migration of compounds from FCM to foods. Due to the tendency to use new polymers and active packaging, it is likely that the most common food packaging components and contaminants will change drastically in the upcoming few years. Therefore, newer and more sophisticated processing and analytical techniques are required in order to better identify and quantify IAS and NIAS. However, this a great challenge due to the number of compounds implicated, the low migration levels, possible reaction and degradation products, and the increasing number and complexity of materials (*e.g.*, new materials, multilayer and multimaterial food packaging, nano-composites, recycled food packaging). Finally, the regulatory bodies related to FCMs need to keep up-dating the regulation in response to the changes imposed by the industry to guarantee food safety.

## CONSENT FOR PUBLICATION

Not applicable.

## CONFLICT OF INTEREST

All authors declare that there is no conflict of interest.

## ACKNOWLEDGEMENTS

This work was supported by the research project "i.FILM – Multifunctional Films for Intelligent and Active Applications" (no. 17921) cofounded by European Regional Development Fund (FEDER) through the Competitiveness and Internationalization Operational Program under the "Portugal 2020" Program, Call no. 33/SI/2015, Co-Promotion Projects. Mariana Andrade is grateful for their research grant (2016/iFILM/BM) in the frame of the iFILM project.

# REFERENCES

[1]     Food And Drug Administration (FDA). Title 21: Food and Drugs. ECFR — Code Fed Regul 2017. https://www.ecfr.gov/cgi-bin/text-idx?gp=&SID=1504141f8e3e0c667eb1af8a74f9969b&mc=true &tpl=/ecfrbrowse/Title21/21tab_02.tpl

[2]     Food And Drug Administration (FDA). Part 175—Indirect Food Additives: Adhesives and Components of Coating. ECFR — Code Fed Regul 2017. https://www.ecfr.gov/cgi-bin/text-idx?SID=1504141f8e3e0c667eb1af8a74f9969b&mc=true&node=pt21.3.175&rgn=div5

[3]     Food And Drug Administration (FDA). Part 176—Indirect Food Additives: Paper and Paperboard Components. ECFR — Code Fed Regul 2017. https://www.ecfr.gov/cgi-bin/text-idx?SID=1504141 f8e3e0c667eb1af8a74f9969b&mc=true&node=pt21.3.176&rgn=div5

[4]     Food And Drug Administration (FDA). Part 177—Indirect Food Additives: Polymers. ECFR — Code Fed Regul 2017. https://www.ecfr.gov/cgi-bin/text-idx?SID=1504141f8e3e0c667eb1af8a74f9969b &mc=true&node=pt21.3.177&rgn=div5

[5]     Food And Drug Administration (FDA). Part 178—Indirect Food Additives: Adjuvants, Production aids, and Sanitizers. ECFR — Code Fed Regul 2017. https://www.ecfr.gov/cgi-bin/text-idx?SID= 1504141f8e3e0c667eb1af8a74f9969b&mc=true&node=pt21.3.178&rgn=div5

[6]     European Parliament and the Council of the European Union. Regulation (EU) No 1935/2004. Off J. Eur Union 2004; 4-17.

[7]     Comission of the European Communities. Commission Regulation (EC) No 2023/2006. Off J. Eur Union 2006; 75-8.

[8]     Commission of the European Communities. Commission Regulation (EU) No 450/2009. Off J. Eur Union 2009; 3-11.

[9]     Commission of the European Communities. Commission Regulation (EU) No 450/2009. Off J. Eur Union 2009; 3-11.

[10]    Commission of the European Communities. Commission Directive 2007/42/EC. Off J. Eur Union 2007; 71-82.

[11]    European Commission. Commission Regulation (EU) N° 10/2011. Off J. Eur Union 2011; 1-89.

[12]    Commission of the European Communities. Commission Regulation (EC) No 282/2008. Off J. Eur Union 2008; 9-18.

[13]    Commission of the European Communities. Commission Directive 2002/72/EC. Off J. Eur Union 2002; 18-57.

[14]    European Parliament and the Council of the European Union. Regulation (EC) No 1333/2008. Off J. Eur Union 2008; 16-33.

[15]    European Parliament and the Council of the European Union. Regulation (EC) No 1334/2008. Off J. Eur Union 2008; 34-49.

[16]    Silva AS, Freire JMC, Franz R, Losada PP. Mass transport studies of model migrants within dry foodstuffs. J Cereal Sci 2008; 48(3): 662-9.
        [http://dx.doi.org/10.1016/j.jcs.2008.02.006]

[17]    Silva AS, Cruz Freire JM, Sendón R, Franz R, Paseiro Losada P. Migration and diffusion of

diphenylbutadiene from packages into foods. J Agric Food Chem 2009; 57(21): 10225-30.
[http://dx.doi.org/10.1021/jf901666h] [PMID: 19839586]

[18]    CEF. Scientific Opinion on the safety assessment of the substances (butadiene, ethyl acrylate, methyl methacrylate, styrene) copolymer either not crosslinked or crosslinked with divinylbenzene or 1,3-butanediol dimethacrylate, in nanoform, for use in food cont. EFSA J 2014; 12(4): 3635.
[http://dx.doi.org/10.2903/j.efsa.2014.3635]

[19]    CEF. Scientific Opinion on the safety evaluation of the substance zinc oxide, nanoparticles, uncoated and coated with [3-(methacryloxy)propyl] trimethoxysilane, for use in food contact materials. EFSA J 2015; 13(4): 1-9.
[http://dx.doi.org/10.2903/j.efsa.2015.4063]

[20]    CEF. Safety assessment of the substance montmorillonite clay modified by dimethyldialkyl(C16-C18)ammonium chloride for use in food contact materials. EFSA J 2015; 13(11): 4285.
[http://dx.doi.org/10.2903/j.efsa.2015.4285]

[21]    CEF. Scientific Opinion on the safety assessment of the substance (methacrylic acid, ethyl acrylate, n-butyl acrylate, methyl methacrylate and butadiene) copolymer in nanoform for use in food contact materials. EFSA J 2015; 13(2): 1-7.
[http://dx.doi.org/10.2903/j.efsa.2015.4008]

[22]    CEF. Safety assessment of the substance zinc oxide, nanoparticles, for use in food contact materials. EFSA J 2016; 14(3)
[http://dx.doi.org/10.2903/j.efsa.2016.4408]

[23]    European Commission. Commission Regulation (EC) No 1282/2011. Off J. Eur Union 2011; 22-9.

[24]    European Commission. Commission Regulation (EU) No 1183/2012. Off J. Eur Union 2012; 11-5.

[25]    Commission E. Commission Regulation (EU) No 202/2014. Off J. Eur Union 2014; 13-5.

[26]    Commission E. Commission Regulation (EU) No 865/2014. Off J. Eur Union 2014; 1-2.

[27]    European Commission. Commission Regulation (EU) No 2015/174. Off J. Eur Union 2015; 2-9.

[28]    European Commission. Commission Regulation (EU) 2016/1416. Off J. Eur Union 2016; 22-41.

[29]    European Commission. Commission Regulation (EU) 2017/752. Off J. Eur Union 2017; 18-23.

[30]    European Commission. Commission Regulation (EU) 2018/79. Off J. Eur Union 2018; 31-4.

[31]    World Health Organization. Endocrine Disrupting Chemicals (EDCs) 2016. http://www.who.int/ceh/risks/cehemerging2/en/

[32]    Commission E. Commission Regulation (EU) 2018/213. Off J. Eur Union 2018; 6-12.

[33]    García-Córcoles MT, Cipa M, Rodríguez-Gómez R, *et al.* Determination of bisphenols with estrogenic activity in plastic packaged baby food samples using solid-liquid extraction and clean-up with dispersive sorbents followed by gas chromatography tandem mass spectrometry analysis. Talanta 2018; 178: 441-8.
[http://dx.doi.org/10.1016/j.talanta.2017.09.067] [PMID: 29136846]

[34]    Gallo P, Di Marco Pisciottano I, Esposito F, *et al.* Determination of BPA, BPB, BPF, BADGE and BFDGE in canned energy drinks by molecularly imprinted polymer cleaning up and UPLC with fluorescence detection. Food Chem 2017; 220: 406-12.
[http://dx.doi.org/10.1016/j.foodchem.2016.10.005] [PMID: 27855918]

[35]    Geens T, Goeyens L, Covaci A. Are potential sources for human exposure to bisphenol-A overlooked? Int J Hyg Environ Health 2011; 214(5): 339-47.
[http://dx.doi.org/10.1016/j.ijheh.2011.04.005] [PMID: 21570349]

[36]    Kitamura S, Suzuki T, Sanoh S, *et al.* Comparative study of the endocrine-disrupting activity of bisphenol A and 19 related compounds. Toxicol Sci 2005; 84(2): 249-59.
[http://dx.doi.org/10.1093/toxsci/kfi074] [PMID: 15635150]

[37]   Brede C, Fjeldal P, Skjevrak I, Herikstad H. Increased migration levels of bisphenol A from polycarbonate baby bottles after dishwashing, boiling and brushing. Food Addit Contam 2003; 20(7): 684-9.
[http://dx.doi.org/10.1080/0265203031000119061] [PMID: 12888395]

[38]   Howdeshell KL, Peterman PH, Judy BM, *et al.* Bisphenol A is released from used polycarbonate animal cages into water at room temperature. Environ Health Perspect 2003; 111(9): 1180-7.
[http://dx.doi.org/10.1289/ehp.5993] [PMID: 12842771]

[39]   Food And Drug Administration (FDA). 21CFR181.27. Title 21 Food Drugs 2017.

[40]   Xue L-L, Chen H-H, Jiang J-G. Implications of glycerol metabolism for lipid production. Prog Lipid Res 2017; 68: 12-25.
[http://dx.doi.org/10.1016/j.plipres.2017.07.002] [PMID: 28778473]

[41]   Christoph R, Schmidt B, Steinberner U, Dilla W, Karinen R. Glycerol Ullmann's Encycl Ind Chem 2006.
[http://dx.doi.org/10.1002/14356007.a12_477.pub2]

[42]   Senturk Parreidt T, Schott M, Schmid M, Müller K. Effect of Presence and Concentration of Plasticizers, Vegetable Oils, and Surfactants on the Properties of Sodium-Alginate-Based Edible Coatings. Int J Mol Sci 2018; 19(3): 742.
[http://dx.doi.org/10.3390/ijms19030742] [PMID: 29509669]

[43]   Zidan SM, Eleowa SA. Banking and use of glycerol preserved full-thickness skin allograft harvested from body contouring procedures. Burns 2014; 40(4): 641-7.
[http://dx.doi.org/10.1016/j.burns.2013.08.039] [PMID: 24070848]

[44]   Marsh K, Bugusu B. Food packaging--roles, materials, and environmental issues. J Food Sci 2007; 72(3): R39-55.
[http://dx.doi.org/10.1111/j.1750-3841.2007.00301.x] [PMID: 17995809]

[45]   Benjamin S, Masai E, Kamimura N, Takahashi K, Anderson RC, Faisal PA. Phthalates impact human health: Epidemiological evidences and plausible mechanism of action. J Hazard Mater 2017; 340: 360-83.
[http://dx.doi.org/10.1016/j.jhazmat.2017.06.036] [PMID: 28800814]

[46]   González-Sálamo J, Socas-Rodríguez B, Hernández-Borges J. Analytical methods for the determination of phthalates in food. Curr Opin Food Sci 2018; 22: 122-36.
[http://dx.doi.org/10.1016/j.cofs.2018.03.002]

[47]   Pantone V, Laurenza AG, Annese C, Fracassi F, Fusco C, Nacci A, *et al.* Methanolysis of epoxidized soybean oil in continuous flow conditions. Ind Crops Prod 2017; 109: 1-7.
[http://dx.doi.org/10.1016/j.indcrop.2017.08.001]

[48]   Bueno-Ferrer C, Garrigós MC, Jiménez A. Characterization and thermal stability of poly(vinyl chloride) plasticized with epoxidized soybean oil for food packaging. Polym Degrad Stabil 2010; 95(11): 2207-12.
[http://dx.doi.org/10.1016/j.polymdegradstab.2010.01.027]

[49]   Yang D, Peng X, Zhong L, *et al.* "Green" films from renewable resources: properties of epoxidized soybean oil plasticized ethyl cellulose films. Carbohydr Polym 2014; 103: 198-206.
[http://dx.doi.org/10.1016/j.carbpol.2013.12.043] [PMID: 24528720]

[50]   Carocho M, Barreiro MF, Morales P, Ferreira ICFR. Adding Molecules to Food, Pros and Cons: A Review on Synthetic and Natural Food Additives. Compr Rev Food Sci Food Saf 2014; 13(4): 377-99.
[http://dx.doi.org/10.1111/1541-4337.12065]

[51]   World Health Organization. Concise International Chemical Assessment Document 26: Benzoic Acid and Sodium Benzoate 2000.

[52]   Del Olmo A, Calzada J, Nuñez M. Benzoic acid and its derivatives as naturally occurring compounds

in foods and as additives: Uses, exposure, and controversy. Crit Rev Food Sci Nutr 2017; 57(14): 3084-103.
[http://dx.doi.org/10.1080/10408398.2015.1087964] [PMID: 26587821]

[53]    Commission Regulation (EU) No 1129/2011. Off J. Eur Union 2011; 1-177.

[54]    Saltmarsh M. Recent trends in the use of food additives in the United Kingdom. J Sci Food Agric 2015; 95(4): 649-52.
[http://dx.doi.org/10.1002/jsfa.6715] [PMID: 24789520]

[55]    Yadav A, Kumar A, Das M, Tripathi A. Sodium benzoate, a food preservative, affects the functional and activation status of splenocytes at non cytotoxic dose. Food Chem Toxicol 2016; 88: 40-7.
[http://dx.doi.org/10.1016/j.fct.2015.12.016] [PMID: 26706697]

[56]    Noorafshan A, Erfanizadeh M, Karbalay-Doust S. Sodium benzoate, a food preservative, induces anxiety and motor impairment in rats. Neurosciences (Riyadh) 2014; 19(1): 24-8.
[PMID: 24419445]

[57]    McCann D, Barrett A, Cooper A, *et al.* Food additives and hyperactive behaviour in 3-year-old and 8/9-year-old children in the community: a randomised, double-blinded, placebo-controlled trial. Lancet 2007; 370(9598): 1560-7.
[http://dx.doi.org/10.1016/S0140-6736(07)61306-3] [PMID: 17825405]

[58]    Pongsavee M. Effect of sodium benzoate preservative on micronucleus induction, chromosome break, and Ala40Thr superoxide dismutase gene mutation in lymphocytes. BioMed Res Int 2015; 2015103512
[http://dx.doi.org/10.1155/2015/103512] [PMID: 25785261]

[59]    Knobeloch L, Salna B, Hogan A, Postle J, Anderson H. Blue babies and nitrate-contaminated well water. Environ Health Perspect 2000; 108(7): 675-8.
[http://dx.doi.org/10.1289/ehp.00108675] [PMID: 10903623]

[60]    Inetianbor JE, Yakubu JM, Ezeonu SC. Effects of Food Additives and Preservatives on Man - a Review. Asian J Sci Technol 2015; 6(2): 1118-35.

[61]    Sanchez-Echaniz J, Benito-Fernández J, Mintegui-Raso S. Methemoglobinemia and consumption of vegetables in infants. Pediatrics 2001; 107(5): 1024-8.
[http://dx.doi.org/10.1542/peds.107.5.1024] [PMID: 11331681]

[62]    Sarasua S, Savitz DA. Cured and broiled meat consumption in relation to childhood cancer: Denver, Colorado (United States). Cancer Causes Control 1994; 5(2): 141-8.
[http://dx.doi.org/10.1007/BF01830260] [PMID: 8167261]

[63]    Volkmer BG, Ernst B, Simon J, *et al.* Influence of nitrate levels in drinking water on urological malignancies: a community-based cohort study. BJU Int 2005; 95(7): 972-6.
[http://dx.doi.org/10.1111/j.1464-410X.2005.05450.x] [PMID: 15839916]

[64]    Sindelar JJ, Milkowski AL. Human safety controversies surrounding nitrate and nitrite in the diet. Nitric Oxide 2012; 26(4): 259-66.
[http://dx.doi.org/10.1016/j.niox.2012.03.011] [PMID: 22487433]

[65]    Carocho M, Morales P, Ferreira ICFR. Natural food additives: Quo vadis? Trends Food Sci Technol 2015; 45(2): 284-95.
[http://dx.doi.org/10.1016/j.tifs.2015.06.007]

[66]    Additives. Watson DH, Ed. Food chemical safety.Cambridge, England: Woodhead Publishing Limited 2001; 2.

[67]    Dainelli D, Gontard N, Spyropoulos D, Zondervan-van den Beuken E, Tobback P. Active and intelligent food packaging: legal aspects and safety concerns. Trends Food Sci Technol 2008; 19: S103-12.
[http://dx.doi.org/10.1016/j.tifs.2008.09.011]

[68] Coles R, McDowell D, Kirwan MJ, Eds. Food Packaging Technology. Blackwell Publishing Ltd 2003.

[69] Rhim J-W, Hong S-I, Ha C-S. Tensile, water vapor barrier and antimicrobial properties of PLA/nanoclay composite films. Lebensm Wiss Technol 2009; 42(2): 612-7.
[http://dx.doi.org/10.1016/j.lwt.2008.02.015]

[70] Vilarinho F, Andrade M, Buonocore GG, Stanzione M, Vaz MF, Sanches Silva A. Monitoring lipid oxidation in a processed meat product packaged with nanocomposite poly(lactic acid) film. Eur Polym J 2018; 98: 362-7.
[http://dx.doi.org/10.1016/j.eurpolymj.2017.11.034]

[71] Jamshidian M, Tehrany EA, Desobry S. Antioxidants Release from Solvent-Cast PLA Film: Investigation of PLA Antioxidant-Active Packaging. Food Bioprocess Technol 2013; 6(6): 1450-63.
[http://dx.doi.org/10.1007/s11947-012-0830-9]

[72] Ribeiro-Santos R, Sanches-Silva A, Motta JFG, Andrade M, Neves I de A, Teófilo RF, *et al.* Combined use of essential oils applied to protein base active food packaging: Study in vitro and in a food simulant. Eur Polym J 2017; 93: 75-86.
[http://dx.doi.org/10.1016/j.eurpolymj.2017.03.055]

[73] Wen P, Zhu D-H, Wu H, Zong M-H, Jing Y-R, Han S-Y. Encapsulation of cinnamon essential oil in electrospun nanofibrous film for active food packaging. Food Control 2016; 59: 366-76.
[http://dx.doi.org/10.1016/j.foodcont.2015.06.005]

[74] Suppakul P, Sonneveld K, Bigger SW, Miltz J. Efficacy of polyethylene-based antimicrobial films containing principal constituents of basil. Lebensm Wiss Technol 2008; 41(5): 779-88.
[http://dx.doi.org/10.1016/j.lwt.2007.06.006]

[75] Sendón R, Sanches-Silva A. Packaging: A Noteworthy Feature in Food Safety.Food Toxicol. 1st ed.. CRC Press, Taylor & Francis Group 2017; pp. 461-90.

[76] Schultes SE. Milady's Standard: Nail Technology. 4th ed., Delmar Learning 2004.

[77] Maitra J, Shukla VK. Cross-linking in Hydrogels - A Review. Am J Pol Sci 2014; 4(2): 25-31.
[http://dx.doi.org/10.5923/j.ajps.20140402.01]

[78] Balaguer MP, Cerisuelo JP, Gavara R, Hernandez-Muñoz P. Mass transport properties of gliadin films: Effect of cross-linking degree, relative humidity, and temperature. J Membr Sci 2013; 428: 380-92.
[http://dx.doi.org/10.1016/j.memsci.2012.10.022]

[79] Azeredo HMC, Waldron KW. Crosslinking in polysaccharide and protein films and coatings for food contact – A review. Trends Food Sci Technol 2016; 52: 109-22.
[http://dx.doi.org/10.1016/j.tifs.2016.04.008]

[80] Reddy N, Li Y, Yang Y. Alkali-catalyzed low temperature wet crosslinking of plant proteins using carboxylic acids. Biotechnol Prog 2009; 25(1): 139-46.
[http://dx.doi.org/10.1002/btpr.86] [PMID: 19224570]

[81] Hirsch JB, Kokini JL. Understanding the Mechanism of Cross-Linking Agents (POCl 3, STMP, and EPI) Through Swelling Behavior and Pasting Properties of Cross-Linked Waxy Maize Starches. Cereal Chem J 2002; 79(1): 102-7.
[http://dx.doi.org/10.1094/CCHEM.2002.79.1.102]

[82] Patil S, Jadge D. Crosslinking Of Polysaccharides: Methods And Applications. Pharm Rev 2008; 6.

[83] Brandsch J, Piringer O. Characteristics of plastic materials Plast Packag Mater Food. 9-45. n.d.

[84] Su W-F. Principles of Polymer Design and Synthesis. Berlin, Heidelberg: Springer Berlin Heidelberg 2013; Vol. 82.
[http://dx.doi.org/10.1007/978-3-642-38730-2]

[85] Lokensgard E. Industrial Plastics: Theory and Applications. 6th ed., Cengage Learning 2016.

[86]    International Life Sciences Institute. Polyethylene terephthalate (PET) for food packaging applications 2000.

[87]    Burton B. Amine Curing of Epoxy Resins: Options and Key Formulation Considerations. Paint Coatings Ind 2006; 22: 68-77.

[88]    Bhunia K, Sablani SS, Tang J, Rasco B. Migration of Chemical Compounds from Packaging Polymers during Microwave, Conventional Heat Treatment, and Storage. Compr Rev Food Sci Food Saf 2013; 12: 523-45.
        [http://dx.doi.org/10.1111/1541-4337.12028]

[89]    Lau O-W, Wong S-K. Contamination in food from packaging material. J Chromatogr A 2000; 882(1-2): 255-70.
        [http://dx.doi.org/10.1016/S0021-9673(00)00356-3] [PMID: 10895950]

[90]    Helmroth IE. Release of additives from packaging plastics. The Netherlands: Wageningen University 2002.

[91]    Seo I, Shin H-S. Determination of toluene and other residual solvents in various food packaging materials by gas chromatography/mass spectrometry (GC/MS). Food Sci Biotechnol 2010; 19: 1429-34.
        [http://dx.doi.org/10.1007/s10068-010-0204-x]

[92]    Fox J. Analysis of Polymer Additives in the Packaging Industry. Univ Florida 2008.

[93]    Piringer OG, Baner AL, Eds. Plastic Packaging. 2008.
        [http://dx.doi.org/10.1002/9783527621422]

[94]    Sanches-Silva A, Andre C, Castanheira I, *et al.* Study of the migration of photoinitiators used in printed food-packaging materials into food simulants. J Agric Food Chem 2009; 57(20): 9516-23.
        [http://dx.doi.org/10.1021/jf8035758] [PMID: 19807101]

[95]    Van Den Houwe K, Evrard C, Van Loco J, Lynen F, Van Hoeck E. Migration of photoinitiators from cardboard into dry food: evaluation of Tenax ® as a food simulant. Food Addit Contam Part A Chem Anal Control Expo Risk Assess 2016; 33(5): 913-20.
        [http://dx.doi.org/10.1080/19440049.2016.1179562] [PMID: 27146794]

[96]    Cai H, Ji S, Zhang J, *et al.* Migration kinetics of four photo-initiators from paper food packaging to solid food simulants. Food Addit Contam Part A Chem Anal Control Expo Risk Assess 2017; 34(9): 1632-42.
        [http://dx.doi.org/10.1080/19440049.2017.1331470] [PMID: 28597726]

[97]    Rimdusit S, Jingjid S, Damrongsakkul S, Tiptipakorn S, Takeichi T. Biodegradability and property characterizations of Methyl Cellulose: Effect of nanocompositing and chemical crosslinking. Carbohydr Polym 2008; 72: 444-55.
        [http://dx.doi.org/10.1016/j.carbpol.2007.09.007]

[98]    Cao N, Fu Y, He J. Mechanical properties of gelatin films cross-linked, respectively, by ferulic acid and tannin acid. Food Hydrocoll 2007; 21: 575-84.
        [http://dx.doi.org/10.1016/j.foodhyd.2006.07.001]

[99]    Miyazaki T, Takeda Y, Akane S, Itou T, Hoshiko A, En K. Role of boric acid for a poly (vinyl alcohol) film as a cross-linking agent: Melting behaviors of the films with boric acid. Polymer (Guildf) 2010; 51: 5539-49.
        [http://dx.doi.org/10.1016/j.polymer.2010.09.048]

[100]   Buchert J, Ercili Cura D, Ma H, *et al.* Crosslinking food proteins for improved functionality. Annu Rev Food Sci Technol 2010; 1: 113-38.
        [http://dx.doi.org/10.1146/annurev.food.080708.100841] [PMID: 22129332]

[101]   Butler MF, Ng Y-F, Pudney PDA. Mechanism and kinetics of the crosslinking reaction between biopolymers containing primary amine groups and genipin. J Polym Sci A Polym Chem 2003; 41:

3941-53.
[http://dx.doi.org/10.1002/pola.10960]

[102] Balaguer MP, Gómez-Estaca J, Gavara R, Hernandez-Munoz P. Biochemical properties of bioplastics made from wheat gliadins cross-linked with cinnamaldehyde. J Agric Food Chem 2011; 59(24): 13212-20.
[http://dx.doi.org/10.1021/jf203055s] [PMID: 22047158]

[103] Kim S, Nimni ME, Yang Z, Han B. Chitosan/gelatin-based films crosslinked by proanthocyanidin. J Biomed Mater Res B Appl Biomater 2005; 75(2): 442-50.
[http://dx.doi.org/10.1002/jbm.b.30324] [PMID: 16047322]

[104] Biscarat J, Charmette C, Sanchez J, Pochat-Bohatier C. Development of a new family of food packaging bioplastics from cross-linked gelatin based films. Can J Chem Eng 2015; 93: 176-82.
[http://dx.doi.org/10.1002/cjce.22077]

[105] Galietta G, Di Gioia L, Guilbert S, Cuq B. Mechanical and Thermomechanical Properties of Films Based on Whey Proteins as Affected by Plasticizer and Crosslinking Agents. J Dairy Sci 1998; 81: 3123-30.
[http://dx.doi.org/10.3168/jds.S0022-0302(98)75877-1]

[106] Sánchez LCA, Real CPV, Perez YB. Effect of an edible crosslinked coating and two types of packaging on antioxidant capacity of castilla blackberries. Food Sci Technol 2014; 34: 281-6.
[http://dx.doi.org/10.1590/fst.2014.0047]

[107] Russo R, Malinconico M, Santagata G. Effect of cross-linking with calcium ions on the physical properties of alginate films. Biomacromolecules 2007; 8(10): 3193-7.
[http://dx.doi.org/10.1021/bm700565h] [PMID: 17803277]

# CHAPTER 14

# Relation of Food Additives with Adverse Health Effects

**Devesh Tewari[1,*], Pooja Patni[2], Sweta Bawari[3] and Archana N. Sah[4]**

[1] *Department of Pharmacognosy, School of Pharmaceutical Sciences, Lovely Professional University, Phagwara, 144411, Punjab, India*

[2] *School of Pharmaceutical Sciences, Lovely Professional University, Phagwara 144411, Punjab, India*

[3] *Department of Pharmaceutical Sciences, Faculty of Technology, Bhimtal Campus, Kumaun University Nainital,263136, Uttarakhand, India*

[4] *School of Pharmacy, Sharda University, Knowledge Park-III, Greater Noida, Uttar Pradesh, 201310, India*

**Abstract:** Food additives are widely used by the food industries for attracting a larger number of consumers by making the food more appealing. Some of the food additives which are used by the food industries are bulking agents, emulsifiers, food colorants, flavoring agents, preservatives, and sweeteners. Despite the beneficial effects of food additives, these additives can also cause serious adverse effects on humans. Some of the most common adverse events include anaphylaxis, asthma, urticaria and/or angioedema. In this chapter, we describe the adverse health events that are caused as a result of different food additives with special reference to allergic, immunologic reactions, asthma, autoimmune diseases, cancer, diabetes and metabolic disorders. Although the animal and *in vitro* studies that examined the adverse health effects of different food additives are available, the clinical studies which examined the adverse health effects of different food additives in a large population group are very limited.

**Keywords:** Artificial additives, Immune response health effects.

## OVERVIEW

Several food additives are utilized in the food industry to enhance the taste and appearance of the food in addition to enhancing the product shelf life. This adds variety and makes food appealing for consumers. Food additives are generally categorized into natural and synthetic types, which include bulking agents, emulsifiers, food colorants, flavoring agents, preservatives, sweeteners, *etc.* Fig. **(1)**.

---

* **Corresponding author Devesh Tewari:** Department of Pharmacognosy, School of Pharmaceutical Sciences, Lovely Professional University, Phagwara, 144411, Punjab, India; Tel: +91-8826235352; E-mail: dtewari3@gmail.com

**Seyed Mohammad Nabavi *et al.* (Eds.)**

Despite the common and wide uses of food additives, their hypersensitivity and other adverse reactions due to food additives are also being reported. Some common adverse reactions from these additives are anaphylaxis, asthma, urticaria and angioedema [1]. The consumption of the food additives can be well understood by an estimation, which suggests that around 10,000 chemicals are added in the food either directly or indirectly as food additives in the USA alone [2, 3]. The literature confirms that most of the adverse events occur due to the use of preservatives, coloring agents and emulsifiers. However, clinical studies in a large population addressing the adverse events that occur as a result of food additives are limited.

The food additives are labelled as E-numbers in the European markets and Switzerland (EU commission, 2011 Regulation EU 1333/2008 on food additives). This means that the food package having E-numbers is indicative of the presence of food additives, and is provided in place of its chemical name [4]. It is also perceived that a product having E- numbers is believed to be less natural in comparison to the product containing identical food additives with the chemical name present in the list of ingredients [4, 5].

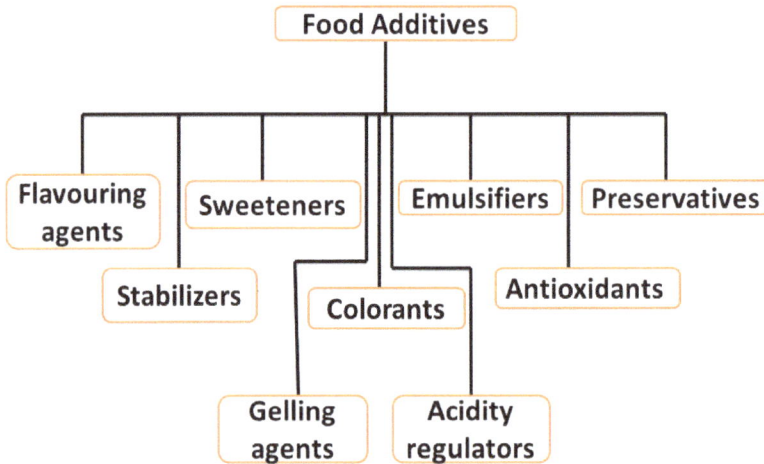

**Fig. (1).** Types of food additives used in different food industries.

In this chapter, we describe the adverse health events that are caused as a result of different food additives with special reference to allergic and immunologic reactions, asthma, autoimmune diseases, cancer, diabetes and metabolic disorders.

## ALLERGIC AND IMMUNOLOGIC REACTIONS

A food colorant is used to color food, making it more appealing. Food colorants are the most important and widely used food additives. Both natural and synthetic food colorants are used to color food. Although natural colorants are the preference of the consumer, synthetic colorants are mainly used by the food industries due to their stability, low price and color strength. Some of the main food colorants include Amaranth, Annatto, Allura Red, Brilliant Blue, Carmine, Erythrosine, Indigotine, Patent Blue, Ponceau 4R, Saffron, Sunset Yellow, Tartrazine, and Turmeric [6].

The food colorants have been reported to exhibit hypersensitivity reactions, which are mainly immune triggered like immediate and delayed type hypersensitivity reactions [7]. Moreover, it is a common belief that these food colorants can produce immune-mediated allergic reactions ranging from urticaria, asthma to anaphylactic shock, often in children [7]. Depending upon their mechanism, the allergic reactions due to additives may be classified as IgE mediated, cell-mediated (non IgE mediated) and mixed IgE/non- IgE-mediated reactions [8]. Several studies have been conducted to understand the prevalence of pseudoallergic reactions globally. A study conducted in Germany by double-blind, placebo-controlled food challenge tests (DBPCFC) on the adult population showed a 0.18% prevalence of pseudoallergic reactions to food additives [9]. Another study showed less than 1% prevalence of food additive sensitivity when evaluated in 100 adult patients with chronic idiopathic urticaria [10]. Similar to the colorants, food preservatives are also a common cause of contact dermatitis and contact allergy. Some preservatives showed adverse health events in females from Singapore in a more frequent manner than in males [11].

## ASTHMA

Food preservatives and colorants have also been correlated to the asthma incidences [12]. It has been reported by the scientific panel of the European Food Safety Authority (EFSA) that allergic reactions such as asthma and urticaria may be produced by Allura Red either alone or more when used in combination with other synthetic coloring agents [13, 14].

The rate of aggravation of asthma in asthmatics by different food additives was believed to be approximately 23-67% of asthmatics. However, double-blind placebo control trials showed the prevalence rate of asthma exacerbations by food additives of less than 5%. The data is available on the implication of monosodium glutamate (MSG), sulphites, and tartrazine in asthma exacerbations [15].

Numerous forms of sulphites are used in food and pharmaceutical industries as additives including inorganic sulfite salts, sodium or potassium metabisulphites ($Na_2S_2O_5$ or $K_2S_2O_5$), sulfur dioxide ($SO_2$), sodium or potassium sulphite ($Na_2S_2O_3$ or $K_2S_2O_3$) and sodium or potassium bisulphite ($NaHSO_3$ or $KHSO_3$). A double-blind trial showed the prevalence of sulphite sensitivity of 0.8% in non-steroid dependent asthmatics and about 8.4% in severe asthmatics [15, 16]. It is an estimate that there is a 3-10% prevalence of sulphite sensitivity in adult asthmatics, which is higher in the moderate-to-severe persistent asthmatics [17].

## AUTOIMMUNE DISEASES

Literature suggested that it is believed by around 30% of patients that their food might cause chronic urticaria. More specifically, a diet rich in natural histamine, spices and seasonings can aggravate the symptoms [18, 19]. Contrarily, in patients with chronic urticaria, food allergies are thought to be rare clinically [20] and some of the agents such as MSG, benzoate, aspartame, salicylate, nitrites and some coloring agents are believed to be responsible for the food reactions [1]. It has also been reported that at least a few chronic urticaria patients had food additives associated symptoms when evaluated by the basophil activation test [21]. Some of the food additives such as prebiotics and probiotics also possess beneficial health effects. Such food additives influence gut microbiota either directly or indirectly and their beneficial effects for the well-being of the host health are well described [22, 23].

## CANCER

In animal studies, altered kidney and liver functions and oxidative stress biomarkers were observed after the intake of tartrazine and azorubine [24]. Reports are also available on the DNA damaging effect of the red food dyes [25]. The food colorants may also arbitrate during the multistep process of carcinogenesis and inflammation which is indicated by the higher tissue concentration of enzymes that are involved in the oxidative mechanism [26]. Some preservatives and coloring agents also showed mutagenic, clastogenic, and cytotoxic effects when observed on human lymphocytes *in vitro* and thus have been inferred to have the potential to cause cancer [27 - 29]. Raposa *et al.* demonstrated that some food additives, more specifically, preservatives and colorants, play a role in the activation of inflammatory pathways. Furthermore, they emphasized on the limited use of preservatives and colorants in the diet [26].

Saccharin, a well-known artificial sweetener, was also reported to be positively associated with the risk of bladder cancer in males [30], however, epidemiological studies in humans did not confirm the bladder cancer-producing effects of saccharin [31]. Therefore, preservatives, colorants and artificial sweeteners have been reported as causative agents of different types of cancer in general, but as far as saccharine is concerned, extensive clinical studies are required.

## DIABETES

Studies conducted in Britain have shown that over half of the population is preferably consuming foodstuffs containing artificial sweetening agents, which are also due to the preference of the consumption of low calorie foods by the general population [32]. The consumption of artificial sweetening agents was also studied in other countries such as Norway and Italy [33, 34] and it was found that the intake of artificial sweeteners was relatively low in these countries.

Different nutrients and food additives such as carbohydrates, nitrosamine compounds and proteins possess the risk of influencing the development of insulin-dependent diabetes in childhood [35]. Another widely utilized food additive is the emulsifier polysorbate-80, which is a ubiquitous constituent of processed foods. It has been shown to enhance the bacterial translocation across the epithelia when observed *in vitro* [36]. Two main commonly used emulsifiers, polysorbate-80 and carboxymethylcellulose in low concentrations, were demonstrated to induce obesity/metabolic syndrome and robust colitis in mice [37]. The metabolic syndrome, which is induced by emulsifiers, is generally considered to be associated with the encroachment of microbiota, enhanced pro-inflammatory potential and change in species composition [37].

Artificial sweeteners are mainly associated with weight gain and metabolic syndromes. Several epidemiological and large scale surveys revealed that there is some sort of a relationship between the consumption of artificial sweeteners and an increase in the body weight or body mass index (BMI) [38 - 41]. Studies are also available on the connection between the consumption of artificial sweeteners and insulin resistance, poor control of glucose in pre-existing diabetic patients and cases of type 2 diabetes [42, 43]. On the other hand, some studies have reported no association of the artificial sweeteners with the incidences of diabetes or glycemic control [44, 45]. The consumption of soft drinks containing artificial sweeteners seems to be escalating in children [46 - 49]. Brown *et al.*, (2010) found a positive relationship between diabetes and the intake of artificial sweeteners in children.

# HYPERKINESIS

The use of food coloring with natural substances as food colorants in ancient Egypt dates back to 1500 B.C., and the regulation to avoid the unsafe and fraudulent use of the food colorants was known since the time of England's King Edward I during the 13th century [51]. The effect of artificial food colorants in the impairment of learning and behavior due to hypersensitivity has been reported in the 1920s [52]. At the annual meeting of the American Medical Association in 1973, a communication was presented by Dr. Benjamin Feingold based upon his own clinical observations, which proposed that the learning problems and pediatric hyperactivity were caused by certain foods and food additives. He also believed that his patients were sensitive towards the food having artificial food colorants, flavors and natural salicylates and therefore, he recommended the diet without these substances [53, 54]. Though Feingold's presentation initially gained extensive media and public attention, however, his work was also criticized by different health professionals [55, 56] and the food industry also reported in 1975 that "no controlled studies have demonstrated that hyperkinesis is related to the ingestion of food additives" [57].

There are reports on some of the artificial colorants such as tartrazine and azorubine that have shown some hyperactivity disorders and attention deficit in children and teenagers [58, 59]. The study by McCann *et al.* reported that artificial colors or sodium benzoate preservatives either used alone or in combination in the diet resulted in the hyperactivity reactions in 3-year and 8 to 9-year-old children [60]. However, EFSA has rejected the suggestions of the study of McCann and co-workers. Though the agency also accepted that the findings may be relevant for some specific groups of people in some populations, but it is not possible to access the overall prevalence in the general populations based on those data [61].

Some reports of various food additives on their health risk assessment are summarized in Table **1**.

Table 1. Food additives with reports on their health risk assessment.

| S. No. | Food Additive | Adverse Effect | Type of Study | References |
|---|---|---|---|---|
| 1. | Sweeteners | | | |
| | Aspartame | Distortion of mood, depression and impairment of cognition | Crossover study in patients of unipolar depression; Double-blind, repeated measures study in healthy adults | [62, 63] |

*(Table 1) cont.....*

| S. No. | Food Additive | Adverse Effect | Type of Study | References |
|---|---|---|---|---|
| | Saccharin | Glucose intolerance | Preclinical study in male C57Bl/6 mice | [64] |
| | Sucralose | Distortion of gut microflora and chronic hepatic inflammation | Preclinical study in male C57Bl/6 mice | [65] |
| **2.** | **Preservatives** | | | |
| | Sodium benzoate | Behavioral changes and hyperactivity; Cytotoxicity and mutagenicity | Double-blind, crossover study in 4 yrs old children; *In vitro* study on ATCC PCS-800-013 human lymphocytes | [58, 66] |
| | Sodium sorbate | Genotoxicity | *In vitro* study on human lymphocytes | [67] |
| **3.** | **Colorants** | | | |
| | Tartrazine | Restlessness, irritability, sleep disturbances and hyperactivity | Double-blind, repeated measures, placebo controlled study in healthy children (2-14 yrs in age) | [68] |
| | Sunset yellow | Hepatotoxicity; Genotoxicity | Preclinical study in Swiss albino rats; *Brassica campestris L.* meristematic cells | [69, 70] |
| | Metanil yellow | Hepatotoxicity | Preclinical study in Swiss albino rats | [69] |
| **4.** | **Emulsifiers** | | | |
| | Carboxymethyl-cellulose | Aberrations in microbiota resulting in intestinal inflammation, anxiety | Preclinical study in wild type C57Bl/6 mice, Tlr5[-l-] and Il10[-l-] engineered mice | [37, 71] |
| | Polysorbate-80 | Aberrations in microbiota resulting in intestinal inflammation, anxiety | Preclinical study in wild type C57Bl/6 mice, Tlr5[-l-] and Il10[-l-] engineered mice | [37, 71] |
| | Carrageenan | Enhances insulin resistance and glucose intolerance, and alters insulin signalling | *In vivo* study in male C57Bl/6J mice and *in vitro* in HepG2 cells | [72] |
| **5.** | **Antioxidants** | | | |
| | Butylated hydroxyanisole | Worsen urticaria | Double blind, placebo controlled study in patients of chronic idiopathic urticaria | [73] |
| | Butylated hydroxytoluene | Worsen urticaria | Double blind, placebo controlled study in patients of chronic idiopathic urticaria | [73] |
| **6.** | **Flavoring agents** | | | |

*(Table 1) cont.....*

| S. No. | Food Additive | Adverse Effect | Type of Study | References |
|--------|---------------|----------------|---------------|------------|
|        | Diacetyl      | Oxidative distress | *In vivo* study in C57/Bl mice | [74] |

## CARDIOVASCULAR DISEASES

Some of the most common food additives are rich in sodium and phosphorus. The use of excess intake of sodium and phosphorus is linked with cardiovascular diseases in chronic kidney diseases [75]. Dietary phosphorus consists of both organic and inorganic phosphorus. The organic esterified phosphorus includes meat, vegetables and dairy products, and the inorganic phosphorus is generally added to the beverages and processed food [75 - 78].

The excess of phosphorus is implicated in the pathogenesis of different unfavourable cardiovascular effects. It has been reported that excess of phosphorus promotes pathologic calcification of heart valve and vascular media [79 - 82] and facilitates in the induction of cardiomyocyte hypertrophy [83 - 85] and it also weakens vascular reactivity through the inhibition of nitric oxide (NO) synthesis when observed in humans and animals [86 - 89].

## CONCLUSION

The consumption of processed food and changes in food habits of the consumers have enhanced the use of food additives. Excessive use of food additives may lead to several complications. Studies herein explained more about the adverse health effects of food additives. Different adverse health effects that are discussed in this chapter include diabetes, allergic reactions, asthma, hyperkinesis, cancer and cardiovascular diseases. Although, animal and *in vitro* studies that examine the adverse health effects of different food additives are available, however, clinical studies on the concerned subject are very limited, or are contradictory. Although, animal and *in vitro* studies are available, clinical studies are limited, especially those, which examine the adverse health effects of different food additives in a large population group. Therefore, large scale studies are required to evaluate the adverse effects of food additives on the human population. The use of food additives is also very frequent in baby foods that raise concerns about the health of infants. There are reports on hypersensitivity reactions and exacerbating allergic conditions in afflicted individuals following the consumption of packaged food containing food additives. Hence, a word of caution for susceptible individuals with a history of allergy on labels of packaged foods would prove to be advantageous in reducing incidences of food additives associated with adverse reactions. Reducing the consumption of packaged food products is the wisest decision any individual can take considering his or her health prospects not only to avoid diseases that surface as a result of the consumption of the food additives but also to avoid the hazards of unhealthy eating habits.

## CONSENT FOR PUBLICATION

Not applicable.

## CONFLICT OF INTEREST

The authors declare no conflict of interest.

## ACKNOWLEDGEMENTS

Declared none.

## REFERENCES

[1]     Simon RA. Adverse reactions to food additives. Curr Allergy Asthma Rep 2003; 3(1): 62-6.
        [http://dx.doi.org/10.1007/s11882-003-0014-9] [PMID: 12542996]

[2]     Karmaus AL, Filer DL, Martin MT, Houck KA. Evaluation of food-relevant chemicals in the ToxCast
        high-throughput screening program. Food Chem Toxicol 2016; 92: 188-96.
        [http://dx.doi.org/10.1016/j.fct.2016.04.012] [PMID: 27103583]

[3]     Neltner TG, Alger HM, Leonard JE, Maffini MV. Data gaps in toxicity testing of chemicals allowed in
        food in the United States. Reprod Toxicol 2013; 42: 85-94.
        [http://dx.doi.org/10.1016/j.reprotox.2013.07.023] [PMID: 23954440]

[4]     Siegrist M, Sütterlin B. Importance of perceived naturalness for acceptance of food additives and
        cultured meat. Appetite 2017; 113 (Suppl. C): 320-6.
        [http://dx.doi.org/10.1016/j.appet.2017.03.019] [PMID: 28315418]

[5]     Evans G, de Challemaison B, Cox DN. Consumers' ratings of the natural and unnatural qualities of
        foods. Appetite 2010; 54(3): 557-63.
        [http://dx.doi.org/10.1016/j.appet.2010.02.014] [PMID: 20197074]

[6]     Batada A, Jacobson MF. Prevalence of artificial food colors in grocery store products marketed to
        children. Clin Pediatr (Phila) 2016; 55(12): 1113-9.
        [http://dx.doi.org/10.1177/0009922816651621] [PMID: 27270961]

[7]     Feketea G, Tsabouri S. Common food colorants and allergic reactions in children: Myth or reality?
        Food Chem 2017; 230: 578-88.
        [http://dx.doi.org/10.1016/j.foodchem.2017.03.043] [PMID: 28407952]

[8]     Sampson HA. Food allergy: a winding road to the present. Pediatr Allergy Immunol 2014; 25(1): 25-6.
        [http://dx.doi.org/10.1111/pai.12202] [PMID: 24588484]

[9]     Zuberbier T, Edenharter G, Worm M, *et al.* Prevalence of adverse reactions to food in Germany - a
        population study. Allergy 2004; 59(3): 338-45.
        [http://dx.doi.org/10.1046/j.1398-9995.2003.00403.x] [PMID: 14982518]

[10]    Rajan JP, Simon RA, Bosso JV. Prevalence of sensitivity to food and drug additives in patients with
        chronic idiopathic urticaria. J Allergy Clin Immunol Pract 2014; 2(2): 168-71.
        [http://dx.doi.org/10.1016/j.jaip.2013.10.002] [PMID: 24607044]

[11]    Cheng S, Leow YH, Goh CL, Goon A. Contact sensitivity to preservatives in Singapore: frequency of
        sensitization to 11 common preservatives 2006-2011. Dermatitis 2014; 25(2): 77-82.
        [http://dx.doi.org/10.1097/DER.0000000000000031] [PMID: 24603520]

[12] Vojdani A, Vojdani C. Immune reactivity to food coloring. Altern Ther Health Med 2015; 21 (Suppl. 1): 52-62.
[PMID: 25599186]

[13] Amchova P, Kotolova H, Ruda-Kucerova J. Health safety issues of synthetic food colorants. Regul Toxicol Pharmacol 2015; 73(3): 914-22.
[http://dx.doi.org/10.1016/j.yrtph.2015.09.026] [PMID: 26404013]

[14] Larsen JC, Mortensen A, Hallas-Møller T. Scientific Opinion on the re-evaluation of Allura Red AC (E 129) as a food additive on request from the European Commission: Question No EFSA-Q-20-8-230 2009.

[15] Bush RK, Montalbano MM. Asthma and food additives. Food Allergy 2008; p. 335.

[16] Bush RK, Taylor SL, Holden K, Nordlee JA, Busse WW. Prevalence of sensitivity to sulfiting agents in asthmatic patients. Am J Med 1986; 81(5): 816-20.
[http://dx.doi.org/10.1016/0002-9343(86)90351-7] [PMID: 3535492]

[17] Vally H, Misso NLA, Madan V. Clinical effects of sulphite additives. Clin Exp Allergy 2009; 39(11): 1643-51.
[http://dx.doi.org/10.1111/j.1365-2222.2009.03362.x] [PMID: 19775253]

[18] Juhlin L. Recurrent urticaria: clinical investigation of 330 patients. Br J Dermatol 1981; 104(4): 369-81.
[http://dx.doi.org/10.1111/j.1365-2133.1981.tb15306.x] [PMID: 7236502]

[19] Maurer M, Ortonne J-P, Zuberbier T. Chronic urticaria: an internet survey of health behaviours, symptom patterns and treatment needs in European adult patients. Br J Dermatol 2009; 160(3): 633-41.
[http://dx.doi.org/10.1111/j.1365-2133.2008.08920.x] [PMID: 19014398]

[20] Kobza Black A, Greaves MW, Champion RH, Pye RJ. The urticarias 1990. Br J Dermatol 1991; 124(1): 100-8.
[http://dx.doi.org/10.1111/j.1365-2133.1991.tb03292.x] [PMID: 1993134]

[21] Kang M-G, Song W-J, Park H-K, Lim K-H, Kim S-J, Lee S-Y, *et al.* Basophil activation test with food additives in chronic urticaria patients. Clin Nutr Res 2014; 27; 3(1): 9-16.
[http://dx.doi.org/10.7762/cnr.2014.3.1.9]

[22] Dahiya DK, Renuka , Puniya M, *et al.* Gut microbiota modulation and its relationship with obesity using prebiotic fibers and probiotics: A review. Front Microbiol 2017; 8: 563.
[http://dx.doi.org/10.3389/fmicb.2017.00563] [PMID: 28421057]

[23] Paula Neto HA, Ausina P, Gomez LS, Leandro JGB, Zancan P, Sola-Penna M. Effects of food additives on immune cells as contributors to body weight gain and immune-mediated metabolic dysregulation. Front Immunol 2017; 8: 1478.
[http://dx.doi.org/10.3389/fimmu.2017.01478] [PMID: 29163542]

[24] Amin KA, Abdel Hameid H II, Abd Elsttar AH. Effect of food azo dyes tartrazine and carmoisine on biochemical parameters related to renal, hepatic function and oxidative stress biomarkers in young male rats. Food Chem Toxicol 2010; 48(10): 2994-9.
[http://dx.doi.org/10.1016/j.fct.2010.07.039] [PMID: 20678534]

[25] Tsuda S, Murakami M, Matsusaka N, Kano K, Taniguchi K, Sasaki YF. DNA damage induced by red food dyes orally administered to pregnant and male mice. Toxicol Sci 2001; 61(1): 92-9.
[http://dx.doi.org/10.1093/toxsci/61.1.92] [PMID: 11294979]

[26] Raposa B, Pónusz R, Gerencsér G, *et al.* Food additives: Sodium benzoate, potassium sorbate, azorubine, and tartrazine modify the expression of NFκB, GADD45α, and MAPK8 genes. Physiol Int 2016; 103(3): 334-43.
[http://dx.doi.org/10.1556/2060.103.2016.3.6] [PMID: 28229641]

[27]   Soares BM, Araújo TMT, Ramos JAB, *et al.* Effects on DNA repair in human lymphocytes exposed to the food dye tartrazine yellow. Anticancer Res 2015; 35(3): 1465-74.
[PMID: 25750299]

[28]   Türkoğlu S. Genotoxicity of five food preservatives tested on root tips of *Allium cepa* L. Mutat Res 2007; 626(1-2): 4-14.
[http://dx.doi.org/10.1016/j.mrgentox.2006.07.006] [PMID: 17005441]

[29]   Mamur S, Yüzbaşioğlu D, Unal F, Yilmaz S. Does potassium sorbate induce genotoxic or mutagenic effects in lymphocytes? Toxicol In Vitro 2010; 24(3): 790-4.
[http://dx.doi.org/10.1016/j.tiv.2009.12.021] [PMID: 20036729]

[30]   Howe GR, Burch JD, Miller AB, *et al.* Artificial sweeteners and human bladder cancer. Lancet 1977; 2(8038): 578-81.
[http://dx.doi.org/10.1016/S0140-6736(77)91428-3] [PMID: 71398]

[31]   Weihrauch MR, Diehl V. Artificial sweeteners--do they bear a carcinogenic risk? Ann Oncol 2004; 15(10): 1460-5.
[http://dx.doi.org/10.1093/annonc/mdh256] [PMID: 15367404]

[32]   Hinson AL, Nicol WM. Monitoring sweetener consumption in Great Britain. Food Addit Contam 1992; 9(6): 669-80.
[http://dx.doi.org/10.1080/02652039209374122] [PMID: 1302206]

[33]   Leclercq C, Berardi D, Sorbillo MR, Lambe J. Intake of saccharin, aspartame, acesulfame K and cyclamate in Italian teenagers: present levels and projections. Food Addit Contam 1999; 16(3): 99-109.
[http://dx.doi.org/10.1080/026520399284145] [PMID: 10492702]

[34]   Ilbäck N-G, Alzin M, Jahrl S, Enghardt-Barbieri H, Busk L. Estimated intake of the artificial sweeteners acesulfame-K, aspartame, cyclamate and saccharin in a group of Swedish diabetics. Food Addit Contam 2003; 20(2): 99-114.
[http://dx.doi.org/10.1080/0265203021000042896] [PMID: 12623659]

[35]   Dahlquist GG, Blom LG, Persson LA, Sandström AI, Wall SG. Dietary factors and the risk of developing insulin dependent diabetes in childhood. Br Med J 1990; 19;300(6735): 1302-6.
[http://dx.doi.org/10.1136/bmj.300.6735.1302]

[36]   Roberts CL, Keita AV, Duncan SH, *et al.* Translocation of Crohn's disease *Escherichia coli* across M-cells: contrasting effects of soluble plant fibres and emulsifiers. Gut 2010; 59(10): 1331-9.
[http://dx.doi.org/10.1136/gut.2009.195370] [PMID: 20813719]

[37]   Chassaing B, Koren O, Goodrich JK, *et al.* Dietary emulsifiers impact the mouse gut microbiota promoting colitis and metabolic syndrome. Nature 2015; 519(7541): 92-6.
[http://dx.doi.org/10.1038/nature14232] [PMID: 25731162]

[38]   Fowler SP, Williams K, Resendez RG, Hunt KJ, Hazuda HP, Stern MP. Fueling the obesity epidemic? Artificially sweetened beverage use and long-term weight gain. Obesity (Silver Spring) 2008; 16(8): 1894-900.
[http://dx.doi.org/10.1038/oby.2008.284] [PMID: 18535548]

[39]   Stellman SD, Garfinkel L. Artificial sweetener use and one-year weight change among women. Prev Med 1986; 15(2): 195-202.
[http://dx.doi.org/10.1016/0091-7435(86)90089-7] [PMID: 3714671]

[40]   Colditz GA, Willett WC, Stampfer MJ, London SJ, Segal MR, Speizer FE. Patterns of weight change and their relation to diet in a cohort of healthy women. Am J Clin Nutr 1990; 51(6): 1100-5.
[http://dx.doi.org/10.1093/ajcn/51.6.1100] [PMID: 2349925]

[41]   Duffey KJ, Popkin BM. Adults with healthier dietary patterns have healthier beverage patterns. J Nutr 2006; 136(11): 2901-7.
[http://dx.doi.org/10.1093/jn/136.11.2901] [PMID: 17056820]

[42]   Mackenzie T, Brooks B, O'Connor G. Beverage intake, diabetes, and glucose control of adults in America. Ann Epidemiol 2006; 16(9): 688-91.
[http://dx.doi.org/10.1016/j.annepidem.2005.11.009] [PMID: 16458538]

[43]   McNaughton SA, Mishra GD, Brunner EJ. Dietary patterns, insulin resistance, and incidence of type 2 diabetes in the Whitehall II Study. Diabetes Care 2008; 31(7): 1343-8.
[http://dx.doi.org/10.2337/dc07-1946] [PMID: 18390803]

[44]   Palmer JR, Boggs DA, Krishnan S, Hu FB, Singer M, Rosenberg L. Sugar-sweetened beverages and incidence of type 2 diabetes mellitus in African American women. Arch Intern Med 2008; 168(14): 1487-92.
[http://dx.doi.org/10.1001/archinte.168.14.1487] [PMID: 18663160]

[45]   Grotz VL, Henry RR, McGill JB, et al. Lack of effect of sucralose on glucose homeostasis in subjects with type 2 diabetes. J Am Diet Assoc 2003; 103(12): 1607-12.
[http://dx.doi.org/10.1016/j.jada.2003.09.021] [PMID: 14647086]

[46]   French SA, Lin B-H, Guthrie JF. National trends in soft drink consumption among children and adolescents age 6 to 17 years: prevalence, amounts, and sources, 1977/1978 to 1994/1998. J Am Diet Assoc 2003; 103(10): 1326-31.
[http://dx.doi.org/10.1016/S0002-8223(03)01076-9] [PMID: 14520252]

[47]   Striegel-Moore RH, Thompson D, Affenito SG, et al. Correlates of beverage intake in adolescent girls: the National Heart, Lung, and Blood Institute Growth and Health Study. J Pediatr 2006; 148(2): 183-7.
[http://dx.doi.org/10.1016/j.jpeds.2005.11.025] [PMID: 16492426]

[48]   Kral TVE, Stunkard AJ, Berkowitz RI, Stallings VA, Moore RH, Faith MS. Beverage consumption patterns of children born at different risk of obesity. Obesity (Silver Spring) 2008; 16(8): 1802-8.
[http://dx.doi.org/10.1038/oby.2008.287] [PMID: 18535546]

[49]   Blum JW, Jacobsen DJ, Donnelly JE. Beverage consumption patterns in elementary school aged children across a two-year period. J Am Coll Nutr 2005; 24(2): 93-8.
[http://dx.doi.org/10.1080/07315724.2005.10719449] [PMID: 15798075]

[50]   Brown RJ, de Banate MA, Rother KI. Artificial sweeteners: a systematic review of metabolic effects in youth. Int J Pediatr Obes 2010; 5(4): 305-12.
[http://dx.doi.org/10.3109/17477160903497027] [PMID: 20078374]

[51]   Burrows Adam JD. Palette of Our Palates: A Brief History of Food Coloring and Its Regulation. Compr Rev Food Sci Food Saf 2009; 8(4): 394-408.
[http://dx.doi.org/10.1111/j.1541-4337.2009.00089.x]

[52]   Nigg JT, Lewis K, Edinger T, Falk M. Meta-analysis of attention-deficit/hyperactivity disorder or attention-deficit/hyperactivity disorder symptoms, restriction diet, and synthetic food color additives. J Am Acad Child Adolesc Psychiatry 2012; 51(1): 86-97.e8.
[http://dx.doi.org/10.1016/j.jaac.2011.10.015] [PMID: 22176942]

[53]   Feingold BF. Hyperkinesis and learning disabilities linked to the ingestion of artificial food colors and flavors. J Learn Disabil 1976; 9(9): 551-9.
[http://dx.doi.org/10.1177/002221947600900902]

[54]   Feingold BF. Hyperkinesis and learning disabilities linked to artificial food flavors and colors. Am J Nurs 1975; 75(5): 797-803.
[PMID: 1039267]

[55]   Lipton MA, Mayo JP. Diet and hyperkinesis--an update. J Am Diet Assoc 1983; 83(2): 132-4.
[PMID: 6875141]

[56]   Mattes JA. The Feingold diet: a current reappraisal. J Learn Disabil 1983; 16(6): 319-23.
[http://dx.doi.org/10.1177/002221948301600602] [PMID: 6886552]

[57]   Arnold LE, Lofthouse N, Hurt E. Artificial Food Colors and Attention-Deficit/Hyperactivity

Symptoms: Conclusions to Dye for. Neurotherapeutics 2012; 3;9(3): 599-609.

[58] Bateman B, Warner JO, Hutchinson E, *et al.* The effects of a double blind, placebo controlled, artificial food colourings and benzoate preservative challenge on hyperactivity in a general population sample of preschool children. Arch Dis Child 2004; 89(6): 506-11.
[http://dx.doi.org/10.1136/adc.2003.031435] [PMID: 15155391]

[59] Aguilar F, Autrup H, Barlow S, Castle L, Crebelli R, Dekant W, *et al.* on the effect of some colors and sodium benzoate on children's behaviour. EFSA J 2007; 2008(660): 1-54.

[60] McCann D, Barrett A, Cooper A, *et al.* Food additives and hyperactive behaviour in 3-year-old and 8/9-year-old children in the community: a randomised, double-blinded, placebo-controlled trial. Lancet 2007; 370(9598): 1560-7.
[http://dx.doi.org/10.1016/S0140-6736(07)61306-3] [PMID: 17825405]

[61] Watson R. European agency rejects links between hyperactivity and food additives. BMJ 2008; 336(7646): 687.
[http://dx.doi.org/10.1136/bmj.39527.401644.DB] [PMID: 18356207]

[62] Walton RG, Hudak R, Green-Waite RJ. Adverse reactions to aspartame: double-blind challenge in patients from a vulnerable population. Biol Psychiatry 1993; 34(1-2): 13-7.
[http://dx.doi.org/10.1016/0006-3223(93)90251-8] [PMID: 8373935]

[63] Lindseth GN, Coolahan SE, Petros TV, Lindseth PD. Neurobehavioral effects of aspartame consumption. Res Nurs Health 2014; 37(3): 185-93.
[http://dx.doi.org/10.1002/nur.21595] [PMID: 24700203]

[64] Suez J, Korem T, Zeevi D, *et al.* Artificial sweeteners induce glucose intolerance by altering the gut microbiota. Nature 2014; 514(7521): 181-6.
[http://dx.doi.org/10.1038/nature13793] [PMID: 25231862]

[65] Bian X, Chi L, Gao B, Tu P, Ru H, Lu K. Gut microbiome response to sucralose and its potential role in inducing liver inflammation in mice. Front Physiol 2017; 8: 487.
[http://dx.doi.org/10.3389/fphys.2017.00487] [PMID: 28790923]

[66] Pongsavee M. Effect of sodium benzoate preservative on micronucleus induction, chromosome break, and Ala40Thr superoxide dismutase gene mutation in lymphocytes. BioMed Res Int 2015; 2015103512
[http://dx.doi.org/10.1155/2015/103512] [PMID: 25785261]

[67] Mamur S, Yüzbaşıoğlu D, Unal F, Aksoy H. Genotoxicity of food preservative sodium sorbate in human lymphocytes in vitro. Cytotechnology 2012; 64(5): 553-62.
[http://dx.doi.org/10.1007/s10616-012-9434-5] [PMID: 22373823]

[68] Rowe KS, Rowe KJ. Synthetic food coloring and behavior: a dose response effect in a double-blind, placebo-controlled, repeated-measures study. J Pediatr 1994; 125(5 Pt 1): 691-8.
[http://dx.doi.org/10.1016/S0022-3476(06)80164-2] [PMID: 7965420]

[69] Saxena B, Sharma S. Food Color Induced Hepatotoxicity in Swiss Albino Rats, Rattus norvegicus. Toxicol Int 2015; 22(1): 152-7.
[http://dx.doi.org/10.4103/0971-6580.172286] [PMID: 26862277]

[70] Dwivedi K, Kumar G. Genetic damage induced by a food coloring dye (sunset yellow) on meristematic cells of *Brassica campestris* L Environ Public Health 2015; 2015

[71] Holder MK, Peters NV, Whylings J, *et al.* Dietary emulsifiers consumption alters anxiety-like and social-related behaviors in mice in a sex-dependent manner. Sci Rep 2019; 9(1): 172.
[http://dx.doi.org/10.1038/s41598-018-36890-3] [PMID: 30655577]

[72] Bhattacharyya S, O-Sullivan I, Katyal S, Unterman T, Tobacman JK. Exposure to the common food additive carrageenan leads to glucose intolerance, insulin resistance and inhibition of insulin signalling in HepG2 cells and C57BL/6J mice. Diabetologia 2012; 55(1): 194-203.
[http://dx.doi.org/10.1007/s00125-011-2333-z] [PMID: 22011715]

[73]    Goodman DL, McDonnell JT, Nelson HS, Vaughan TR, Weber RW. Chronic urticaria exacerbated by the antioxidant food preservatives, butylated hydroxyanisole (BHA) and butylated hydroxytoluene (BHT). J Allergy Clin Immunol 1990; 86(4 Pt 1): 570-5.
[http://dx.doi.org/10.1016/S0091-6749(05)80214-3] [PMID: 2229816]

[74]    Jedlicka LDL, Silva JDC, Balbino AM, *et al.* Effects of Diacetyl Flavoring Exposure in Mice Metabolism. BioMed Res Int 2018; 20189875319
[http://dx.doi.org/10.1155/2018/9875319] [PMID: 30065948]

[75]    Gutiérrez OM. Sodium- and phosphorus-based food additives: persistent but surmountable hurdles in the management of nutrition in chronic kidney disease. Adv Chronic Kidney Dis 2013; 20(2): 150-6.
[http://dx.doi.org/10.1053/j.ackd.2012.10.008] [PMID: 23439374]

[76]    Sherman RA, Mehta O. Phosphorus and potassium content of enhanced meat and poultry products: implications for patients who receive dialysis. Clin J Am Soc Nephrol 2009; 4(8): 1370-3.
[http://dx.doi.org/10.2215/CJN.02830409] [PMID: 19628683]

[77]    Sherman RA, Mehta O. Dietary phosphorus restriction in dialysis patients: potential impact of processed meat, poultry, and fish products as protein sources. Am J Kidney Dis 2009; 54(1): 18-23.
[http://dx.doi.org/10.1053/j.ajkd.2009.01.269] [PMID: 19376617]

[78]    Uribarri J, Calvo MS. Hidden sources of phosphorus in the typical American diet: does it matter in nephrology? Semin Dial 2003; 16(3): 186-8.
[http://dx.doi.org/10.1046/j.1525-139X.2003.16037.x] [PMID: 12753675]

[79]    Giachelli CM, Jono S, Shioi A, Nishizawa Y, Mori K, Morii H. Vascular calcification and inorganic phosphate. Am J Kidney Dis 2001; 38(4) (Suppl. 1): S34-7.
[http://dx.doi.org/10.1053/ajkd.2001.27394] [PMID: 11576919]

[80]    Mathew S, Tustison KS, Sugatani T, Chaudhary LR, Rifas L, Hruska KA. The mechanism of phosphorus as a cardiovascular risk factor in CKD. J Am Soc Nephrol 2008; 19(6): 1092-105.
[http://dx.doi.org/10.1681/ASN.2007070760] [PMID: 18417722]

[81]    Lau WL, Pai A, Moe SM, Giachelli CM. Direct effects of phosphate on vascular cell function. Adv Chronic Kidney Dis 2011; 18(2): 105-12.
[http://dx.doi.org/10.1053/j.ackd.2010.12.002] [PMID: 21406295]

[82]    El-Abbadi MM, Pai AS, Leaf EM, *et al.* Phosphate feeding induces arterial medial calcification in uremic mice: role of serum phosphorus, fibroblast growth factor-23, and osteopontin. Kidney Int 2009; 75(12): 1297-307.
[http://dx.doi.org/10.1038/ki.2009.83] [PMID: 19322138]

[83]    Ayus JC, Mizani MR, Achinger SG, Thadhani R, Go AS, Lee S. Effects of short daily versus conventional hemodialysis on left ventricular hypertrophy and inflammatory markers: a prospective, controlled study. J Am Soc Nephrol 2005; 16(9): 2778-88.
[http://dx.doi.org/10.1681/ASN.2005040392] [PMID: 16033855]

[84]    Galetta F, Cupisti A, Franzoni F, *et al.* Left ventricular function and calcium phosphate plasma levels in uraemic patients. J Intern Med 2005; 258(4): 378-84.
[http://dx.doi.org/10.1111/j.1365-2796.2005.01544.x] [PMID: 16164578]

[85]    Neves KR, Graciolli FG, dos Reis LM, Pasqualucci CA, Moysés RMA, Jorgetti V. Adverse effects of hyperphosphatemia on myocardial hypertrophy, renal function, and bone in rats with renal failure. Kidney Int 2004; 66(6): 2237-44.
[http://dx.doi.org/10.1111/j.1523-1755.2004.66013.x] [PMID: 15569312]

[86]    Shuto E, Taketani Y, Tanaka R, *et al.* Dietary phosphorus acutely impairs endothelial function. J Am Soc Nephrol 2009; 20(7): 1504-12.
[http://dx.doi.org/10.1681/ASN.2008101106] [PMID: 19406976]

[87]    Takeda E, Taketani Y, Nashiki K, *et al.* A novel function of phosphate-mediated intracellular signal transduction pathways. Adv Enzyme Regul 2006; 46: 154-61.

[http://dx.doi.org/10.1016/j.advenzreg.2006.01.003] [PMID: 16846635]

[88]   Kööbi P, Vehmas TI, Jolma P, *et al.* High-calcium vs high-phosphate intake and small artery tone in advanced experimental renal insufficiency. Nephrol Dial Transplant 2006; 21(10): 2754-61.
       [http://dx.doi.org/10.1093/ndt/gfl270] [PMID: 16837509]

[89]   Gutiérrez OM. The connection between dietary phosphorus, cardiovascular disease, and mortality: where we stand and what we need to know. Adv Nutr 2013; 4(6): 723-9.
       [http://dx.doi.org/10.3945/an.113.004812] [PMID: 24228204]

# CHAPTER 15

# Membranes and Membrane Operations in Functional Food Production

**Carmela Conidi, Francesco Galiano, Alfredo Cassano* and Alberto Figoli***

*Institute on Membrane Technology, National Research Council, ITM-CNR, via P. Bucci, 17/C, I-87036 Rende, Cosenza, Italy*

**Abstract:** This chapter focuses on the recent advances in the use of membrane processes for the recovery of biologically active compounds (BACs) from agro-food products and by-products. The fundamentals of typical membrane operations, as well as of membrane preparation, are firstly presented. Then, typical case studies for the recovery of polyphenols, peptides, carotenoids and tocopherols are presented and discussed. Multistep membrane processes for the separation, purification and concentration of BACs from their original sources are specifically designed based on laboratory experimental data. These processes provide concentrated fractions for the formulation of functional foods within a biorefinery strategy, with significant economic and environmental advantages over conventional methodologies.

**Keywords:** Agro-food production, Biologically active compounds, Functional foods, Membrane separation.

## INTRODUCTION

The purification of biologically active compounds (BACs) from food products or food processing streams has gained a great interest in the few years due to the growing interest of consumers towards functional foods and nutraceutical products. According to a new market report published by Transparency Market Research, the global nutraceuticals market was valued at US$ 165.62 billion in 2014 and is expected to reach US$278.96 billion by 2021, growing at a Compound Annual Growth Rate (CAGR) of 7.3% from 2014 to 2021 [1]. BACs are generally present in complex multi-component matrices; therefore, these molecules have to be fractionated and purified with appropriate separation technologies able to preserve their bioactivity at low energy, capital and labour costs. Membrane separation processes represent a valid alternative to convention-

* **Corresponding authors A. Figoli and A. Cassano:**Institute on Membrane Technology, National Research Council, ITM-CNR, *via* P. Bucci, 17/C, I-87036 Rende, Cosenza, Italy; E-mails: a.figoli@itm.cnr.it and a.cassano@itm.cnr.it

***Seyed Mohammad Nabavi et al.* (Eds.)**

al technologies for the separation of antioxidant compounds [2]. These processes are based on the use of permselective barriers that allow the transmission of specific feed components while retaining others. In particular, pressure-driven membrane operations, such as microfiltration (MF), ultrafiltration (UF), nanofiltration (NF), reverse osmosis (RO) and osmotic membrane distillation (OMD) have been widely investigated for the recovery, separation and concentration of BACs from aqueous and alcoholic processing streams of agro-food products and by-products [3, 4]. These processes are characterized by low operating and maintenance costs, mild operative conditions for temperature and pressure, easy control, scale-up and highly selective separations. In addition, they do not require any extraction mass agents or the use of chemical additives avoiding products contaminations and preserving the biological activity of target compounds [5]. This chapter offers an overview of membrane processes for the separation, concentration and purification of BACs of interest for the production of functional foods. Fundamentals of membrane separation processes and general aspects of membrane preparation are firstly introduced. Then, specific applications for the recovery of BACs from agro-food products and by-products are presented and discussed highlighting typical advantages and drawbacks over conventional separation technologies.

## MEMBRANE PROCESSES

### Pressure-driven Membrane Operations

Pressure-driven membrane operations are based on the use of permselective barriers (membranes) that allow the diffusion of specific feed components under a hydrostatic pressure difference applied between the two sides of the membrane. As a result, the feed solution is converted into a *permeate* stream containing all components which have permeated the membrane and a *retentate* containing all compounds rejected by the membrane. The degree of rejection depends on the properties of the membrane such as the pore size, the charge and the surface properties.

Pressure-driven membrane processes include MF, UF, NF, and RO. These processes are classified according to the pore size, the pressure exerted through the membrane and the separation mechanism [6]. The filtration capability of pressure-driven membrane processes is presented in Fig. (**1**).

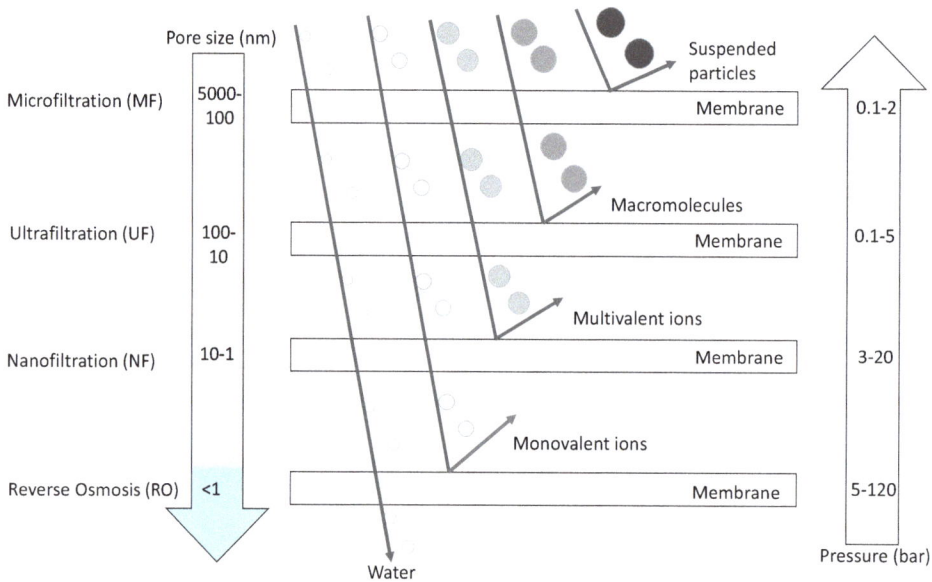

**Fig. (1).** Filtration capability of pressure-driven membrane processes.

MF membranes are typically used to separate particles with a diameter of 0.1-5 μm from a solvent and from low molecular weight compounds. The driving force used in MF processes is of the order of 0.5-2 bar.

The UF process is based on the use of asymmetric membranes with a pore size in the skin layer of 10-100 nm. Usually, dissolved molecules or small particles not larger than 0.1 μm in diameter are retained. UF membranes are characterized by the molecular weight cut-off (MWCO), defined as the equivalent molecular weight of the smallest species that exhibit 90% rejection. The MWCO of UF membranes is between $10^3$ and $10^6$ Dalton. Hydrostatic pressures typically used in UF are of 1-5 bar. The separation capability of MF and UF membranes is mainly affected by size, shape and charge of particles being filtered; however, membrane-solute interactions, presence of other solutes and operating parameters play a key role in the retention capabilities of these membranes (*i.e.*, membranes with similar MWCO and different material exhibit different solute rejection).

NF is a membrane process situated between the separation capabilities of UF and RO membranes. It is essentially used to fractionate solutes based on cation or anion valency and also to separate various organic solutes with low molecular weights. The separation mechanism is based on steric, Donnan and dielectric exclusion effects. The pore size of NF membranes is in the range of 10-30 Å. Hydrostatic pressures used in the process can vary from 15 bar to 20 bar.

RO membranes are generally used to separate low molecular weight compounds from a relatively pure solvent. The particle size range for RO applications is between 0.1 and 1 nm and solutes with a molecular weight greater than 300 Da are separated. The hydrostatic pressures to obtain significant transmembrane flux can vary from 10 to 100 bar depending upon the osmotic pressure of the feed mixture.

Pressure-driven membrane operations are generally operated according to a cross-flow filtration in comparison with the conventional method of perpendicular (or dead-end) filtration. In the traditional filtration, the incoming stream flows perpendicularly to the filter media producing a cake layer of retained particles on the membrane surface whose thickness affects strongly the permeation rate.

In the cross-flow system, the feed solution is filtered tangentially to the membrane surface and particles are continually swept away from the membrane surface keeping the cake layer thickness relatively thin. Unlike traditional filtration, the cross-flow filtration performs self-cleaning, allowing longer operating times.

In the last 30 years, pressure-driven membrane processes have been widely developed in the food industry for several reasons: i) in comparison to other traditional techniques (chromatography, thermal processes, *etc.*) membrane separations are easy to scale-up, flexible and safe for the application in food industry; ii) they are considered as green processes with a low environmental impact (no chemical additives are required in the process, no pollutants are generated); iii) they can combine different processes in one single step guaranteeing both high performances and food quality [7].

### *Osmotic Membrane Distillation*

The osmotic membrane distillation (OMD) is a membrane contactor technique, also known as osmotic evaporation, membrane evaporation, isothermal membrane distillation or gas membrane extraction. OMD can be carried out at ambient temperature and, for this reason, it is very well appreciated for the concentration of heat-sensitive compounds such as juices [8].

In OMD, a hydrophobic macroporous membrane is located between two aqueous solutions with different water activity. A volatile compound, generally represented by water, is removed from the feed side, in a vapour phase, and then condensed in the permeate side constituted by a hypertonic solution. The vapour pressure difference between the two sides of the membrane represents the driving force for the permeation of the vapour. The water transport through the membrane can be summarized in three steps: 1) evaporation of the water from the feed side; 2) water transport, as a vapour, through the membrane's pores; 3) condensation of permeated water on the permeate side Fig. (**2**).

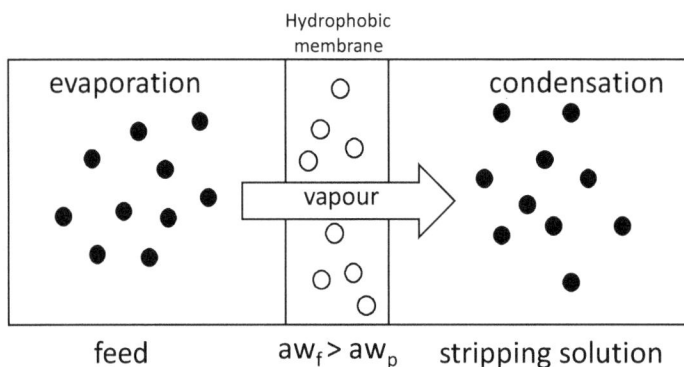

**Fig. (2).** Schematic representation of membrane osmotic distillation (aw, water activity; f, feed; p, permeate).

Membranes used in OMD are typically hydrophobic in nature; polymers with low surface free energy such as polyethylene (PE), polytetrafluoroethylene (PTFE), polypropylene (PP) and polyvinylidene fluoride (PVDF) are used for this purpose. However, OMD membranes can be also realised by grafting on the surface of hydrophilic ceramic membranes, molecules containing hydrophobic fluorocarbon chains like fluoroalkyl silanes or by coating the surface of alumina membranes with a thin lipid film. Stripping solutions used in OMD should be thermally stable and also preferably no-toxic, no-corrosive and low cost. A number of salts such as $MgSO_4$, NaCl, $CaCl_2$, $MgCl_2$, $KH_2PO_4$, and $K_2HPO_4$ are suitable. NaCl has a relatively low-temperature solubility coefficient, while $CaCl_2$ is sensitive to precipitation in the presence of $CO_2$. These salts are quite corrosive to ferrous alloys at elevated temperatures. Potassium salts of ortho- and pyro-phosphoric acid offer several advantages, including low equivalent weight, high water solubility, steep positive temperature coefficients of solubility and safe use in foods and pharmaceuticals [9].

### *Membrane Modules*

At the industrial level, in order to achieve the desired separation, hundreds or thousands of square meters of the membrane is required. To minimise the volume area and to pack the membranes in a smaller unit, membranes are integrated into the so-called *membrane modules*. On a large industrial scale, membrane modules are available in three basic designs: plate and frame, spiral-wound and tubular. They are quite different in their design, mode of operation, production costs and energy requirement for pumping the feed solution through the module [10]. In *plate and frame* modules, flat membranes are layered together with spacers and permeate collectors. The feed is forced to pass perpendicularly or tangentially through the membrane, depending on the configuration of the module: dead-end or cross-flow, respectively. Then, the permeate is collected through a central manifold.

In spiral-wound modules, the flat membranes, together with feed and porous spacers, are rolled up around a central collector and housed in an outer tubular shell. Spiral-wound modules are principally applied in pervaporation and water desalination guaranteeing high permeate fluxes and low operational costs.

*The tubular* modules comprise hollow fibers (0.05-0.4 mm), capillary (0.5-3.0 mm) and tubular type (0.5-2.0 cm) configurations depending on the dimension of the inner diameter applied. In hollow fiber or capillary configuration, a bundle of hundreds or thousands of fibers is located within a pressure vessel. The feed flows radially or tangentially to the membranes and the permeate is collected at the other side of the open fiber end. In tubular systems, the membranes are not self-supporting. Thus, they are formed on the inside of the tube that acts as a support, which is usually made of porous fiber. The feed flows inside the lumen of the membranes while the permeate is collected in the outer shell. The main advantages of tubular modules are the lower propensity to fouling formation due to the high diameter and the easy procedure needed for cleaning. They find principal applications in MF and UF processes.

## Membrane Preparation

### *Conventional Preparation Techniques*

The majority of commercially available polymeric membranes are prepared by phase inversion process. A polymer solution is firstly prepared by dissolving a polymer in a suitable solvent obtaining a homogenous single-phase system. The phase separation process includes the inversion of the single-phase system in a two phase system consisting of a polymer-rich phase, constituting the matrix of the membrane, and a liquid rich phase, constituting the pores of the final membrane. Depending on how the phase separation process occurs, different techniques can be identified: non-solvent induced phase separation (NIPS), evaporation induced phase separation (EIPS), thermally induced phase separation (TIPS) and vapour induced phase separation (VIPS) Fig. (**3**) [11].

NIPS is the most widespread technique adopted for the preparation of polymeric membranes by phase inversion process due to its versatility and the possibility of preparing a large variety of membranes by varying the operating parameters. NIPS is based on the immersion of the cast polymer film in a coagulation bath, represented by a non-solvent (generally water), responsible for the demixing of the polymer solution and the subsequent precipitation of the polymer. The exchange, in fact, between solvent and non-solvent leads to the formation of the membrane. NIPS technique is generally adopted for the preparation of membranes with an asymmetric and porous structure.

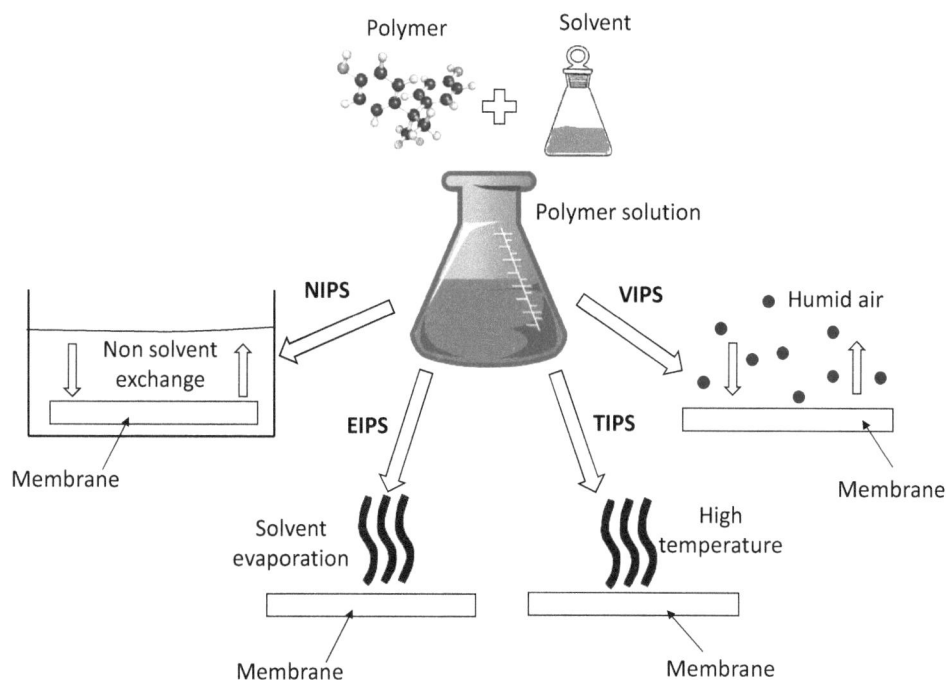

**Fig. (3).** Preparation of polymeric membranes by phase inversion processes.

EIPS technique involves the evaporation of a volatile solvent (such as acetone or chloroform) from a starting polymer solution followed by the precipitation of the polymer and the formation of the final membrane. A homogeneous single-phase solution is firstly prepared by dissolving a polymer in a proper volatile solvent (or a mixture of solvents). The polymer solution is then cast on a suitable support and, becoming thermodynamically unstable, it forms, due to evaporation, a two-phase solution. EIPS technique generally leads to the formation of membranes with a dense structure due to the fact that the phase inversion process is much slower than NIPS.

In the TIPS process, the phase separation occurs because of a temperature change. A polymer is solubilised in a solvent (identified as a latent solvent) at an elevated temperature and cast on cold support. The cast solution is then cooled down allowing the precipitation of the polymer and the formation of the membrane. The latent solvent is then removed by solvent extraction leading to the formation of dense or microporous membranes [12].

In the VIPS process, finally, the cast film is exposed to humid air before the immersion in a coagulation bath. The vapour phase consists of a non-solvent (typically water) often saturating the environment. The precipitation of the polymer and the formation of the membrane occur because of the exchange between the solvent and non-solvent. This technique allows the production of porous membranes without a dense top layer.

## *Preparation of Membranes with Antifouling Properties*

One of the main bottlenecks acting on the majority of membrane processes is the phenomenon of fouling. Fouling occurs due to the deposition of inorganic or organic particles present in the feed solution onto the membrane surface causing a decline of permeate flux and negatively affecting the quality of the filtrate. Moreover, fouling formation negatively influences the economic impact of the process decreasing the membrane life cycle and requiring continuous costs related to membrane cleanings. As shown in Fig. (**4**), there are four main mechanisms concerning fouling formation: 1) Standard pore blocking: it is characterised by the infiltration of foulant particles in the membrane pores causing a pore size reduction; 2) Complete bore blocking: it is characterised by a total obstruction of membrane pores due to foulant particles deposition. This situation is encountered when the particles have a dimension higher than the pores of the membrane; 3) Intermediate blocking: it is characterised by the bridging of the foulant particles at the pore entry obstructing the entrance but not completely closing it; 4) Cake layer formation: it is characterised by a severe deposition of particles at membrane surface forming a cake layer taking over the whole membrane and, thus, controlling the transport and the rejection [13].

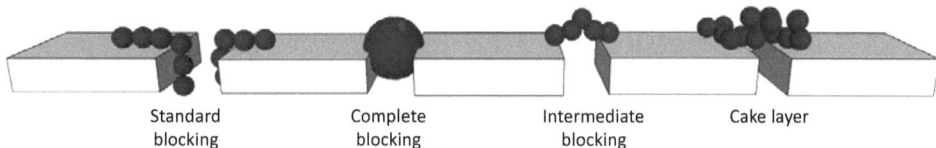

Standard Complete Intermediate Cake layer
blocking blocking blocking

**Fig. (4).** Fouling mechanisms.

In food processing, the problem of fouling is often encountered in driven membrane processes and principally due to the deposition and accumulation of proteins, polysaccharides and other macromolecules on the membrane surface. Several authors studied the mechanism of fouling formation in different membrane applications related to food processing, such as the clarification of blood orange juice [14], the ultrafiltration of apple juice [15], the clarification of pineapple juice [16] and the MF of surimi wash water [17].

Several strategies have been applied so far in order to mitigate the onset of fouling on the membrane surface. The choice of the appropriate membrane material, module, membrane cleaning and set-up configuration can help to alleviate the fouling formation [18]. One of the main approaches adopted for fouling remediation consists of the modification of the membrane surface. Indeed, hydrophobic membranes are known to be more affected by fouling phenomena due to the higher propensity of foulant particles to interact with surfaces by establishing hydrophobic interactions. The hydrophilization of membrane surfaces, therefore, plays a crucial role in the production of membranes with improved properties in terms of fouling formation and fouling remediation. The main concept is based on the introduction of hydrophilic groups (such as -OH and -NH$_2$ groups) directly in the polymer structure (in order to obtain a more hydrophilic material) or by modifying the surface after membrane preparation by coating or grafting hydrophilic materials. The quaternary phosphonium and ammonium-based polymer coatings have been used by Hatakeyama *et al.* [19] for the production of surfaces more resistant to protein adsorption (bovine serum albumin and fibrinogen). A series of coating materials based on crosslinked poly(ethylene glycol) diacrylate (XLPEGDA) were also developed by Ju *et al.* [20] for the production of anti-fouling membranes. Recently, Galiano *et al.* [21] reported the successful use of a polymerised bicontinuous microemulsion (PBM) coating to be applied to the UF-PES membrane with antifouling and biofouling properties. In both cases, the anti-fouling potential of the produced coatings was directly related to both improved hydrophilic moiety and smoothness of the membrane surface.

The presence of additives, such as nanoparticles, has also been widely investigated for the production of membranes with lower fouling tendency. TiO$_2$ nanoparticles were, for instance, dispersed and incorporated in PES ultrafiltration membranes by Razmjou *et al.* [22]. Produced mixed matrix membranes exhibited higher flux recovery (84%) and improved antifouling properties in comparison to control membranes. Cao *et al.* [23] obtained similar results about the antifouling effects of TiO$_2$ nanoparticles in PVDF membranes.

## Recovery of Bioactive Compounds by Membrane Operations

Several studies have confirmed the efficiency of membrane technology for the separation, fractionation, purification and concentration of different classes of BACs from several natural products. Membrane separation processes are among the key physicochemical and non-destructive techniques applied to separate macromolecules and micromolecules derived from different waste streams and respective extracts [24]. They stand out as alternatives to conventional processes for the chemical, pharmaceutical, biotechnological and food industries due to their advantages such as high efficiency, simple equipment, easy scale-up and low energy consumption [25]. In addition, the membrane technology can operate under mild conditions of temperature and pressure, therefore, preserving the biological activity of the compounds to be recovered and the properties of the original product. They do not require any extraction mass agents such as solvents, avoiding product contaminations and the need for subsequent purification.

Pressure-driven membrane processes are consolidated systems in the food and beverage industries for the treatment of several products and by-products. Other membrane processes, such as OMD, have also been successfully investigated in the same area. These processes, mostly in a sequential form or combined with other separation technologies, offer new and many opportunities in terms of competitiveness, improvement of quality and environmental friendliness.

MF and UF are typically applied for the primary treatment, while purification and concentration steps are usually performed by NF, RO and OMD processes [26, 27]. The solution properties, charges of ionic species and the type of membrane used, affect the behaviour and the efficiency of the separation and concentration methods. Table **1** summarizes some examples of pressure-driven membrane operations for the separation of BACs from different agro-food products and by-products. Specific applications of membrane processes for the recovery of phenolic compounds, peptides and carotenoids are reported. The obtained synergistic effects in the development of formulations for functional foods production are showed.

## *Polyphenols*

The extraction, purification and concentration of polyphenolic compounds from different vegetables matrix by membranes separation technologies have been largely investigated in the last years. In particular, MF, UF and NF are successfully used to concentrate and selectively fractionate different classes of polyphenols including flavonoids and soluble anthocyanins from aqueous or hydroalcoholic plant extracts or fruit juices [28 - 30].

Polyphenols are usually extracted by conventional solvents: hot water, methanol, ethanol, acetone and ethyl acetate. These procedures are often multistage, laborious and consume time and energy. In addition, they produce oxidation of phenols leading to a decreased yield of these compounds in the extracts. Therefore, it is necessary to develop innovative and sustainable procedures to produce such value-added chemicals in a more efficient and environmentally friendly mode without affecting their stability [31]. The potential of membrane operations, also in integrated systems, for the purification and concentration of phenolic compounds, has been largely investigated.

**Table 1. Membrane operations for the separation of BACs from different agro-food sources.**

| Bioactive compounds | Target compounds | Sources | Membrane processes |
|---|---|---|---|
| *Flavonoids* | Quercetin, catechin | Apple juice, tea, red wine | MF, UF, NF, RO |
| | Narirutin, naringin, hesperidin, neohesperidin | Citrus juices | MF, UF, NF, RO |
| | Apigenin, luteolin | Artichoke wastewaters | UF, NF, RO |
| | Cyanidin, cyanin, myrtillyn | Blood orange, pomegranate juices | MF, UF, NF, RO |
| *Carotenoids* | α-carotene, β-carotene | Palm oil, carrot juice | MF, NF |
| | Lycopene, lutein | Carrot, kiwifruit, tomato juices | MF, UF |
| *Phenolic acids* | Caffeic acid, chlorogenic acid, p-coumaric acid, ferulic acid | Apple juice, olive mill and artichoke wastewaters | MF, UF, NF, RO |
| | Citric acid | Citrus juices | MF, UF, NF, RO |
| | Ellagic acid | Black-berry juices | UF, NF |
| | Tyrosol, hydroxytyrosol oleuropein, gallic acid | Olive mill wastewaters | MF, UF, NF, RO |
| *Proteins* | α-lactalbumin, β-lactalbumin, bovine serum albumin (BSA) | Whey, milk | MF, UF, NF |
| | Immunoglobulins | Egg yolk | UF |
| | Phycocyanin | Marine organisms (microalgae) | UF, NF, RO |
| *Omega 3-fatty acids* | Linoleic acid | Fish processing wastes | MF, UF, NF |

Mello *et al.* [32] studied the NF process for the concentration of flavonoids and phenolic acids in aqueous and ethanolic propolis extracts using a polyamide (PA) membrane with a MgSO4 rejection of 98%. The process was investigated in terms of productivity (permeate flux) and product quality. The NF membrane concentrated all phenolic compounds from aqueous extracts (retention towards flavonoids of 100%); on the other hand, 90% of flavonoids were retained for ethanolic extracts. According to the obtained results, NF was considered as a good and efficient alternative to propolis extracts concentration.

Recently, Syed *et al.* [33] evaluated an integrated NF/RO process for the fractionation of bioactive monomeric flavan-3-olds in grape pomace. In the first step, the grape pomace extracts were processed with different flat-sheet NF membranes in order to identify a suitable protocol for the fractionation of phenolic compounds. Selected membranes with different pore size, material and chemical nature, were evaluated for their productivity, operating mode (NF) *versus* diafiltration (DF) and selectivity towards compounds of interest.

Experimental results showed that a membrane with an MWCO of 900 Da (Duramen 900 in modified polyimide from Evonik) produced high permeation fluxes and better purification of different classes of phenolics when compared to the other selected membranes. The NF permeate, enriched in optimized fractionated extracts, was further concentrated by an RO membrane in PA thin film composite (99.4% salt rejection). The RO process produced a washing solution (permeate) that can be reused during the DF process and a retentate fraction enriched in monomeric and oligomeric flavan-3-ols. This fraction is of interest for the production of functional foods or pharmaceutical formulations.

Membrane technologies also appear as an attractive approach for the recovery and concentration of anthocyanins from different vegetables matrix. Anthocyanins are phenolic compounds responsible for the bright and attractive orange, red, purple, and blue colours of most fruits, vegetables, flowers and some cereal grains.

Anthocyanin-rich extracts are increasingly attractive to the food industry as natural alternatives to synthetic dyes, because of their colouring properties. In addition, anthocyanins exhibit a strong antioxidant activity, which helps to prevent neuronal diseases, cardiovascular illnesses, cancer, diabetes, inflammation, and many other diseases [34, 35].

Kalbasi and Cisneros-Zevallos [36] studied the effect of PVDF UF flat sheet membranes with different MWCO (1000, 500, 250, 100, 30 and 10 kDa) on the recovery of polymeric and monomeric anthocyanins from Concord grape juice, as well as their effects on colour and antioxidant potential. The selected membranes were also compared in terms of productivity, fouling index and resistances. A decrease in permeate fluxes was observed by decreasing the MWCO while membrane resistance increased exponentially with fouling. UF membranes with a MWCO of 100 kDa concentrated polymeric anthocyanins in the retentate fractions, while monomeric anthocyanins were recovered in the permeate stream. A correlation between the number of polyphenols and TAA was also observed.

Cissé *et al.* [37] evaluated the potential of flat-sheet UF and NF membranes of different materials (PA thin-film composite and PES) and MWCO (from 0.15 to 150 kDa) to concentrate anthocyanins from *Hibiscus sabdariffa* L. roselle extract.

The performance of the membranes at different transmembrane pressure (TMP) values (from 0.5 to 3.0 MPa) was also evaluated in terms of permeate fluxes and retentions towards total soluble solids, acidity and total anthocyanins. The results indicated that an increase of retention for analysed compounds was observed by increasing the TMP for both UF and NF membranes. Higher permeate fluxes and higher retention towards anthocyanins (of about 95%) were measured by NF membranes with a MWCO in the range of 0.15-0.3 kDa working at a TMP of 2-3 MPa. An industrial trial, using a spiral-wound NF membrane, showed that anthocyanins in roselle extracts can be concentrated from 4 to 25 g of total soluble solids per 100 g, increasing 6 times the anthocyanins concentration. Similarly, in the process investigated by Couto *et al.* [38], different NF membranes in flat-sheet configuration with different MWCO and polymeric material were evaluated in terms of productivity and concentration of anthocyanins in the treatment of clarified açai juice. In general, the NF 270 membrane, a composite membrane with a PA top layer and a polysulphone (PSU) microporous support, presented the highest value of permeate flux in the treatment of açai juice, low index of fouling and anthocyanins retention of about 99%. Therefore, the produced retentate fraction, enriched in anthocyanins, can be considered of interest for nutraceutical applications. Conidi *et al.* [39] investigated a membrane-based process with NF membranes for the separation and concentration of phenolic compounds from orange press liquors. The authors evaluated the performance of spiral-wound NF membranes with different MWCO (250, 300, 400 and 1000 Da) and polymeric material (PA, polypiperazine amide (PPA) and PES) in order to identify a suitable membrane to separate phenolic compounds from sugars. The obtained results showed a reduction in the average rejection for sugars by increasing the MWCO of the selected membranes while the rejection for anthocyanins remained higher than 89% for all the NF membranes investigated. A PSU membrane with an MWCO of 1,000 Da showed the lowest average rejection for sugar compounds and rejections for anthocyanins and flavonoids of 89.2% and 70%, respectively. Recently, the same authors investigated the recovery and concentration of phenolic compounds in pomegranate juice by using UF and NF membranes [40]. In this approach, the raw juice was firstly clarified using UF hollow fiber membranes (cellulose triacetate, 150 kDa, FUC 1582, Mycrodin Nadir) under selected operating conditions (TMP 0.6 bar; axial feed flow rate, 400 l/h; temperature, 25 °C). The clarified juice was treated with flat-sheet UF and NF membranes with different MWCO (from 1,000 to 4,000 Da) and polymeric material in order to purify BACs from sugars. The selected membranes were compared in terms of productivity, fouling index and retention towards polyphenols, anthocyanins, total antioxidant activity (TAA) and sugars. The Desal GK membrane, a thin film composite membrane with a MWCO of 2000 Da, showed higher permeate fluxes, lower fouling index and the highest selectivity when compared with the other selected membranes. In particular, high retentions for anthocyanins, total polyphenols and TAA (in the range 80-95%) were measured. As reported in Table **2**, the observed retention for glucose and fructose was in the range 1-3%. Improved purification of BACs was obtained combining the concentration step with DF in a discontinuous way. In particular, the clarified juice was firstly concentrated in batch concentration mode and up to a volume reduction factor (VRF) of 5. Successively, the retentate was diluted with purified water and the permeate was removed separately.

The retentate stream, enriched in anthocyanins and other phenolic compounds, exhibited a high antioxidant activity. Consequently, it was considered useful for the formulation of nutraceutical products or as a natural colorant in alternative to synthetic ones.

Table 2. Rejection coefficient (expressed as %) of UF and NF membranes towards sugars and phenolic compounds of pomegranate juice.

| Analysed compounds | Membrane type | | | |
|---|---|---|---|---|
| | Etna 01 PP (1,000 Da) | PES004 (4,000 Da) | MPF-36 (1,000 Da) | Desal GK (2,000 Da) |
| Glucose | 3.31±4.96 | 4.18±0.46 | 3.86±1.20 | 1.61±0.01 |
| Fructose | 2.36±0.04 | 3.17±0.84 | 9.92±1.11 | 2.17±0.84 |
| Total polyphenols | 85.22±0.23 | 94.97±0.01 | 97.50±0.02 | 88.25±0.34 |
| TAA | 57.11±2.72 | 85.61±0.87 | 95.23±0.90 | 78.15±3.72 |
| Cyanidin 3,5-O-diglucoside | 72.52±0.45 | 98.54±0.48 | 99.54±0.13 | 92.77±0.48 |
| Cyanidin 3-O-glucoside | 67.52±1.58 | 90.44±0.81 | 98.88±0.13 | 82.17±0.08 |
| Delphinidin 3-O-glucoside | 69.95±1.53 | 93.99±3.40 | 98.94±0.39 | 83.60 ±0.46 |
| Pelargolidin 3,5-O-diglucoside | 84.11±2.52 | 63.13±0.23 | 80.42±4.95 | 79.90±0.81 |

Permeate and diafiltrate fractions enriched in sugar compounds were proposed for their reuse as food additives or as bases for soft drinks. The membrane-based process for the clarification and fractionation of pomegranate juice is described in Fig. (**5**) .

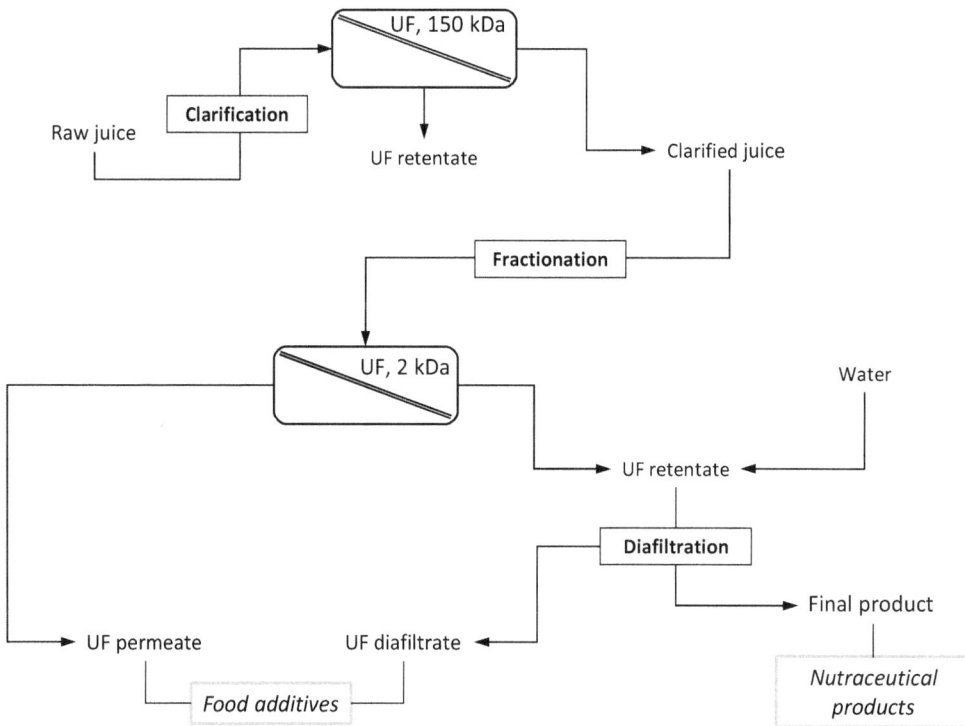

**Fig. (5).** Integrated membrane process for the recovery of phenolic compounds from pomegranate juice (UF, ultrafiltration) (adapted from Conidi *et al.*, 2017).

Recently, Galiano *et al.* [41] evaluated the quality of pomegranate juice -in terms of total phenols, flavonoids, anthocyanins and ascorbic acid content- clarified by using hollow fiber PVDF and PSU membranes prepared in the laboratory through the phase inversion technique. PVDF membranes presented lower retention towards healthy phytochemicals in comparison to PSU membranes. Accordingly, the juice clarified with PVDF membranes showed the best antioxidant activity. Moreover, the treatment with PVDF membranes produced a clarified juice with 2.9-times fold higher α-amylase inhibitory activity in comparison to PSU (IC$_{50}$ values of 75.86 *vs.* 221.31 μg/mL, respectively). These results highlight the great potential of the clarified juice as a source of functional constituents.

The recovery and concentration of anthocyanins from different vegetable sources have been also investigated by using membrane operations in a sequential design. In order to overcome the drawbacks of individually operated membrane process such as low flux of OMD, limitations of achieving higher concentration in RO and also to improve the productivity, Patil and Raghavarao [42] evaluated the performance of a hybrid membrane process on large scale for the concentration of anthocyanins from red radishes (*Raphanus sativus* L.).

In the proposed application, the aqueous extract of fresh red radishes was firstly clarified with a PVDF UF membrane having an MWCO of 10 kDa, in order to remove tannins, proteins and suspended solids. The UF treatment produced a clear solution with a soluble solids content of 1 °Brix. The clarified solution was then submitted to a pre-concentration step performed by RO operated with a PA membrane (NaCl rejection 99%) and to a final OMD concentration step by using a PP membrane with a pore size of 0.2 μm and $CaCl_2$ as stripping solution.

Soluble solids and anthocyanin content of the final concentrated extract resulted of 26 °Brix and 9.8 g/L, respectively (about 25-fold increase in concentration in comparison to the initial extract).

Kozák *et al.* [43] proposed a similar approach, on laboratory and large scale, for the concentration of anthocyanins in blackcurrant juice. The process involved an MF step to clarify the juice, followed by a RO unit to pre-concentrate the juice up to 26 °Brix and a final OD process to concentrate the juice up to 72 °Brix. During the different processes, the operating parameters were optimized, working at a laboratory scale. The large scale measurements were carried out on the basis of the laboratory results. The investigated process allowed to obtain a concentrated juice with a content of anthocyanins three times higher than the raw juice and good preservation of the color and flavor intensity. Concentrated orange press liquors up to 47 °Brix were also produced on laboratory scale through a combination of UF (clarification), NF (pre-concentration) and OMD (concentration). The anthocyanin content of the concentrated orange press liquor was more than seven times higher than that measured in the starting solution [44]. The concentrated fraction was considered of interest for the production of functional foods or in food coloring as an alternative to the use of artificial colorants.

The general flow sheet for the recovery, purification and concentration of phenolic compounds from vegetable sources through a combination of membrane operations is illustrated in Fig. (**6**).

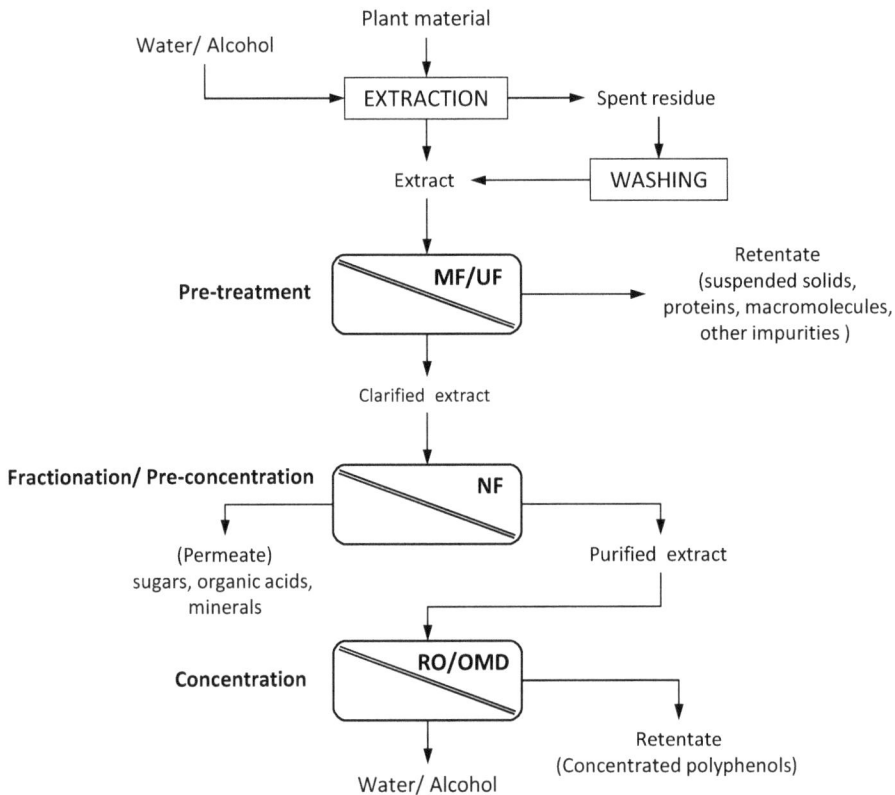

**Fig. (6).** General flow sheet for the recovery of phenolic compounds from vegetable sources by membrane processing (MF, ultrafiltration; UF, ultrafiltration; NF, nanofiltration; RO, reverse osmosis; OMD, osmotic membrane distillation).

## Peptides

In recent years, the interest for health-promoting functional foods, dietary supplements and pharmaceutical preparations containing these BACs has markedly increased. Therefore, several studies have been performed on the production and purification of bioactive peptides derived from the hydrolysis of different proteins including whey, casein, egg-white, meat and fish proteins and vegetable sources [45 - 47]. Bioactive peptides based on their structural properties, amino-acid composition and sequences, have been shown to possess a wide range of functional properties including antioxidant, anti-hypertensive, antimicrobial, immune-modulatory, prebiotic, mineral binding, anti-thrombotic and hypocholesterolemic effects [48 - 50].

Conventional methods for the separation and recovery of bioactive peptides involve selective precipitation, crystallization, chromatography techniques such as ion exchange, affinity binding, size exclusion and hydrophobic interactions [51, 52]. These techniques have different disadvantages for large-scale applications due to high costs and low yield of products. Among membrane processes, pressure-driven membrane operations provide a sustainable industrial technology for the separation and purification of peptides. In particular, these processes have been used, separately or in combination, to fractionate different peptides with the desired molecular weights and functional properties. In addition, they can also control the molecular weight distribution and the charge of specific peptides [53].

UF and NF membranes are applied in whey processing in order to increase the protein content and to isolate many valuable bioactive proteins/peptides as α-lactoglobulin, β-lactoglobulin, bovine serum albumin (BSA), immunoglobulin (Ig), lactoferrin and glycomacropeptide [54, 55].

Metsämuuronen and Nyström [56] evaluated the performance of flat-sheet UF membranes with different membrane material (regenerated cellulose, polyamide, PES and PSU) and MWCO (from 100 to 20 kDa) in the production of fractions enriched in α-lactoglobulin from diluted whey solutions. The effect of pH and temperature on the selectivity towards α-lactoglobulin was also investigated. Among the different tested membranes, the highest selectivity of α-lactoglobulin/β-lactoglobulin (about 66) was achieved by using cellulose regenerate 30 kDa membranes at pH 4.3 and 25 °C. A combination of UF and NF membranes was investigated by Butylina *et al.* [57] to fractionate and purify peptides from sweet whey. During the UF process, a regenerated cellulose membrane with an MWCO of 10 kDa was used. This step allowed to concentrate all the analyzed proteins (lysozyme, BSA, lactoferrin, α-lactoglobulin and β-lactoglobulin) on the retentate side. The resulting permeate fractions were then processed with a sulphonated polyethersulphone NTR 7450 membrane of 1 kDa in order to purify lactose from small peptides/amino acids. The selectivity of peptides to lactose was 6.5 and 0.8 for acidic (pH 3) and basic conditions (pH 9.5), respectively. The investigated UF/NF process allowed to separate and isolate a peptidic fraction with peptides having a molar mass range of 500-1800 Da. Recently, Arrutia *et al.* [58] evaluated the potential of membrane processes for the fractionation and purification of whey proteins. In this approach, concentrated whey proteins were, at first, hydrolyzed with trypsin and the obtained peptides were separated by UF and NF membranes in order to improve or define the biological properties of the obtained peptides. Selected UF and NF membranes having different MWCO (in the range 1 to 5 kDa) made in polyethersulphone (PES) were tested at three different pH values (2, 6 and 8) and compared in terms of separation performances. According to the obtained results, both membranes showed a good performance in the purification of acidic peptides from anionic and neutral peptides and a better separation factor working at basic pH values; a higher selectivity and peptide transmission were obtained with the PES 5 kDa membrane. The recovery of bioactive peptides by membrane operations from sea-food products and by-products has also been investigated. In particular, fish peptides obtained by enzymatic hydrolysis have been processed by pressure-driven membrane operations in order to produce fractions enriched in bioactive peptides for the production of valuable food ingredients [59 - 61].

Vandanjon *et al.* [62], studied a sequence of UF and NF processes for producing isolate fractions enriched in bioactive peptides with molecular weights in the range of 100-500 and 1000-3500 Da from white fish fillet hydrolysates. Two different UF membranes (PSU with a MWCO of 8 kDa and modified PES of 4 kDa) and a NF membrane PA of 300 Da) were used. Selected membranes were combined into two different sequences for the treatment of raw hydrolysates with different chemical compositions. In the first approach hydrolysates containing peptides with molecular weight greater than 3,500 Da were pretreated with the 8 kDa UF membrane; the UF permeate was processed with the 4 kDa membrane and the produced permeate was finally treated by NF. Another sequential design involved the UF membrane of 4 kDa and the NF membrane for treating fish protein hydrolysates having peptides with molecular weight lower than 3500 Da. Both processes are schematically represented in Fig. (**7**). The investigated processes allowed to produce enriched fractions of BACs of specific molecular weights of interest for the formulation of functional foods.

Similar results were reported by Saidi *et al.* [63] in the treatment of fish protein hydrolysates from tuna dark muscle, by using UF and NF membranes. In particular, fractions enriched in bioactive peptides having molecular weights in the range 1-4 kDa were produced and a better purification was obtained working in a DF mode. The produced fractions (NF retentate and NF permeate) were proposed to be used as a source of high nutritional quality. Different authors have also investigated the efficiency of membrane processing in the fractionation/concentration of protein derived from vegetable food matrix [64].

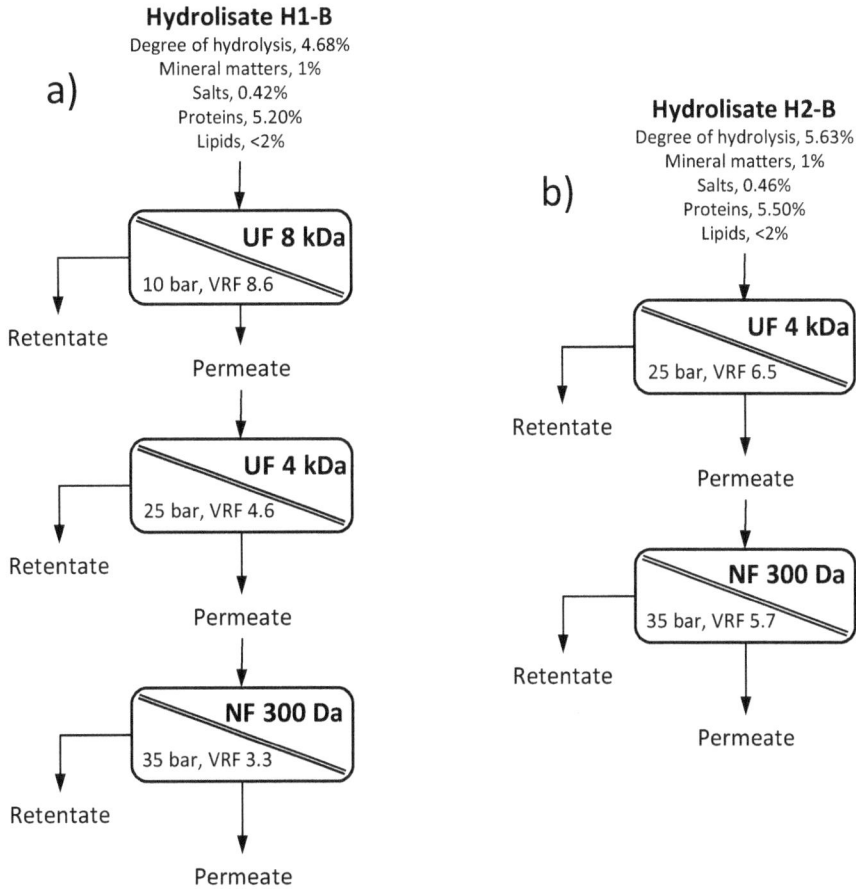

**Fig. (7).** Sequence of membrane operations for the fractionation/concentration of two different with fish hydrolysates; a) H1-B; b) H2-B (UF, ultrafiltration; NF, nanofiltration; VRF, volume reduction factor) (adapted from Vandanjon *et al.*, 2009).

In particular, UF membranes have been widely applied to produce bioactive soy peptide fractions from soy protein hydrolysates. Enzymatic hydrolysis coupled with membrane fractionation of soy peptides might result in releasing and enhancing their biological activity and could be used as a potential nutraceutical for the prevention of different diseases [65].

Park *et al.* [66] investigated the antioxidant activity of soy protein hydrolysate obtained by enzymatic hydrolysis of soy protein. After the enzymatic process, the resulting bioactive soy peptides were isolated by using UF membranes with an MWCO in the range of 3-30 kDa to obtain four different fractions (<3, 3-10, 10-

30 and 30 kDa). The antioxidant activities of the UF fractions were significantly higher as compared to those of the initial hydrolysate, especially for the fraction of 3 kDa. Similar results were reported by Roblet *et al.* [67] in the treatment of soy protein with PES membranes of 10 kDa. In particular, the influence of UF fractionation and membrane configuration (spiral-wound and hollow-fiber) on the bioactivity of soy protein hydrolysate with pepsin-pancreatin enzyme was evaluated. UF permeate fractions exhibited high antioxidant as compared to soy hydrolysate. As a consequence, UF soy peptides fractions having low molecular weight were the most effective as antioxidants.

### *Carotenoids and Tocopherols*

Carotenoids are natural pigments responsible for the yellow, orange and red colors in various fruits and vegetables. In the food industry, the primary uses of carotenoids are as food colorants. The discovery of health-related properties attributed to carotenoids such as those related to the, reduction in the risk of cancer, cardiovascular diseases, osteoporosis, and diabetes, increase their possible uses in the pharmaceutical field [68]. On the other hand, tocopherols (Vitamin E) and tocotrienols, have antioxidant action in protecting cell membranes against reactive lipid radicals and cancer preventive activities [69]. Membrane separation processes have been increasingly used for extraction, purification and concentration of carotenoids such as β-carotene, lycopene and lutein from different vegetable sources, including vegetable oils, in substitution of traditional technologies. Carotenoids and tocopherols can be recovered from red palm oil through a preliminary transesterification, which converts them into smaller and more soluble methyl esters followed by a NF process to separate carotenes from the methyl esters [70, 71]. A three-stage NF process to separate β-carotene from palm methyl esters was suggested by Darnoko and Cheryan [71]. In this approach, based on the use of a flat-sheet NF membrane (DS7, GE Osmonics), the permeate from the initial separation step is used as a feed of the next membrane step. The investigated process allowed to produce a concentrate stream containing 1.19 g/L carotene and a decolorized palm methyl ester stream containing less than 0.1 g/L beta-carotene.

A combination of solvent extraction with membrane processing was investigated by Tsui and Cheryan [72] in order to obtain enriched extracts of lutein and zeaxanthin from corn residues. UF membranes of 1,000-2,000 Da were used to separate ethanol-soluble proteins and other large solutes from ethanol extracts of corn. The UF permeate, enriched in xanthophyll, was concentrated by using NF membranes with the MWCO of 300 Da.

Membrane processes are also attractive technologies for the production of concentrated fractions of carotenoids from fruit juices and aqueous extracts. In particular, MF and UF membranes have been investigated for the concentration of lycopene from melon juice [73, 74], papaya [75] and aqueous extracts of cashew apple [76]. Despite having low molecular weight, lycopene is retained by MF and UF membranes since it binds to other larger molecules such as proteins, lipids and pectin [77]. These processes increase the lycopene concentration in the retentate up to 10 times, yielding a product that may have different applications in the food and pharmaceutical industries.

The recovery and concentration of carotenoids in watermelon juice has also been investigated by using membrane operations in a sequential design. In particular, an integrated membrane process based on the use of MF and RO membranes was investigated by Oliveira *et al.* [78]. In the first step, the juice was pre-concentrated by using MF tubular ceramic membranes ($\alpha$-Al$_2$O$_3$ membranes of 0.2 µm, Pall Corporation, Membralox® Ceramic Membrane Products, Port Washington, NY, USA) under selected operating conditions (TMP, 2 bar; temperature, 35 °C). The retentate fraction presented a lycopene content 5.6 higher than the feed juice, which was very close to the volumetric concentration factor achieved in the process. In order to purify lycopene from sugars and total soluble solids, MF experiments were also performed in a DF mode. The DF step allowed to reduce soluble compounds in the MF retentate of about 8.5 times with respect to the fresh juice. In particular, glucose, fructose and sucrose decreased by 71%, 40% and 54%, respectively, when compared to the fresh juice. The MF retentate was then concentrated with a plate and frame RO membrane (polyamide composite, NaCl rejection 98%) operating at 35 °C, a TMP of 60 bar and a feed flow rate of 650 L/h. This step produced a concentrated solution with a dark red colour, lycopene content 17.7 times higher than the fresh juice and a high antioxidant capacity (5.66 µmol Trolox/100 g), indicating its suitability as a natural antioxidant or colorant.

## CONCLUDING REMARKS

The interest in the recovery of high-value components in the functional food and nutraceutical industry has remarkably increased in the last decade. The use of membrane technologies in this field offers interesting advantages over conventional separation processes in terms of minimal thermal damage of treated solutions, high quality of final products and low energy consumption.

In this chapter, the use of pressure-driven membrane operations and osmotic membrane distillation for the separation and concentration of phenolics, peptides and carotenoids from agro-food products and by-products has been discussed. The proposed applications clearly indicate that separation processes must be evaluated individually according to the molecule physicochemical characteristics and complexity of the original extracts. Similarly, processing parameters, membrane material and membrane types should be optimized case by case. In addition, the development of emerging membrane technologies such as pervaporation, membrane emulsification, biocatalytic membrane reactors, forward osmosis and electrodialysis will stimulate further growth of membrane technology for the recovery of electrically charged compounds (electrodialysis), the production of highly concentrated extracts under mild operating conditions (forward osmosis), conversion of exogenous substrates into valuable food ingredients (biocatalytic membrane reactors) and preparation of emulsions (membrane emulsification).

Finally, membrane processes as low-energy processes with high selectivity can play a key role in the development of a new biorefinery concept based on the simultaneous production of natural antioxidants of nutraceutical interest, macromolecules (such as biopolymers) and biofuels (*i.e.*, bioethanol and biogas) from agro-food wastes and by-products.

## NOMENCLATURE

| | |
|---|---|
| **BACs** | Biologically Active Compounds |
| **BSA** | Bovine Serum Albumine |
| **DF** | Diafiltration |
| **EIPS** | Evaporation Induced Phase Separation |
| **MF** | Microfiltration |
| **MWCO** | Molecular Weight Cut-Off |
| **NF** | Nanofiltration |
| **NIPS** | Non Solvent Induced Phase Separation |
| **OMD** | Osmotic Membrane Distiliation |
| **PA** | Polyamide |
| **PE** | Polyethylene |
| **PES** | Polyethersulphone |
| **PP** | Polypropylene |
| **PPA** | Polypiperazine Amide |
| **PSU** | Polysulphone |
| **PTFE** | Polytetrafluoroethylene |
| **PVDF** | Polyvinylidene Fluoride |
| **RO** | Reverse Osmosis |
| **TAA** | Total Antioxidant Activity |
| **TIPS** | Thermally Induced Phase Separation |

| | |
|---|---|
| **UF** | Ultrafiltration |
| **VIPS** | Vapour Induced Phase Separation |
| **VRF** | Volume Reduction Factor |

**Subscripts**

| | |
|---|---|
| **f** | feed |
| **p** | permeate |

## CONSENT FOR PUBLICATION

Not applicable.

## CONFLICTS OF INTEREST

The authors declare that there are no conflicts of interest.

## ACKNOWLEDGEMENTS

Declared none.

## REFERENCES

[1] Transparency Market Research. Nutraceuticals Market - Global Industry Analysis, Size, Share, Growth and Forecast, 2015-2021. Albany, NY: Transparency Market Research 2015.

[2] Akin O, Temelli F, Köseoğlu S. Membrane applications in functional foods and nutraceuticals. Crit Rev Food Sci Nutr 2012; 52(4): 347-71.
[http://dx.doi.org/10.1080/10408398.2010.500240] [PMID: 22332598]

[3] Conde E, Diaz-Reinoso B, Gonzales-Munos MJ, Moure A, Dominguez H, Parajo JC. Recovery and concentration of antioxidants from industrial effluents and from processing streams of underutilized vegetal biomass. Food Public Health 2013; 3(2): 69-91.

[4] Galanakis C. Recovery of high added-value components from food wastes: conventional, emerging technologies and commercialized applications. Trends Food Sci Technol 2012; 26(2): 68-87.
[http://dx.doi.org/10.1016/j.tifs.2012.03.003]

[5] Drioli E, Romano M. Progress and new perspectives on integrated membrane operations for sustainable industrial growth. Ind Eng Chem Res 2001; 40(5): 1277-300.
[http://dx.doi.org/10.1021/ie0006209]

[6] Van der Bruggen B, Vandecasteele C, Van Gestel T, Doyen W, Leysen R. A review of pressure-driven membrane processes in wastewater treatment and drinking water production. Environ Prog 2003; 22(1): 46-56.
[http://dx.doi.org/10.1002/ep.670220116]

[7] Daufin G, Escudier JP, Carrère H, Bérot S, Fillaudeau L, Decloux M. Recent and emerging applications of membranes in the food and dairy industry. Food Bioprod Process 2001; 79(C2): 89-102.
[http://dx.doi.org/10.1205/096030801750286131]

[8] Savaş Bahçeci K, Gül Akıllıoğlu H, Gökmen V. Osmotic and membrane distillation for the concentration of tomato juice: effects on quality and safety characteristics. Innov Food Sci Emerg Technol 2015; 31: 131-8.

[http://dx.doi.org/10.1016/j.ifset.2015.07.008]

[9]     Hogan PA, Canning RP, Peterson PA, Johnson RA, Michaels AS. A new option: osmotic distillation. Chem Eng Prog 1998; 94(7): 49-61.

[10]    Figoli A, Santoro S, Galiano F, Basile A. Pervaporation membranes: preparation, characterization and application.Pervaporation, Vapour Permeation and Membrane Distillation. 1st ed. Cambridge: Woodhead Publishing 2015; pp. 19-63.
        [http://dx.doi.org/10.1016/B978-1-78242-246-4.00002-7]

[11]    Figoli A, Simone S, Drioli E. Polymeric Membranes.Membrane Fabrication. 1st ed. Boca Raton: CRC Press 2015; pp. 3-44.
        [http://dx.doi.org/10.1201/b18149-3]

[12]    Li D, Krantz WB, Greenberg AR, Sani RL. Membrane formation *via* thermally induced phase separation (TIPS): Model development and validation. J Membr Sci 2006; 279(1-2): 50-60.
        [http://dx.doi.org/10.1016/j.memsci.2005.11.036]

[13]    Guo W, Ngo HH, Li J. A mini-review on membrane fouling. Bioresour Technol 2012; 122: 27-34.
        [http://dx.doi.org/10.1016/j.biortech.2012.04.089] [PMID: 22608938]

[14]    Cassano A, Marchio M, Drioli E. Clarification of blood orange juice by ultrafiltration: analyses of operating parameters, membrane fouling and juice quality. Desalination 2007; 212(1-3): 15-27.
        [http://dx.doi.org/10.1016/j.desal.2006.08.013]

[15]    de Bruijn J, Venegas A, Borquez R. Influence of crossflow ultrafiltration on membrane fouling and apple juice quality. Desalination 2002; 148(1-3): 131-6.
        [http://dx.doi.org/10.1016/S0011-9164(02)00666-5]

[16]    de Barros STD, Andrade CMG, Mendes ES, Peres L. Study of fouling mechanism in pineapple juice clarification by ultrafiltration. J Membr Sci 2003; 215(1-2): 213-24.
        [http://dx.doi.org/10.1016/S0376-7388(02)00615-4]

[17]    Huang L, Morrissey MT. Fouling of membranes during microfiltration of surimi wash water: Roles of pore blocking and surface cake formation. J Membr Sci 1998; 144(1-2): 113-23.
        [http://dx.doi.org/10.1016/S0376-7388(98)00038-6]

[18]    Mohammad AW, Ng CY, Lim YP, Ng GH. Ultrafiltration in food processing industry: review on application, membrane fouling, and fouling control. Food Bioprocess Technol 2012; 5(4): 1143-56.
        [http://dx.doi.org/10.1007/s11947-012-0806-9]

[19]    Hatakeyama ES, Ju H, Gabriel CJ, *et al.* New protein-resistant coatings for water filtration membranes based on quaternary ammonium and phosphonium polymers. J Membr Sci 2009; 330(1-2): 104-16.
        [http://dx.doi.org/10.1016/j.memsci.2008.12.049]

[20]    Ju H, McCloskey BD, Sagle AC, Kusuma VA, Freeman BD. Preparation and characterization of crosslinked poly(ethylene glycol) diacrylate hydrogels as fouling-resistant membrane coating materials. J Membr Sci 2009; 330(1-2): 180-8.
        [http://dx.doi.org/10.1016/j.memsci.2008.12.054]

[21]    Galiano F, Figoli A, Deowan SA, *et al.* A step forward to a more efficient wastewater treatment by membrane surface modification *via* polymerizable bicontinuous microemulsion. J Membr Sci 2015; 482: 103-14.
        [http://dx.doi.org/10.1016/j.memsci.2015.02.019]

[22]    Razmjou A, Mansouri J, Chen V. The effects of mechanical and chemical modification of TiO2 nanoparticles on the surface chemistry, structure and fouling performance of PES ultrafiltration membranes. J Membr Sci 2011; 378(1-2): 73-84.
        [http://dx.doi.org/10.1016/j.memsci.2010.10.019]

[23]    Cao X, Ma J, Shi X, Ren Z. Effect of $TiO_2$ nanoparticle size on the performance of PVDF membrane. Appl Surf Sci 2006; 253(4): 2003-10.
        [http://dx.doi.org/10.1016/j.apsusc.2006.03.090]

[24]   Galanalis CM. Separation of functional macromolecules and micromolecules: from ultrafiltration to the border of nanofiltration. Trends Food Sci Technol 2015; 42(1): 44-63.
[http://dx.doi.org/10.1016/j.tifs.2014.11.005]

[25]   Li J, Chase HA. Applications of membrane techniques for purification of natural products. Biotechnol Lett 2010; 32(5): 601-8.
[http://dx.doi.org/10.1007/s10529-009-0199-7] [PMID: 20049625]

[26]   Díaz-Reinoso B, Gonzáles-Lopez N, Moure A, Domínguez H, Parajó JC. Recovery of antioxidants from industrial waste liquors using membranes and polymeric resins. J Food Eng 2010; 96(1): 127-33.
[http://dx.doi.org/10.1016/j.jfoodeng.2009.07.007]

[27]   Conidi C, Rodriguez-Lopez AD, Garcia-Castello EM, Cassano A. Purification of artichoke polyphenols by using membrane filtration and polymeric resins. Separ Purif Tech 2015; 144: 153-61.
[http://dx.doi.org/10.1016/j.seppur.2015.02.025]

[28]   Cassano A, Drioli E, Eds. Integrated membrane operations in the food production. Berlin: Walter de Gruyter 2014.

[29]   Sarmento LAV, Machado RAF, Petrus JCC, Tamanini TR, Bolzan A. Extraction of polyphenols from cocoa seeds and concentration through polymeric membranes. J Supercrit Fluids 2008; 45(1): 64-9.
[http://dx.doi.org/10.1016/j.supflu.2007.11.007]

[30]   Prudêncio APA, Prudêncio ES. Phenolic composition and antioxidant activity of the aqueous extract of bark from residues from mate tree (*Ilex paraguariensis* St. Hil.) bark harvesting concentrated by nanofiltration. Food Bioprod Process 2012; 90(C3): 399-405.
[http://dx.doi.org/10.1016/j.fbp.2011.12.003]

[31]   Azmir J, Zaidul ISM, Rahman MM, *et al.* Techniques for extraction of bioactive compounds from plant materials: A review. J Food Eng 2013; 117(4): 426-36.
[http://dx.doi.org/10.1016/j.jfoodeng.2013.01.014]

[32]   Mello BCBS, Petrus JCCC, Hubinger MD. Concentration of flavonoids and phenolic compounds in aqueous and ethanolic propolis extracts through nanofiltration. J Food Eng 2010; 96(4): 533-9.
[http://dx.doi.org/10.1016/j.jfoodeng.2009.08.040]

[33]   Syed UT, Brazinha C, Crespo JG, Ricardo-da-Silva JM. Valorization of grape pomace: Fractionation of bioactive flavan-3-ols by membrane processing. Separ Purif Tech 2017; 172: 404-14.
[http://dx.doi.org/10.1016/j.seppur.2016.07.039]

[34]   Nichenametla SN, Taruscio TG, Barney DL, Exon JH. A review of the effects and mechanisms of polyphenolics in cancer. Crit Rev Food Sci Nutr 2006; 46(2): 161-83.
[http://dx.doi.org/10.1080/10408390591000541] [PMID: 16431408]

[35]   Castañeda-Ovando A, Pacheco-Hernández ML, Páez-Hernández ME, Rodríguez JA, Galán-Vidal CA. Chemical studies of anthocyanins: A review. Food Chem 2009; 113(4): 859-71.
[http://dx.doi.org/10.1016/j.foodchem.2008.09.001]

[36]   Kalbasi A, Cisneros-Zevallos L. Fractionation of monomeric and polymeric anthocyainins from Concord grape (Vitis labrusca L.) juice by membrane ultrafiltration. J Agric Food Chem 2007; 55(17): 7036-42.
[http://dx.doi.org/10.1021/jf0706068] [PMID: 17665929]

[37]   Cissé M, Vaillant F, Pallet D, Dornier M. Selecting ultrafiltration and nanofiltration membranes to concentrate anthocyanins from roselle extract (*Hibiscus sabdariffa* L.). Food Res Int 2011; 44(9): 2607-14.
[http://dx.doi.org/10.1016/j.foodres.2011.04.046]

[38]   Couto DS, Dornier M, Pallet D, *et al.* Evaluation of nanofiltration membranes for the retention of anthocyanins of açai (*Euterpe oleracea Mart.*) juice. Desalination Water Treat 2011; 27(1-3): 108-13.
[http://dx.doi.org/10.5004/dwt.2011.2067]

[39] Conidi C, Cassano A, Drioli E. Recovery of phenolic compounds from orange press liquor by nanofiltration. Food Bioprod Process 2012; 90(C4): 867-74.
[http://dx.doi.org/10.1016/j.fbp.2012.07.005]

[40] Conidi C, Cassano A, Caiazzo F, Drioli E. Separation and purification of phenolic compounds from pomegranate juice by ultrafiltration and nanofiltration membranes. J Food Eng 2017; 195: 1-13.
[http://dx.doi.org/10.1016/j.jfoodeng.2016.09.017]

[41] Galiano F, Figoli A, Conidi C, *et al.* Functional properties of *Punica granatum* L. juice clarified by hollow fiber membranes. Processes (Basel) 2016; 4(3): 1-16.
[http://dx.doi.org/10.3390/pr4030021]

[42] Patil G, Raghavarao KSMS. Integrated membrane process for the concentration of anthocyanin. J Food Eng 2007; 78(4): 1233-9.
[http://dx.doi.org/10.1016/j.jfoodeng.2005.12.034]

[43] Kozák Á, Bánvölgyi SZ, Vincze I, Kiss I, Békássy Molnár E, Vatai G. Comparison of integrated large-scale and laboratory scale membrane processes for the production of black currant juice concentrate. Chem Eng Prog 2008; 47(7): 1171-7.
[http://dx.doi.org/10.1016/j.cep.2007.12.006]

[44] Cassano A, Conidi C, Ruby-Figueroa R. Recovery of flavonoids from orange press liquor by an integrated membrane process. Membranes (Basel) 2014; 4(3): 509-24.
[http://dx.doi.org/10.3390/membranes4030509] [PMID: 25116725]

[45] de Castro RJS, Sato HH. Biologically active peptides: Processes for their generation, purification and identification and applications as natural additives in the food and pharmaceutical industries. Food Res Int 2015; 74: 185-98.
[http://dx.doi.org/10.1016/j.foodres.2015.05.013] [PMID: 28411983]

[46] Rizzello CG, Tagliazucchi D, Babini E, Rutella GS, Saa DLT, Gianotti A. Bioactive peptides from vegetable food matrices: Research trends and novel biotechnologies for synthesis and recovery. J Funct Foods 2016; 2016(27): 549-69.
[http://dx.doi.org/10.1016/j.jff.2016.09.023]

[47] Arroume N, Froidevaux R, Kapel R, *et al.* Food peptides: purification, identification and role in the metabolism. Curr Opin Food Sci 2016; 7: 101-7.
[http://dx.doi.org/10.1016/j.cofs.2016.02.005]

[48] Agyei D, Danquah MK. Industrial-scale manufacturing of pharmaceutical-grade bioactive peptides. Biotechnol Adv 2011; 29(3): 272-7.
[http://dx.doi.org/10.1016/j.biotechadv.2011.01.001] [PMID: 21238564]

[49] Agyei D, Danquah MK. Rethinking food-derived bioactive peptides for antimicrobial and immunomodulatory activities. Trends Food Sci Technol 2012; 3(2): 62-9.
[http://dx.doi.org/10.1016/j.tifs.2011.08.010]

[50] Dhaval A, Yadav N, Purwar S. Potential applications of food derived bioactive peptides in management of health. Int J Pept Res Ther 2016; 22(3): 377-98.
[http://dx.doi.org/10.1007/s10989-016-9514-z]

[51] Mora L, Escudero E, Fraser PD, Aristoy MC, Toldrá F. Proteomic identification of antioxidant peptides from 400 to 2500 Da generated in Spanish dry-cured ham contained in a size-exclusion chromatography fraction. Food Res Int 2014; 56: 68-76.
[http://dx.doi.org/10.1016/j.foodres.2013.12.001]

[52] Guo L, Hou H, Li B, Zhang Z, Wang S, Zhao X. Preparation, isolation and identification of iron-chelating peptides derived from Alaska pollock skin. Process Biochem 2013; 48(5-6): 988-93.
[http://dx.doi.org/10.1016/j.procbio.2013.04.013]

[53] Harnedy PH, FitzGerald RJ. Bioactive peptides from marine processing waste and shellfish: A review. J Funct Foods 2012; 4(1): 6-24.

[http://dx.doi.org/10.1016/j.jff.2011.09.001]

[54]    Atra R, Vatai G, Bekassy-Molnar E, Balint A. Investigation of ultra- and nanofiltration for utilization of whey protein and lactose. J Food Eng 2005; 67(3): 325-32.
[http://dx.doi.org/10.1016/j.jfoodeng.2004.04.035]

[55]    Bazinet L, Firdaous L. Membrane processes and devices for separation of bioactive peptides. Recent Pat Biotechnol 2009; 3(1): 61-72.
[http://dx.doi.org/10.2174/187220809787172623] [PMID: 19149724]

[56]    Metsämuuronen S, Nyström M. Enrichment of α-lactalbumin from diluted whey with polymeric ultrafiltration membranes. J Membr Sci 2009; 337(1-2): 248-56.
[http://dx.doi.org/10.1016/j.memsci.2009.03.052]

[57]    Butylina S, Luque S, Nyström M. Fractionation of whey-derived peptides using a combination of ultrafiltration and nanofiltration. J Membr Sci 2006; 280(1-2): 418-26.
[http://dx.doi.org/10.1016/j.memsci.2006.01.046]

[58]    Arrutia F, Rubio R, Riera FA. Production and membrane fractionation of bioactive peptides from a whey protein concentrate. J Food Eng 2016; 184: 1-9.
[http://dx.doi.org/10.1016/j.jfoodeng.2016.03.010]

[59]    Chabeaud A, Vandanjon L, Bourseau P, Jaouen P, Chaplain-Derouiniot M, Guerard F. Performances of ultrafiltration membranes for fractionating a fish protein hydrolysate: application to the refining of bioactive peptidic fractions. Separ Purif Tech 2009; 66(3): 463-71.
[http://dx.doi.org/10.1016/j.seppur.2009.02.012]

[60]    Chabeaud A, Vandanjon L, Bourseau P, Jaouen P, Guérard F. Fractionation by ultrafiltration of a saithe protein hydrolysate (Pollachius virens): Effect of material and molecular weight cut-off on the membrane performances. J Food Eng 2009; 91(3): 408-14.
[http://dx.doi.org/10.1016/j.jfoodeng.2008.09.018]

[61]    Bourseau P, Vandanjona L, Jaouen P, *et al.* Fractionation of fish protein hydrolysates by ultrafiltration and nanofiltration: impact on peptidic populations. Desalination 2009; 244(1-3): 303-20.
[http://dx.doi.org/10.1016/j.desal.2008.05.026]

[62]    Vandanjon L, Grignon M, Courois E, Bourseau P, Jaouen P. Fractionating white fish fillet hydrolysates by ultrafiltration and nanofiltration. J Food Eng 2009; 95(1): 36-44.
[http://dx.doi.org/10.1016/j.jfoodeng.2009.04.007]

[63]    Saidi S, Deratani A, Belleville MP, Amar RB. Production and fractionation of tuna by-product protein hydrolysate by ultrafiltration and nanofiltration: impact on interesting peptides fractions and nutritional properties. Food Res Int 2014; 65: 453-61.
[http://dx.doi.org/10.1016/j.foodres.2014.04.026]

[64]    Saxena A, Tripathi BP, Kumar M, Shahi VK. Membrane-based techniques for the separation and purification of proteins: an overview. Adv Colloid Interface Sci 2009; 145(1-2): 1-22.
[http://dx.doi.org/10.1016/j.cis.2008.07.004] [PMID: 18774120]

[65]    Tsou MJ, Kao FJ, Tseng CK, Chiang WD. Enhancing the anti-adipogenic activity of soy protein by limited hydrolysis with Flavourzyme and ultrafiltration. Food Chem 2010; 122(1): 243-8.
[http://dx.doi.org/10.1016/j.foodchem.2010.02.070]

[66]    Park SY, Lee JS, Baek HH, Lee HG. Purification and characterization of antioxidant peptides from soy protein hydrolysate. J Food Biochem 2010; 34: 120-32.
[http://dx.doi.org/10.1111/j.1745-4514.2009.00313.x]

[67]    Roblet C, Amiot J, Lavigne C, *et al.* Screening of *in vitro* bioactivities of a soy protein hydrolysate separated by hollow fiber and spiral-wound ultrafiltration membranes. Food Res Int 2012; 46(1): 237-49.
[http://dx.doi.org/10.1016/j.foodres.2011.11.014]

[68]    Jomova K, Valko M. Health protective effects of carotenoids and their interactions with other

biological antioxidants. Eur J Med Chem 2013; 70: 102-10.
[http://dx.doi.org/10.1016/j.ejmech.2013.09.054] [PMID: 24141200]

[69]　Järvinen R, Erkkilä AT. Tocopherols: physiology and health effects Reference Module in Food Science, Encyclopedia of Food and Health. Elsevier 2016.

[70]　Chiu CM, Coutinho CD, Gonçalves LAG. Carotenoids concentration of palm oil using membrane technology. Desalination 2009; 245(1-3): 783-6.
[http://dx.doi.org/10.1016/j.desal.2009.03.002]

[71]　Darnoko D, Cheryan M. Carotenoids from red palm methyl esters by nanofiltration. J Am Oil Chem Soc 2006; 83(4): 365-70.
[http://dx.doi.org/10.1007/s11746-006-1214-y]

[72]　Tsui EM, Cheryan M. Membrane processing of xanthophylls in ethanol extracts of corn. J Food Eng 2007; 83(4): 590-5.
[http://dx.doi.org/10.1016/j.jfoodeng.2007.03.041]

[73]　Vaillant F, Cisse M, Chaverri M, *et al.* Clarification and concentration of melon juice using membrane processes. Innov Food Sci Emerg Technol 2005; 6(2): 213-20.
[http://dx.doi.org/10.1016/j.ifset.2004.11.004]

[74]　Gomes FS, Costa PA, Campos MBD, Tonon RV, Couri S, Cabral LMC. Watermelon juice pre-treatment with microfiltration process for obtaining lycopene. Int J Food Sci Technol 2013; 48: 601-8.
[http://dx.doi.org/10.1111/ijfs.12005]

[75]　Paes J, da Cunha CR, Viotto LA. Concentration of lycopene in the pulp of papaya (*Carica papaya* L.) by ultrafiltration on a pilot scale. Food Bioprod Process 2015; 96: 296-305.
[http://dx.doi.org/10.1016/j.fbp.2015.09.003]

[76]　de Abreu FP, Dornier M, Dionisio AP, Carail M, Caris-Veyrat C, Dhuique-Mayer C. Cashew apple (*Anacardium occidentale* L.) extract from by-product of juice processing: a focus on carotenoids. Food Chem 2013; 138(1): 25-31.
[http://dx.doi.org/10.1016/j.foodchem.2012.10.028] [PMID: 23265451]

[77]　Hurst WJ, Ed. Methods of Analysis for Functional Foods and Nutraceuticals. Boca Raton: CRC Press 2002.
[http://dx.doi.org/10.1201/9781420014679]

[78]　Oliveira CS, Gomes FS, Silva LFMS, Godoy RLO, Tonon RV, Cabral LMC. Integrated membrane separation processes aiming to concentrate and purify lycopene from watermelon juice. Innov Food Sci Emerg Technol 2016; 38: 149-54.
[http://dx.doi.org/10.1016/j.ifset.2016.09.025]

# CHAPTER 16

# Controversies Regarding Food Additives and Future Trends

**Ana Sanches Silva[1,2,*], Dalia Sánchez-Machado[3], Jaime López-Cervantes[3]** and **Seyed M. Nabavi[4,*]**

[1] *National Institute for Agricultural and Veterinary Research (INIAV), I.P., Vairão, Vila do Conde, Portugal*

[2] *Center for Study in Animal Science (CECA), University of Oporto, Oporto, Portugal*

[3] *Instituto Tecnológico de Sonora, 5 de Febrero 818 Sur, Ciudad Obregón, Sonora, Mexico*

[4] *Applied Biotechnology Research Center, Baqiyatallah University of Medical Sciences, Tehran14359-16471, Iran*

**Abstract:** Nowadays food additives are far more than just salt, vinegar, herbs and spices. These compounds are essential to preserve and enhance the original characteristics of foods in order to make them more appealing, nutritious, safe, convenient and affordable. They also have an outstanding role in the production of greater quantities of food with high-quality standards and in the obtainment of food to promote well-being and health. This chapter focuses on the main controversies of food additives, namely the duality between natural and synthetic antioxidants and provides insight into their future trends. Although natural additives are generally preferred, they can also present drawbacks such as low availability, high price, low potency, low food compatibility and difficulty to predict the effect due to their multiple activities. In fact, new food processing technologies are expected to slow down food additives use, but, on the other hand, new additives, will replace the current ones in order to improve the characteristics of foods, increase food safety and improve the health and well-being of consumers.

**Keywords:** Controversies, Food additives, Future trends, Human health.

## INTRODUCTION

Different factors, including world population growth, changes in lifestyle patterns (*e.g.* limited time to prepare meals), demand for nutritious, safe, colourful, flavourful, affordable and convenient food and high-quality standards, have

* **Corresponding authors Ana Sanches Silva and Seyed M. Nabavi:** National Institute for Agricultural and Veterinary Research (INIAV), I.P., Vairão, Vila do Conde, Portugal Center for Study in Animal Science (CECA), University of Oporto, Oporto, Portugal; E-mail: ana.silva@iniav.pt or anateress@gmail.com and Applied Biotechnology Research Center, Baqiyatallah University of Medical Sciences, Tehran14359-16471, Iran; E-mail: nabavi208@gmail.com

caused an exponential increase in the use of food additives, especially in processed food [1]. This type of food, not only includes food which encompasses the use of different food additives but also food that was submitted to a treatment such as cooling, freezing, heating, milling, smoking, canning, fermentation, freeze-drying and drying.

Food technologists are not confined to salt, vinegar, herbs and spices to preserve and improve the flavour of food. Advances in technologies, have led to increasing use of food preservation methods (*e.g.* refrigeration, freezing, modified atmosphere packaging) and to wider use of a greater variety of additives [2]. Fig. (**1**) depicts the main causes that lead to an exponential use of food additives. More than 2500 substances can be used as food additives to produce a technological effect [3]. Regarding the definition of food additives, the European Parliament and the Council of the European Union, the US Food and Drug Administration (FDA), the Food Agricultural and Organization (FAO) and World Health Organization (WHO), have recognized three definitions, which essentially agree to the same concept. According to the Regulation (EC) no.1333/2008 and the Joint FAO/WHO Expert Committee on Food Additives (JECFA), a *food additive* is any substance not normally consumed as food itself and not normally used as a characteristic ingredient of food, whether or not it has nutritive value. The intentional addition of the additive to food during the preparation, manufacture, processing, treatment, packaging, transport or storage to achieve a technological purpose for the food, results or may be reasonably expected to result, in it or its by-products becoming directly or indirectly a component of such food [4, 6]. According to the FDA and the International Food Information Council (IFIC), a food additive is 'any substance the intended use of which results or may reasonably be expected to result - directly or indirectly - in a component or otherwise affecting the characteristics of any food.' In fact, this definition includes any substance used in the production, processing, treatment, packaging, transportation or storage of food. The legal definition aims to impose a premarket approval requirement and excludes ingredients generally recognized as safe (GRAS) and colour additives and pesticides where other premarket approval requirements are applied [5]. The term does not include contaminants or substances added to food for maintaining or improving nutritional qualities [6].

Fig. (**2**) depicts the groups and main sub-groups of food additives based on the FDA. Direct food additives are those added to a food for a specific purpose. Most of the food additives are direct additives and can be identified on the foods label. Indirect food additives become part of the food due to its packaging, storage or other handling and are found in trace amounts. More than 3000 food additives are allowed in the United States and they are included in the database "Everything Added to Food in the United States" [5]. The main functional classes of food additives according to Regulation (EC) no. 1333/2008 [4] and FDA and IFIC [5] are compiled in Table **1**.

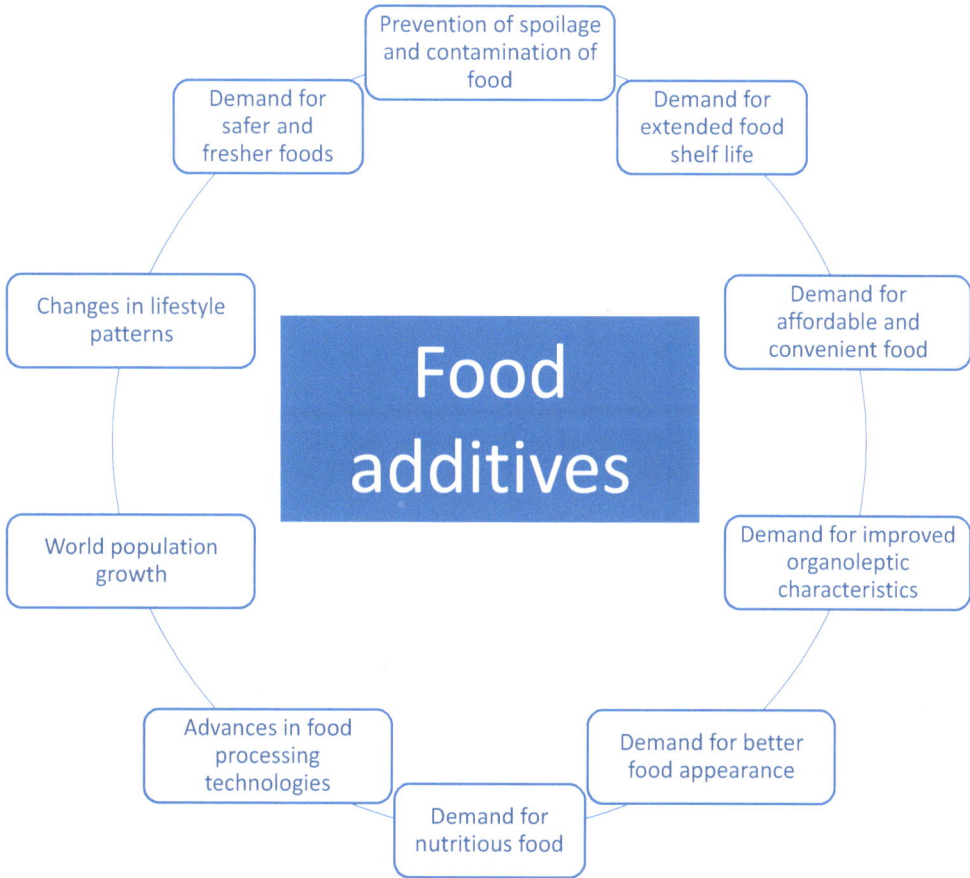

**Fig. (1).** Main causes of the exponential use of food additives.

Although it is common to add additives to food, it is highly controversial due to the relation of some additives, especially of those synthetic, to adverse health effects (*e.g.* phosphate-containing food additives have been related to chronic kidney disease) [7]. According to a survey carried out on 430 consumers in Seoul, Korea, consumers are particularly reluctant regarding preservatives, colorants and artificial sweeteners in foods [1]. In this survey, lack of knowledge regarding food additives was perceived, but after the information campaign, knowledge scores improved significantly from 67.3 to 91.9%.

Time limitations and lack of nutrition knowledge drive consumers to use heuristics to make food decisions. It is worth to highlight that the lack of nutrition information leads many times to associate the code of food additives to the absence of naturalness. A negative spillover effect can be observed from food additives perceived or evaluated as negative to other food additives. This code, E-code (which comprises "E" which stands for Europe and a number) was given in the European Union and Switzerland. Moreover, according to a study carried out by Siegrist and Sutterlin [8], consumers base their food-related choices on symbolic information and this can lead to biased judgments and decisions. In this line, the results of a Swiss study to evaluate consumer's perception of artificial food additives concluded that different factors affect the acceptance of food additives including the knowledge of regulation, risk and benefit perceptions as well as the preference for natural products [9]. This highlights the importance of communicating risks and benefits of food additives to consumers in the same way they can do correct food choices based on reliable data.

The main goal of this chapter is to address the actual controversies of food additives and to gain insight into their future trends.

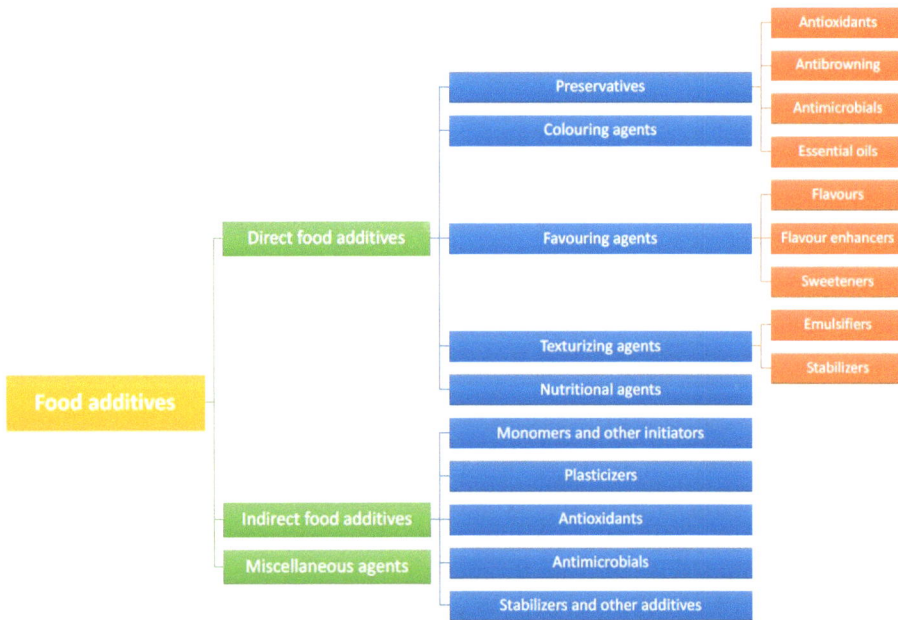

**Fig. (2).** Groups and main sub-groups of food additives.

## CONTROVERSIES OF FOOD ADDITIVES

It is obvious that food additives represent a great advance of food industry due to all the advantages they bring to food such as to allow the adequate supply of food to people according to the worldwide growing population (it is expected that in

2050 there will be 9 billion people) because additives reduce food losses [10].

Some of the facts mostly contributing to the controversy around food additives are: the lack of worldwide common legislation and the fact that consumers consider food additives, especially synthetic ones, as unhealthy, unnatural and with potential Public Health risk [9]. In this line, some foods labels mention in the label information that "no synthetic additives" were used or that just "natural additives" have been used to appeal consumers [11]. However, some natural food additives lack to prove their safety. Antioxidants that have been focused by numerous research studies worldwide in the last decades due to their putative health effects, fail to prove their effectiveness after being ingested, due to their low absorption, and prooxidant effects and it is difficult to determine their ideal dosage. Moreover, some do not pass through the blood-brain barrier. Prooxidant effect depends on the concentration of antioxidants and neighbouring molecules and in some cases can be beneficial for human health because it can increase the antioxidant defence and xenobiotic-metabolising enzymes. In fact, *in vivo* studies with laboratory mice revealed that mice are more sensitive to antioxidants than humans [12].

Therefore, more research studies are required to increase the knowledge on the bioavailability, mechanisms of action, metabolism, ideal dosages, biological activities of antioxidants and food additives in general [13]. Moreover, the possible reactions with food components, toxicity, synergy with other compounds, adverse effects and safe dosages of natural additives must be evaluated [11].

Although at first-sight, consumers prefer natural food additives, due to their putative health benefits or no association with adverse health effects. These can present some drawbacks:

i. **Low Potency**: A limitation can be the amount that is required to obtain a technological effect. If the amount is too high, it might negatively affect the organoleptic characteristics of food and be rejected by the consumers. Therefore, the evaluation of the ratio potency/effectiveness of the food additives is of major importance because this can also have an implication on the safety of the final product.
ii. **Lack of availability**: Some sources of natural additives are not available permanently and/or available in high amounts. Moreover, their intense use causes imbalance in the ecosystem.
iii. **Synergistic effects**: These effects make difficult to predict the effect of natural compounds on the food and, may invalidate their use.
iv. **Compatibility**: The lack of compatibility with food components may invalidate their use.

v. **Stability**: Some natural food additives present lower stability than corresponding synthetic molecules. However new industrial techniques can improve it.

vi. **Price**: Generally, the price of natural food additives is higher than the corresponding synthetic option, and this is a limitation for their industrial use.

Fig. (**3**) presents the major pros and cons of both synthetic and natural additives

## FUTURE TRENDS OF FOOD ADDITIVES

In the future, there will be the tendency to use less resources to produce greater quantities of food and to produce new foods equilibrated in terms of nutrients and bioactive components, in order to promote well-being and health [10].

The main players in the definition of the future of food additives are consumers, the food industry, regulatory bodies and food and packaging scientific research. Consumers prefer natural foods, *i.e*, those grown and produced in a traditional way and free from food additives [14]. Moreover, within foods with food additives, consumers prefer natural food additives because they are perceived as healthier [15]. Therefore, there is a clear tendency for substituting synthetic food additives by natural compounds, which are not associated with health concerns. In the case of antioxidants there is a tendency for substituting butylated hydroxytoluene (BHT), butylated hydroxyanisole (BHA), tert-butylhydroquinone (TBHQ) and propyl gallate (PG), the main synthetic molecules used as antioxidants by the food industry, by natural antioxidants such as carotenoids, polyphenols, ascorbic acid and tocopherols [16, 17]. In fact, this is a way to get back to the origins and use those additives that were considered primitive additives, more efficiently.

In this line, the scientific community, as well as the food industry, are merging efforts to develop new products or systems in order to minimize the use of synthetic food additives and promote the use of natural compounds such as essential oils, vitamins, plant extracts and bioactive compounds [18 - 22].

New food processing technologies are also emerging, and it is also expected that they will continue to develop in order to reduce the need for food additives, producing minimally processed food. These include UV radiation, Pulsed Electric Field (PEF), High-Pressure Processing (HPP), 3D printing, Cold Atmospheric Pressure Plasma (CAPP) and Low Energy Electron Beam (LEEB) [23 - 28].

New delivery systems such as microencapsulation and nanoencapsulation or active packaging are expected to continue to have a great development because they allow the continuous release of food additives [20, 29]. Encapsulation can minimize the lack of stability of some natural food pigments and colorants (*e.g.* anthocyanins, betanin, carotenoids and chlorophylls) [39]. On the other hand, active packaging allows reducing the direct incorporation of additives to foods which simplifies the food processing and allows having a controlled release of food additives to the surface of the food, which is where the degradation reactions begin [18]. Edible coatings are also emerging due to the interest in materials that do not pose any environmental concern. Edible coatings are generally applied to fruits and vegetables but can also be applied to processed food. Moreover, this concept can be designed in order to have an active function, *i.e.* as active edible coatings. Among edible coatings, the use of layer by layer approach is very recent and is based on the deposition of different biopolymers in an alternate way, allowing to improve the properties and bioactivities of the coatings [31].

New and more effective food additives, preferably from natural origin, will continue to be developed and produced. This will require the constant update/revision of regulations in order to avoid any fraud, or food adulteration and to ensure that acceptable daily intake (ADI) of food additives ensures safety. Therefore, new analytical techniques will be required in order to easily detect multiple food additives in complex matrices like foods and if they comply with the restricted maximum levels. In some cases, these food additives may be found at very low detection limits such in the case of indirect additives.

**Table 1. Classes of food additives according to Regulation (EC) no. 1333/2008 [4] and to FDA and IFIC [5].**

| Classes according to Regulation (EC) no. 1333/2008 | Classes according to FDA and IFIC |
|---|---|
| **Acidity regulators** | Anti-caking agents |
| **Acids** | Colour Additives |
| **Anti-caking agents** | Dough Strengtheners and Conditioners |
| **Anti-foaming agents** | Emulsifiers |
| **Antioxidants** | Enzyme Preparations |
| **Bulking agents** | Fat Replacers |
| **Carriers** | Firming Agents |
| **Colours** | Flavour Enhancers |
| **Emulsifiers** | Flavours and Spices |
| **Emulsifying salts** | Gases |
| **Firming agents** | Humectants |
| **Flavour enhancers** | Leavening Agents |
| **Flour treatment agents** | Nutrients |

| Classes according to Regulation (EC) no. 1333/2008 | Classes according to FDA and IFIC |
|---|---|
| **Foaming agents** | pH Control Agents and acidulants |
| **Gelling agents** | Preservatives |
| **Glazing agents (including lubricants)** | Stabilisers and Thickeners, Binders, Texturisers |
| **Humectants** | Sweeteners |
| **Modified starches** | Yeast Nutrients |
| **Packaging gases** | |
| **Preservatives** | |
| **Propellants** | |
| **Raising agents** | |
| **Sequestrants** | |
| **Stabilisers** | |
| **Sweeteners** | |
| **Thickeners** | |

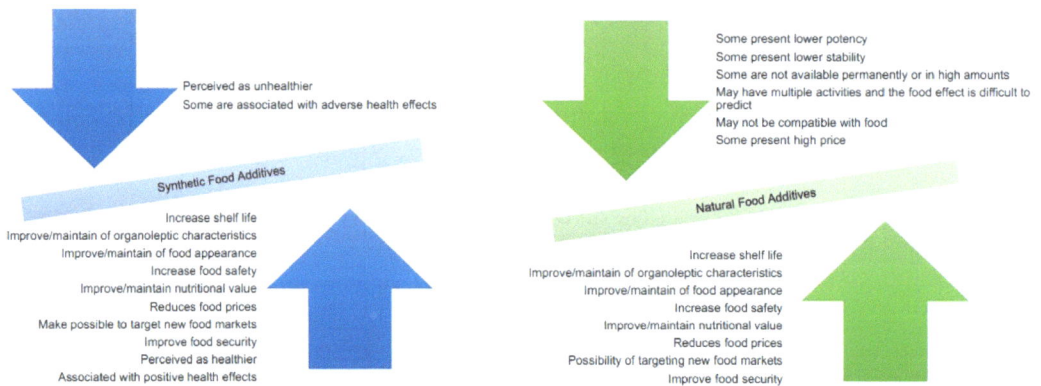

**Fig. (3).** Main pros and cons of synthetic and natural food additives.

Future trends can also include the use of biotechnology to produce food additives, development of vaccines for intolerants or the use of DNA recombinant technologies [3].

In the future, it is foreseen that specific measures can be taken in order to better inform consumers about natural food additives and possibly legislation exclusively dedicated to natural food additives can come in force.

## CONCLUDING REMARKS

It is undeniable that food additives are essential elements in today's society due to their technological, convenient and appealing benefits.

Important challenges for food additives are expected in the future, as addressed in this chapter. On the one hand, new food processing technologies will try to slow down its use, on the other hand, new additives will replace the current ones in order to improve the characteristics of foods, increase food safety and improve the health and well-being of consumers. A sound alliance between scientific research in this area and a dynamic and supportive food industry is essential to face the legal and market challenges. Future food additives trends will most probably use biotechnology for their production, develop vaccines for intolerants or use DNA recombinant technologies. In the future, it will be important to carry out randomized large-scale clinical studies to evaluate the long-term health effects of food additives and their mixtures and to address their interactions with food components.

## CONSENT FOR PUBLICATION

Not applicable.

## CONFLICT OF INTEREST

The authors declare that there are no conflicts of interest

## ACKNOWLEDGEMENTS

Declared none.

## REFERENCES

[1]     Shim SM, Seo SH, Lee Y, Moon GI, Kim MS, Park JH. Consumers' knowledge and safety perceptions of food additives: Evaluation on the effectiveness of transmitting information on preservatives. Food Control 2011; 22(7): 1054-60.
[http://dx.doi.org/10.1016/j.foodcont.2011.01.001]

[2]     Sanches-Silva A, López-Hernández J, Paseiro-Losada P. Modified atmosphere packaging and temperature effect on potato crisps oxidation during storage. Anal Chim Acta 2004; 524: 185-9.
[http://dx.doi.org/10.1016/j.aca.2004.06.010]

[3]     Carocho M, Barreiro MF, Morales P. *Ferreira ICFR*. Adding molecules to food, pros and cons: A review on synthetic and natural food additives. Compr Rev Food Sci Food Saf 2014; 13(4): 377-99.
[http://dx.doi.org/10.1111/1541-4337.12065]

[4]     Regulation (EC) No. 1333/2008 of the European Parliament and of the Council of 16 December 2008 on food additives. Off J Eur Union 2008; 354: 16-33.

[5]     FDA & IFIC. US Food and Drug Administration (FDA) and the International Food Information Council (IFIC) Food ingredients and colours 2010. Available from: https://www.fda.gov/downloads/ Food/IngredientsPackagingLabeling/ucm094249.pdf

[6]     Codex Alimentarius. General Standard for Food Additives CODEX STAN 192-1995 1995. Available from: http://www.fao.org/fao-who-codexalimentarius/sh-proxy/en/?lnk=1&url=https%253A%252F %252Fworkspace.fao.org%252Fsites%252Fcodex%252FStandards%252FCODEX%2BSTAN%2B19 2-1995%252FCXS_192e.pdf

[7]     Winger RJ, Uribarri J, Lloyd L. Phosphorus-containing food additives: An insidious danger for people with chronic kidney disease. Trends Food Sci Technol 2012; 24(2): 92-102.
[http://dx.doi.org/10.1016/j.tifs.2011.11.001]

[8]     Siegrist M, Sütterlin B. Importance of perceived naturalness for acceptance of food additives and cultured meat. Appetite 2017; 113: 320-6.
[http://dx.doi.org/10.1016/j.appet.2017.03.019] [PMID: 28315418]

[9]     Bearth A, Cousin ME, Siegrist M. The consumer's perception of artificial food additives: Influences on acceptance, risk and benefit perceptions. Food Qual Prefer 2014; 38: 14-23.
[http://dx.doi.org/10.1016/j.foodqual.2014.05.008]

[10]    Augustin MA, Riley M, Stockmann R, et al. Role of food processing in food and nutrition security. Trends Food Sci Technol 2016; 56: 115-25.
[http://dx.doi.org/10.1016/j.tifs.2016.08.005]

[11]    Carocho M, Morales P, Ferreira ICFR. Natural food additives: Quo vadis? Trends Food Sci Technol 2015; 45(2): 284-95.
[http://dx.doi.org/10.1016/j.tifs.2015.06.007]

[12]    Carocho M, Ferreira ICFR. A review on antioxidants, prooxidants and related controversy: natural and synthetic compounds, screening and analysis methodologies and future perspectives. Food Chem Toxicol 2013; 51(1): 15-25.
[http://dx.doi.org/10.1016/j.fct.2012.09.021] [PMID: 23017782]

[13]    Cerqueira FM, De Medeiros MHG, Augusto O. Antioxidantes dietéticos: Controvérsias e perspectivas. Quim Nova 2007; 30(2): 441-9.
[http://dx.doi.org/10.1590/S0100-40422007000200036]

[14]    Román S, Sánchez-Siles LM, Siegrist M. The importance of food naturalness for consumers: Results of a systematic review. Trends Food Sci Technol 2017; 67: 44-57.
[http://dx.doi.org/10.1016/j.tifs.2017.06.010]

[15]    Martins N, Roriz CL, Morales P, Barros L, Ferreira ICFR. Food colorants: Challenges, opportunities and current desires of agro-industries to ensure consumer expectations and regulatory practices. Trends Food Sci Technol 2016; 52: 1-15.
[http://dx.doi.org/10.1016/j.tifs.2016.03.009]

[16]    Sanches-Silva A, Cruz JM, Sendón-García R, Paseiro-Losada P. Determination of butylated hydroxytoluene in food samples by high-performance liquid chromatography with ultraviolet detection and gas chromatography/mass spectrometry. J AOAC Int 2007; 90(1): 277-83.
[PMID: 17373461]

[17]    Sanches-Silva A, Costa HS, Bueno-Solano C, et al. Determination of α-tocopherol in shrimp waste to evaluate its potential to produce active packaging. Ital J Food Sci 2011; SLIM2010: 139-41.

[18]    Sanches-Silva A, Ribeiro T, Albuquerque TG, et al. Ultra-high pressure LC for astaxanthin determination in shrimp by-products and active food packaging. Biomed Chromatogr 2013; 27(6): 757-64.
[http://dx.doi.org/10.1002/bmc.2856] [PMID: 23225623]

[19]    Sanches-Silva A, Ribeiro T, Albuquerque TG, et al. Ultra-high pressure LC determination of glucosamine in shrimp by-products and migration tests of chitosan films. J Sep Sci 2012; 35(5-6): 633-40.
[http://dx.doi.org/10.1002/jssc.201100855] [PMID: 22517638]

[20]    Ribeiro-Santos R, Andrade M, Sanches-Silva A. Application of Encapsulated Essential Oils as Antimicrobial Agents in Food Packaging. Curr Opin Food Sci 2017; 14: 78-84.
[http://dx.doi.org/10.1016/j.cofs.2017.01.012]

[21]    Ribeiro-Santos R, Sanches-Silva A, Gomes Motta JF, et al. Whey protein active films incorporated with a blend of essential oils: characterization and effectiveness packaging. Packag Technol Sci 2018;

31: 27-40.
[http://dx.doi.org/10.1002/pts.2352]

[22]   Lado BH, Yousef AE. Alternative food-preservation technologies: efficacy and mechanisms. Microbes Infect 2002; 4(4): 433-40.
[http://dx.doi.org/10.1016/S1286-4579(02)01557-5] [PMID: 11932194]

[23]   de Boer A, Bast A. Demanding safe foods – Safety testing under the novel food regulation (2015/2283). Trends Food Sci Technol 2018; 72: 125-33.
[http://dx.doi.org/10.1016/j.tifs.2017.12.013]

[24]   Pereira RN, Vicente AA. Environmental impact of novel thermal and non-thermal technologies in food processing. Food Res Int 2010; 43: 1936-43.
[http://dx.doi.org/10.1016/j.foodres.2009.09.013]

[25]   Freitas A, Moldão-Martins M, Costa HS, Albuquerque TG, Valente A, Sanches-Silva A. Effect of UV-C radiation on bioactive compounds of pineapple (*Ananas comosus* L. Merr.) by-products. J Sci Food Agric 2015; 95(1): 44-52.
[http://dx.doi.org/10.1002/jsfa.6751] [PMID: 24852602]

[26]   Lipton JI, Cutler M, Nigl F, Cohen D, Lipson H. Additive manufacturing for the food industry. Trends Food Sci Technol 2015; 43(1): 114-23.
[http://dx.doi.org/10.1016/j.tifs.2015.02.004]

[27]   Islam MS, Patras A, Pokharel B, *et al.* UV-C irradiation as an alternative disinfection technique: Study of its effect on polyphenols and antioxidant activity of apple juice. Innov Food Sci Emerg 2016; 34: 344-51.
[http://dx.doi.org/10.1016/j.ifset.2016.02.009]

[28]   Hertwig C, Meneses N, Mathys A. Cold atmospheric pressure plasma and low energy electron beam as alternative nonthermal decontamination technologies for dry food surfaces: A review. Trends Food Sci Technol 2018; 77: 131-42.
[http://dx.doi.org/10.1016/j.tifs.2018.05.011]

[29]   Ribeiro-Santos R, Sanches-Silva A, Gomes Motta JF, *et al.* Potential of migration of active compounds from protein based films with essential oils to a food and a food simulant. Packag Technol Sci 2017; 30: 791-8.
[http://dx.doi.org/10.1002/pts.2334]

[30]   Rodriguez-Amaya DB. Natural food pigments and colorants. Curr Opin Food Sci 2016; 7: 20-6.
[http://dx.doi.org/10.1016/j.cofs.2015.08.004]

[31]   Arnon-Rips H, Poverenov E. Improving food products' quality and storability by using Layer by Layer edible coatings. Trends Food Sci Technol 2018; 75: 81-92.
[http://dx.doi.org/10.1016/j.tifs.2018.03.003]

# SUBJECT INDEX

## A

Ability 20, 22, 24, 64, 65, 67, 68, 84, 89, 120, 122, 123, 125, 130, 131, 136, 138
   colorant 130
   functional 130
   health impairment 123
   health-promoting 120
   intolerance 136
   powerful antioxidant 68
Acceptable daily intakes (ADI) 9, 130, 133, 134, 135, 136, 137, 138, 139, 140, 192, 193, 195, 204
Acidifying agents 72, 234, 236, 238, 242
Acidity 71, 72, 73, 255, 296
Acidity regulator and 237, 238
   chelating agent 237
   flavor enhancer 238
   structure stabilizer 237
   taste enhancer 237
Acidity regulators 1, 2, 7, 69, 234, 237, 238, 319
Acids 3, 7, 10, 23, 27, 28, 29, 40, 43, 44, 45, 49, 65, 66, 67, 69, 70, 71, 72, 73, 74, 85, 91, 125, 130, 133, 135, 136, 173, 175, 198, 200, 202, 206, 215, 224, 236, 237, 238, 253, 254, 256, 257, 259, 294, 319
   butyric 69
   caffeic 44, 45, 67, 294
   caprylic 89
   carminic 28, 29, 125, 130, 133, 135, 136
   carnosic 23, 65, 66
   chlorogenic 44, 66, 294
   cinnamic 45, 49
   coumaric 45
   ferulic 44, 45, 259, 294
   fumaric 74, 236, 237
   lactic 70, 71, 72, 175, 215, 224
   malic 40, 72, 73, 175, 236, 237, 257
   malonic 43
   nosiduronic 200
   oxalic 43, 175
   phthalic 253, 254

   piliformic 85
   polylactic 256
   pulvinic 91
   pyruvic 175
   rosmarinic 23, 65, 67
   sorbic 3, 10, 40
   succinic 65, 73, 74, 238
   sulfamic 206
   vanillic 66
Acrylic resins 258
Action 21, 72, 74, 85, 94
   antifungal 85
   biopreservative 94
   destructive 21
   synergistic 72, 74
Activity 6, 9, 41, 43, 44, 47, 64, 67, 69, 83, 85, 86, 87, 88, 89, 90, 91, 92, 93, 95, 130, 133, 213, 240, 252
   antidermatophytic 91
   anti-leishmanial 90
   antimicrobial pesticide 91
   antiviral 88, 89
   bactericidal 83, 91, 92, 93
   biopesticidal 92
   biopreservative 93
   emulsifying 213
   estrogenic 252
   fungistatic 85, 95
   inhibiting enzyme 41
   optimal catalytic 43
   pesticidal 92
   phenylalanine ammonia lyase 44
   toxicological 240
Acute otitis media (AOM) 84
Additives 1, 2, 4, 8, 9, 11, 12, 18, 19, 24, 30, 31, 42, 62, 69, 72, 105, 134, 158, 186, 220, 234, 255, 260, 285, 287, 313, 315, 317, 318
   chemical 18, 19, 30, 42, 285, 287
   flavoring 2
   human 9
   natural 31, 105, 313, 317, 318
   natural antioxidant 62
   nutritional 24, 62, 134

# B

*Bacillus cereus* 20, 90, 94, 106, 107
*Bacillus liqueniformis* 107
*Bacillus megatherium* 107
*Bacillus spizizenii* 106
*Bacillus subtilis* 83, 85, 106, 107
*Bacillus thuringiensis* 92
Bactericides 95
Bacteriocins 93, 94, 95
Bacteriolytic enzymes 94
Bakery products 215, 217
  making high-quality 217
  production of 217
  yeast-leavened 215
Beverages 3, 5, 25, 27, 30, 46, 94, 130, 131,
    132, 183, 185, 186, 203, 235, 236, 237,
    238
  alcohol-containing 94
  calorie-free 186
  dairy 236
  fruit 46
  lactic acid 235
  malt 185
  nutraceutical 25
  powdered artificial 30
Biologically active compounds (BACs) 284,
    285, 292, 297, 300, 302
Bladder tumors, urinary 205
Blood 29, 201, 292, 294
  oxygenated 29
Blood-brain barrier 317
Blood glucose 199
Blood urea 239, 240, 241
  concentration 241
  nitrogen (BUN) 239, 241
Body mass index (BMI) 273
Bovine serum albumin (BSA) 49, 292, 294,
    301
Bronchitis 31, 84
  chronic 31
Browning of food 37
Browning process 38, 39, 41, 44, 51
Browning reactions 24, 37, 38, 39, 40, 41, 42,
    45, 46, 47, 48, 49, 50, 51
  catalysed 50
  enzymatic 46
  fast 39
  non-enzymatic 24, 38, 40

reduced 37
reverse 45
Butoconazole nitrate (BN) 85

# C

Camphor 21
Cancer 1, 4, 7, 111, 205, 251, 269, 270, 272,
    273, 276, 295, 304
  breast 111, 251
  colon 111
*Candida albicans* 86, 87, 91, 106, 107
*Candida krusei* 85
*Canna indica* 126
Carbocyclic nucleoside 88
Carcinogenic effects 135, 136
Carcinogenicity 205, 223
Cardiomyocyte hypertrophy 276
Cardiovascular illnesses 295
Carmine dyes 136
Carmines 4, 28, 132,136, 137, 271
  containing 136
  indigo 132, 135, 137
Cellulose 31, 197, 236, 257, 301
  interacting crystalline 236
  regenerated 301
Cheese 19, 26, 29, 72, 73, 93, 94, 110, 132,
    158, 192, 217, 218
  enzyme-modified 29
  yogurt 192
Chlorophyll 2, 25, 28, 29, 125, 130, 319
  green pigment 130
  pigments 28
Cinnamic 21, 29
  alcohol 29
  aldehyde 21
*Cinnamomum burmannii* 128
*Cinnamomum cassia* 106, 109, 110
*Cinnamomum osmopholeum* leaf 91
*Clostridium botulinum* 91, 255
*Clostridium perfringens* 91
*Clostridium tyrobutyricum* 94
Cold atmospheric pressure plasma (CAPP)
    318
Compound annual growth rate (CAGR) 234,
    284
Compounds 2, 3, 16, 20, 21, 22, 24, 47, 48,
    50, 65, 66, 67, 69, 71, 74, 94, 173, 176,
    181, 213, 258, 261, 273, 287, 293, 317
  alcoholic 50

www.ingramcontent.com/pod-product-compliance
Lightning Source LLC
Chambersburg PA
CBHW050805220326
41598CB00006B/122